Human Cancer Diagnosis and Detection Using Exascale Computing

Scrivener Publishing
100 Cummings Center, Suite 541J
Beverly, MA 01915-6106

Publishers at Scrivener
Martin Scrivener (martin@scrivenerpublishing.com)
Phillip Carmical (pcarmical@scrivenerpublishing.com)

Human Cancer Diagnosis and Detection Using Exascale Computing

Edited by

Kapil Joshi
Department of Computer Science & Engineering, Uttaranchal Institute of Technology, Dehradun, India

and

Somil Kumar Gupta
School of Computing, DIT University, Dehradun, India

Scrivener Publishing

WILEY

This edition first published 2024 by John Wiley & Sons, Inc., 111 River Street, Hoboken, NJ 07030, USA and Scrivener Publishing LLC, 100 Cummings Center, Suite 541J, Beverly, MA 01915, USA

For more information about Scrivener publications please visit www.scrivenerpublishing.com.

Wiley Global Headquarters
111 River Street, Hoboken, NJ 07030, USA

For details of our global editorial offices, customer services, and more information about Wiley products visit us at www.wiley.com.

Library of Congress Cataloging-in-Publication Data

ISBN 978-1-394-19767-5

Cover image: Pixabay.Com
Cover design by Russell Richardson

Set in size of 11pt and Minion Pro by Manila Typesetting Company, Makati, Philippines

Printed in the USA

10 9 8 7 6 5 4 3 2 1

Contents

Preface

The treatment of cancer has remained a top priority in the vast field of medical science and technology. Successful diagnosis and treatment of cancer is one of the major challenges of medical science. Millions of people throughout the world have been affected by cancer, and in many aspects. To deal with this challenge, the science and technology community has developed many cutting-edge mechanisms over time that have improved and developed new methods of cancer diagnosis and detection.

Exascale computing has the potential to increase our ability in terms of computation to develop efficient methods for a better healthcare system. This technology promises to revolutionize cancer diagnosis and detection, ushering in an era of unprecedented precision, speed, and efficiency. The fusion of exascale computing with the field of oncology has the potential to redefine the boundaries of what is possible in the fight against cancer.

This book is a comprehensive exploration of this transformative unification of science, medicine, and technology. In the pages that follow, we delve deeply into the realm of exascale computing and its profound implications for cancer research and patient care.

This volume serves as a bridge between the worlds of computational science and clinical oncology. It joins experts from diverse fields who have dedicated their careers to pushing the boundaries of what is achievable in the realm of cancer diagnosis and detection. Authors of different chapters within this book have given significant insight into the challenges posed by cancer and the innovative solutions that exascale computing offers.

The chapters that follow cover a wide range of topics, from the fundamentals of exascale computing and its application to cancer genomics to the development of advanced imaging techniques and machine learning algorithms. We explore the integration of data analytics, artificial intelligence, and high-performance computing to move cancer research to the next phase.

Our goal in presenting this book is not only to educate and inform, but also to inspire. We aim to empower researchers, clinicians, and technologists with the knowledge and tools needed to advance the cause of cancer diagnosis and detection. By leveraging the unprecedented computational capabilities of exascale computing, we have the opportunity to accelerate discoveries, optimize treatments, and ultimately save lives.

We acknowledge that our understanding of cancer is still evolving, and the challenges ahead are formidable. However, with the synergy of human intellect and exascale computing, we have the potential to make profound strides in the battle against this devastating disease. Together, we can transform the future of cancer diagnosis and detection, offering hope to countless individuals and their families.

We invite you to delve into the pages herein and join us on this remarkable expedition at the intersection of science, technology, and medicine. Together, we can illuminate new pathways in the fight against cancer and usher in an era of hope, healing, and discovery.

We are deeply grateful to all authors for their excellent contributions to this book. We also highly appreciate the dedicated support and valuable assistance rendered by Martin Scrivener and the Scrivener Publishing team during the publication of this book.

1

Evaluating the Impact of Healthcare 4.0 on the Performance of Hospitals

Pramod Kumar[1], Nitu Maurya[2], Keerthiraj[3], Somanchi Hari Krishna[4*], Geetha Manoharan[5] and Anupama Bharti[6]

[1]*Faculty of Commerce and Management, Assam Down Town University, Sankar Madhab Path, Gandhi Nagar, Panikhaiti, Guwahati, Assam, India*
[2]*Management, KCC Institute of Legal and Higher Education, Noida, India*
[3]*Political Science, School of Liberal Arts, Alliance University, Bengaluru, Karnataka, India*
[4]*Department of Business Management, Vignana Bharathi Institute of Technology, Aushapur Village Ghatkesar Mandal Malkangiri Medchal Dist, Telangana, India*
[5]*School of Business, SR University, Warangal, Telangana, India*
[6]*Department of Sociology and Social Work, Himachal Pradesh University, Shimla, India*

Abstract

In this evaluation, we identify innovation packages and associated implementation barriers that might be considered to be part of Healthcare 4.0 (H4.0) and investigate their impact on performance enhancement in a sample hospital setting. In order to determine how to proceed, we conducted a cross-sectional review with 181 hospital directors from various nations who have already proactively begun implementing H4.0. Using multivariate statistical methods, the gathered data were examined. According to the findings, H4.0 technologies may be divided into two groups based on how they are used in hospitals. Using the sociotechnical systems theory, common hurdles to H4.0 adoption were empirically divided into two types. H4.0 technology bundles had a good and noticeable impact on how well hospitals performed. It is essential to continuously consider both H4.0 technologies and obstacles since their collaboration with H4.0 barriers adversely affected performance improvement. Our discoveries will help hospital management in

**Corresponding author*: harikrishnasomanchi@gmail.com
Pramod Kumar: ORCID: 0000-0002-1971-4770
Keerthiraj: ORCID: https://orcid.org/0000-0002-2536-8579

Kapil Joshi and Somil Kumar Gupta (eds.) Human Cancer Diagnosis and Detection Using Exascale Computing, (1–18) © 2024 Scrivener Publishing LLC

expecting likely deterrents to the reception of H4.0, empowering more proactive endeavors to further develop performance and give superior grade, sensibly estimating healthcare in the age of the fourth modern unrest.

Keywords: Healthcare 4.0, hospital, technologies, performance of hospital, barriers

1.1 Introduction

Healthcare 4.0 addresses a significant change in the way healthcare frameworks are viewed. It draws inspiration from Industry 4.0, the fourth industrial revolution [1]. The fourth industrial revolution was propelled by globalization, increased seriousness, advances in information and communications technology (ICT), and market expansion [2]. Because of Industry 4.0, the association went through a computerized change. Steam power was the primary cause of the modern uprising, whereas power molded the second. The third modern upset began in the 1970s as a result of advancements in processing innovation. The fourth industrial revolution was sparked by advances in ICT technologies, which included fully computerized and clever manufacturing processes suitable for independent communication and control among many corporate levels of an association [2–4]. Industry 4.0 features include ongoing information exchange and flexible manufacturing as a result of vertical, horizontal, and end-to-end integration [5]. End-to-end integration is the automated management of a product over its entire life cycle. Vertical integration is the coordination of every authoritative action. Horizontal integration is the combination of all worthy chain parts. In a cycle that consolidates item-focused esteem creation, a progression of exercises is carefully connected together. Examples include analyzing customer needs, developing items, manufacturing them, offering services, maintaining them, and recycling them [3, 6]. According to the definition of Industry 4.0, "Industry 4.0 refers to the integration of Internet of Things (IoT) technologies into industrial value creation, enabling manufacturers to harness fully digitalized, connected, smart, and decentralised value chains, able to deliver greater flexibility and robustness to firm competitiveness and enable them to build flexible and adaptable business structures, [acquiring] the permanent ability for internal evolutionary developments in order to collaborate more effectively with other companies" [2, 7, 8].

Real-time healthcare customization is made possible by H4.0 [9], transforming organizations from hospital-centered to patient-centered ones where many departments collaborate effectively to enhance patient health [10].

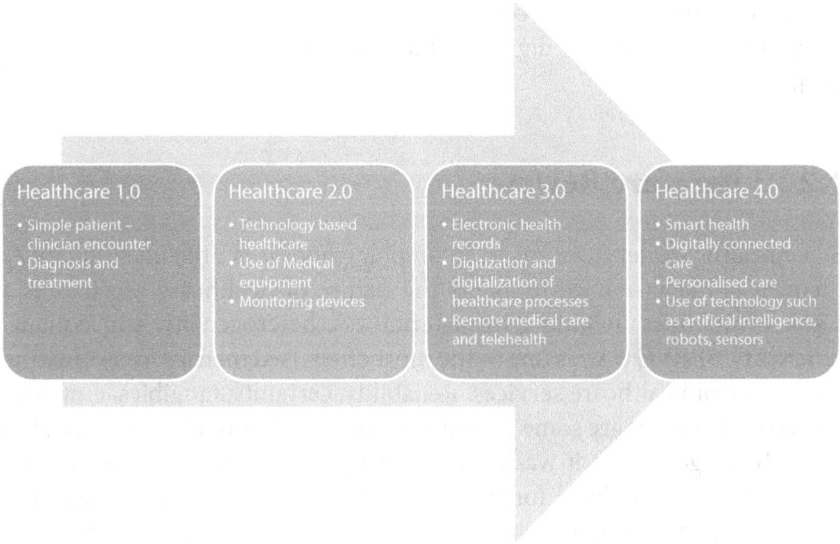

Figure 1.1 Changing healthcare systems [9].

Figure 1.1 shows the Changing healthcare systems from healthcare 1.0 to HealthCare 4.0. Hospital staff members can share and use intra- and inter-hospital services [11, 12] as well as hospital supporting procedures [13, 14] with ease thanks to H4.0. While incorporating new technologies into medical procedures may have a good short-term effect on hospitals' outputs, the long-term effects of doing so may not be immediately obvious [58].

The technologies that should be considered when implementing H4.0 and how they could interact to increase performance in healthcare frameworks are the subject of current research [15, 16]. Similar to this, agreement has not yet been achieved on how exactly H4.0 technologies affect hospitals' performance [17]. The digital transformation of healthcare has produced a variety of outcomes [18], especially when one takes into account the role of obstacles brought about by financial and political interests, as well as requests from associations, affiliations, and lobbyists [14].

The phrase "Industry 4.0" was first used in Germany in 2011 as part of a strategic drive to use technology to transform. Our study is based on the sociotechnical systems theory [19], which holds that an organization develops through the right interaction of its social and technical elements, which enhances performance. Sociotechnical systems are a method for organizing complex organizational activity that takes into account how people and technology interact at work [20]. We propose to explore H4.0 taking into account both social and technological components crucial to its implementation, which could help endeavors to be connected to the reception of state of the digital technologies in healthcare organizations [59].

1.2 Literature Review

Since healthcare services are an intangible good, it is difficult to quantify them. It is likewise hard to assess the nature of healthcare services as a result of qualities including immaterialness, heterogeneity, and concurrence [21]. SERVQUAL is one of the most often used metrics for evaluating the quality of healthcare services. Reliability, certainty, tangibles, empathy, and responsiveness are some of its dimensions. This model, in any case, has a disadvantage in that it was created for a general help environment and should be contextualized for the utilization environment [22]. Although there have been numerous studies to gauge the quality of healthcare services [23, 24], Dagger, Sweeney, and Johnson's model is one of the most widely used. The term "interpersonal quality" refers to the relationships and dyadic communication that have grown between the patient and the consideration supply. It is largely influenced by behavior, communication, and relationships. The expression "relationship" alludes to the degree and nature of the bond that has been laid out between a specialist organization and a customer, whereas the terms "manner" and "communication" describe the information exchanged between a provider and a customer, as well as their level of interaction and two-way communication, respectively [25]. The technical quality includes two aspects. The first and second dimensions are, respectively, the output obtained and the service provider's technical expertise. Technical competency is determined by the knowledge, experience, credentials, or skill of the provider. The service outcome gives an account of how the service procedure went [60], arising from contacts with a service provider throughout a single or series of service encounters [25, 26].

ICT has been utilized all the more every now and then to help the viability, effectiveness, and quality of healthcare systems [27]. The phrase "Healthcare 4.0" refers to a number of integrated ICT, electronics, and microstructure developments that take into account more effective restorative plans and support functions [28]. The availability of less expensive ICTs that can diagnose problems and offer quick findings and remedies, the shrinking size of ICTs, and improved capacities for data acquisition and management are only a few reasons why ICT usage may be increasing [29]. Healthcare 4.0 is reportedly a transition of healthcare systems [30]. ICT is used in both the hospital's administrative and medical practices [28]. Lower costs, remote sensor networks for further developed straightforwardness, electronic wellbeing record frameworks, portable wellbeing applications, further developed finding and patient consideration rehearsals [61], support for customized medication possibilities, more limited pausing and lead times, empowering cooperative healthcare, and better help for training and education are only a couple of the advantages of ICT use in healthcare frameworks [25]. The capacity of the healthcare framework to create the ideal outcomes ought to be evaluated in view of its impact on the type of healthcare services. Studies [25, 31–33] have shown the significance of Healthcare 4.0, but no studies have looked at how it will raise the standard of healthcare services. This paper analyzes how Healthcare 4.0 will impact several facets of the standard of medical treatment through a thorough review of the literature [62].

Many studies identify comparable technologies that fall under the H4.0 implementation umbrella. The list includes the Internet of Things, cloud computing, wearable biomedical sensors, and machine learning as enabling influences of an informed perspective on health [34]. Big data analytics is included in the H4.0 portfolios of several studies. Others studied how various technologies were used in healthcare systems, including 3D printing [35], collaborative robots [36], augmented reality [37], and remote monitoring [38]. Despite variations in citation rates, literature research points to the complementary roles that these technologies play.

I4.0 is the continual revolution of conventional industrial and manufacturing procedures using the most cutting-edge smart technology. I4.0 is focused on using large-scale interconnectivity technology deployments to enable better communication, self-monitoring, and higher automation. It also includes smart devices that can evaluate and diagnose problems without requiring human intervention [40]. The term "I4.0" describes a great degree of product personalization under extremely flexible production circumstances [41]. The idea of H4.0 was created as a result of applying I4.0's technology and design ideas to the healthcare industry [42]. The implementation of digital technology is what spurs the H4.0 approach, which necessitates critical adjustments in healthcare organizations on both the technical and social fronts [43]. With the advent of H4.0, hospitals now have a higher level of automation and connection, which improves both patient care and operational procedures [15].

1.3 Methodology

The research's methodological approach was empirical because it was exploratory in character. Empirical research, in Goodwin's opinion, is the most effective way to learn from direct or indirect experience or observation [44]. The previously mentioned research questions can be addressed by measuring empirical information obtained from non-irregular respondents who meet specific prerequisites, which is a typical methodology in investigations of a comparable sort [45]. Due to its many potential benefits, including its elevated degree of representativeness, minimal expense, expected measurable importance, and normalized excitement for all respondents, the study strategy is a typical pick among the information assortment approaches open for empirical examination. Four fundamental components make up the methodology described in this study (see Figure 1.2):

- Sample selection and characterization
- Creation of data-collecting tools and metrics
- Confirmation of the reliability and validity of the constructs
- Data analysis. Detailed information on these steps is provided in the following sections.

1.3.1 Selection of the Sample and Characterization

Hospitals from Argentina, Brazil, India, Italy, Mexico, and the USA partook in a worldwide report. We utilized a non-irregular procedure with some foreordained choice measures. To start with, respondents need to

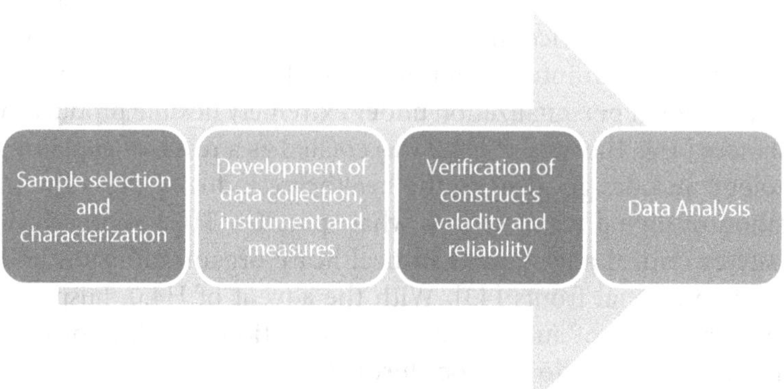

Figure 1.2 Research process.

have significant positions of authority in their hospitals (center or senior administration), which ought to give them the capacity to picture and comprehend the hospital they address and its unmistakable characteristics [53]. Because of the great degree of intricacy imbued in healthcare organization associations, we likewise searched out a few respondents from various foundations and divisions inside every organization. Such a requirement needs to present a more complete picture of the entire hospital and its H4.0 execution experience [46] given that the evidence on the use of new ICTs may span from regulatory processes to medical treatment. Many respondents per hospital greatly improve the internal validity and reliability of our study and lessen issues caused by single-respondent bias. Notwithstanding the absence of an obviously characterized choice measure for hospitals, we got information from hospitals with different logical qualities. The study's clinics generally and methodically recorded their exhibition results consistently, taking into consideration more profound information on every respondent's viewpoint while addressing the inquiry [54].

As compared with studies that also used surveys as their primary data source, the last example had 181 reactions from 18 hospitals in six nations, with a response rate that is exceptionally high (i.e., 67.8%) [47]. The majority of responders (87.8%) and hospitals (88.9%) were situated in emerging economies. Participants had an average of 57.5% clinical experience in their departments, 69.6% were in supervisor or coordinator roles, and 81.2% had been in their positions for more than 2 years. Also, the majority of responders (61.3% and 59.7%) worked in teaching hospitals, many of which (51.9%) had more than 20 years of history, and 75.7% and 77.9% of responders, respectively, came from institutions with less than 2,000 staff and more than 150 beds.

1.3.2 Creation of a Data-Gathering Tool and Measures

The application form comprised four sections. It first established the demographic profile of the sample by collecting information on the traits of the respondents, their departments, and hospitals. ICT technologies were utilized as a substitute for H4.0 execution since certain respondents probably would not know all about the idea [48]. To check the reception level, we utilized a five-point Likert scale with a scope of 1 (not used) to 5 (completely embraced). The last part of the study requested that respondents rate how their hospitals' performance has changed over the past 3 years. As per specialists, reactions are bound to be exact when execution changes are utilized as an intermediary for an association's prosperity, especially when the example is essentially comprised of center directors [49]. Five pointers were used to decide the degree of execution improvement.

1.3.3 Inspection of the Conceptions' Reliability and Validity

We performed three exploratory factor analyses (EFAs) employing principal component (PC) extraction to assess components using review results. Specialists regularly use EFA to recognize the hidden ideas basic in a bunch of noticed factors [55]. It should be employed in cases like ours where there is no prior knowledge of the components or patterns underlying the observed variables.

Operational performance improvement metrics were used to run the first EFA. Using a varimax turn of the axes, which had an eigenvalue of 3.47 and represented 69.30% of the complete change in the answers, we had the option to achieve critical loadings for the five presentation pointers in the main PC. The Cronbach's alpha test aftereffect equal to 0.885 exhibited great unwavering quality in reaction to the review's development, which has an alpha limit of 0.6 or higher [50].

Using feedback on the degree of acceptance of the nine technologies included in the questionnaire, a second EFA was conducted. The objective was to locate H4.0 technology bundles. By rotating with a varimax, we were able to keep two PCs with eigenvalues greater than 1.

The third EFA used responses to the criticality level of eight execution barriers for H4.0. To extract the two components, we use an EFA with varimax rotation and eigenvalues of at least 1. The empirical validation of the two bundles was achieved through barrier variable loading on single components [56]. As suggested by the STS theory, we classified barrier bundles as either social or technological in accordance with their nature, as H4.0 indicates significant changes to how healthcare organizations function. Social hurdles, such as a lack of skilled team members or a strategy that is not in line with the hospital's strategy, are emotional or intangible issues that may impede the adoption of H4.0.

1.3.4 Data Evaluation

In this step, we initially isolated perceptions into bunches as per the degree of handling activation, correspondence, and detecting innovation reception. To do this, the middle reaction values of each group were utilized as the models to distinguish between low and high adopters. Of the 92 observations, 89 had adoption levels that were higher than the cutoff point and were categorized as "high adopters," whereas the remaining observations had adoption levels that were lower than the cutoff point [57]. The remaining observations were classified as "high adopters" in the processing-actuation study, whereas 88 respondents were labeled as "low adopters" since their adoption rates were below the bundle's cutoff.

Comparable advances were taken to characterize perceptions as indicated by H4.0 barriers. In light of the middle reaction upsides of the specialized and social barriers packs, respondents were divided into "lowly constrained" and "highly constrained" groups. Technical challenges were rated as lowly constrained for 80 perceptions and extremely constrained for 101; interpersonal challenges were rated as lowly constrained for 80 perceptions and very constrained for 101.

Using one-way ANOVA, the effect of H4.0 innovation acceptance on the improvement of hospitals' performance was investigated (dependent variable) [39]. The objective was to assess H1. A two-way ANOVA was used to evaluate the relationships between H4.0 innovations and barriers to hospitals' exhibition improvement. The Kolmogorov–Smirnov test was used to determine if the residuals from the one- and two-way ANOVA models were ordinarily distributed. The results demonstrated that the errors were independently distributed and on a regular basis.

We ignored the fundamental impact, as Montgomery would have proposed, when both the primary and collaboration impacts were critical. Considering that a base example size is not expected to do ANOVAs [50], the way that we did not test the entire factorial model (counting higher-request communications) because of the little example size is significant.

1.4 Result and Discussion

The results of the ANOVA are displayed in Table 1.1, and they all anticipated that the performance of hospitals will be much enhanced by H4.0 technology. In fact, according to our research, both H4.0 technology bundles and hospital performance are positively associated. In fact, the hospitals' average performance improvement levels (0.382 and 0.321, respectively) were higher than those of low adopters in terms of detecting correspondence and handling incitation. Given the widespread belief that IT integration enables quicker and more effective operations in healthcare companies, these results are relatively predictable. Our results also support research from studies, which did exploratory tests specifically regions/treatments inside a clinic [51]. Consequently, when their principal impacts are considered, H4.0 advances in all actuality do appear to work on hospitals' performance all in all.

Table 1.1 Results of ANOVA.

Independent variable	*F*-value of hospital performance
Sensing communication	12.30
Processing actuation	8.64
Sensing communication × technical barriers	3.70
Sensing communication × social barriers	0.06
Processing actuation × technical barriers	0.04
Processing actuation × social barriers	5.32

Two links stand out when analyzing the relationships between H4.0 technologies and constraints: i) the relationship between processing-actuation technologies and social constraints and ii) the relationship between sensing-communication technologies and technical constraints. Using a 90% confidence range, the marginal means of the interactions are estimated. After examining how closely sensing-communication technologies and technical obstacles are related, we come to the conclusion that there is a significant difference between hospitals that adopt sensing-communication technologies at a low rate and those that do so at a high rate, with the latter performing significantly better, when hospital leaders do not view technical barriers as a significant obstacle to the implementation of H4.0 (lowly constrained). These results suggest that a higher level of technical hurdles reduces the beneficial effect of sensing-communication technologies on hospitals' performance.

This is consistent with the findings of some studies that highlighted the possibility that some technical obstacles, such as IT infrastructure and information security threats, could undermine the projected benefits of the deployment of H4.0 [52]. While healthcare rules and accrediting bodies differ, hospitals that make a major effort to attain compliance are subject to a variety of obligations. Such initiatives are typically time- and money-consuming, and they frequently make it difficult for hospitals to build an effective information and communication system. Our findings corroborate previous findings and show that technical obstacles must be removed in order to fully implement H4.0, particularly when implementing technologies aimed at gathering and disseminating health-related data. All in all, hospitals that need to work on their tasks, administrations, and treatments using sensing-communication technologies

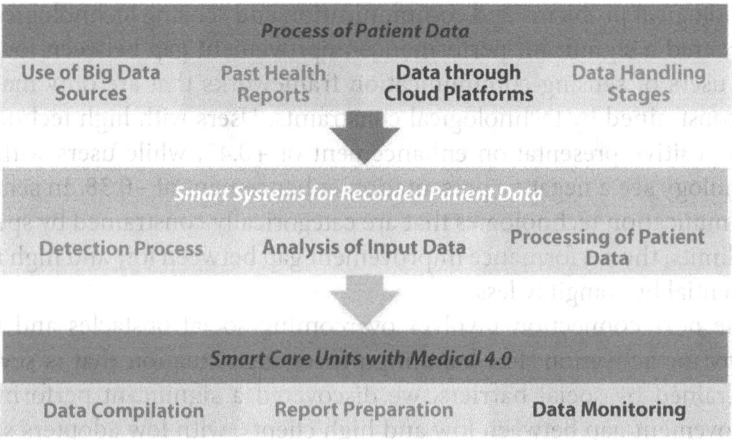

Figure 1.3 Healthcare 4.0 technologies for hospitals [63].

may initially have to dispense with the inborn specialized obstacles to understand the advantages of this digital change completely. Figure 1.3 shows the healthcare 4.0 technologies used in hospitals.

1.5 Conclusion

In this article, we looked at how H4.0 technologies, impediments, and their interactions affect the hospitals' ability to perform better. Two key conclusions are suggested by this research. Initially, two distinct bundles of H4.0 technologies might be created. The most frequent obstacles to the deployment of H4.0 might potentially be divided into two bundles. Second, there is a positive and strong correlation between the performance of hospitals and these H4.0 technology packages. It is crucial to take into account both H4.0 technologies and barriers in order to comprehend how they will affect hospitals because their interaction with H4.0 obstacles was proven to be vital for performance improvement.

The exploration's discoveries show that executing H4.0 innovation from the two packs improves hospitals' execution, supporting H1. Unexpected effects on execution are noted while examining the relationship between H4.0 technology packs and technical and social hurdles. Nonetheless, the strength of the relationship impacts may vary depending on the improvements and constraints taken into account.

In order to explain the performance improvement of hospitals, two distinct forms of interactions stood out as important. The first one focuses on technological problems and communication and sensing technologies. We discovered a significant performance improvement gap between low and high users of sensing-communication frameworks that are only marginally constrained by technological constraints. Users with high technology see a positive presentation enhancement of +0.45, while users with low technology see a negative presentation enhancement of −0.38. In sensing-communication technologies that are categorically constrained by specialized limits, the performance improvement gap between low and high users is essential but tangibly less.

The next connection involves overcoming social obstacles and technology for activation. For handling processing-actuation that is severely constrained by social barriers, we discovered a significant performance improvement gap between low and high clients, with low adopters showing a negative improvement of −0.48 and high adopters showing a positive rise of +0.39. In hospitals with a few social restrictions, the performance gap between low and high adopters is statistically insignificant and much less. This surprising finding suggests that the benefits of this technology package become more obvious when hospitals have trouble implementing H4.0 since they miss the mark on vital information, abilities, mentalities, values, and needs. This startling decision to some extent supports the central idea of sociotechnical frameworks hypothesis, which the one-sided or individual support of social or technical parts might deliver accidental communications that adversely affect organizational performance. When taking into account the relationship between societal boundaries and processing-actuation technologies, it seems to be especially obvious.

Future research that makes use of computational simulation tools will also be able to look at how H4.0 implementation could help hospitals function under difficult conditions.

References

1. Jayaraman, P.P., Forkan, A.R.M., Morshed, A., Haghighi, P.D., Kang, Y., Healthcare 4.0: A review of frontiers in digital health. *Wiley Interdiscip. Rev. Data Min. Knowl. Discov.*, 10, 2, e1350, 2020.
2. Piccarozzi, M., Aquilani, B., Gatti, C., Industry 4.0 in Management studies: A systematic literature review. *Sustainability*, 10, 10, 3821, 2018.
3. Sony, M. and Aithal, P.S., Developing an industry 4.0 readiness model for indian engineering industries. *Int. J. Manag. Technol. Soc. Sci.*, 5, 2, 141–153, 2020.

4. Sony, M., Antony, J., Mc Dermott, O., Garza-Reyes, J.A., An empirical examination of benefits, challenges, and critical success factors of industry 4.0 in manufacturing and service sector. *Technol. Soc.*, 67, 101754, 2021.
5. Sony, M., Industry 4.0 and lean management: A proposed integration model and research propositions. *Prod. Manuf. Res.*, 6, 1, 416–432, 2018.
6. Wang, S., Wan, J., Li, D., Zhang, C., Implementing smart factory of industrie 4.0: An outlook. *Int. J. Distrib. Sens. Netw.*, 12, 1, 3159805, 2016.
7. Prause, G. and Atari, S., On sustainable production networks for Industry 4.0. *Entrepreneurship Sustain. Issues*, 4, 4, 421–431, 2017.
8. Koether, R., *Taschenbuch Der Logistik*, Carl Hanser Verlag GmbH & Co. KG, München, Germany, 2018.
9. Li, J. and Carayon, P., Healthcare 4.0: A vision for smart and connected healthcare. *IISE Trans. Healthc. Syst. Eng.*, 11, 3, 1–10, 2021.
10. Alloghani, M., Al-Jumeily, D., Hussain, A., Aljaaf, A., Mustafina, J., Petrov, E., Healthcare Services Innovations based on the state of the art Technology Trend Industry 4.0, in: *2018 11th International Conference on Developments in eSystems Engineering (DeSE)*, IEEE, pp. 64–70, 2018.
11. Ali, O., Shrestha, A., Soar, J., Wamba, S., Cloud computing-enabled healthcare opportunities, issues, and applications: A systematic review. *Int. J. Inf. Manag.*, 43, 46–158, 2018.
12. Alharbi, F., Atkins, A., Stanier, C., Al-Buti, H., Strategic value of cloud computing in healthcare organisations using the Balanced Scorecard approach: A case study from a Saudi hospital. *Proc. Comput. Sci.*, 98, 332–339, 2016.
13. Ciuti, G., Caliò, R., Camboni, D., Neri, L., Bianchi, F., Arezzo, A., Magnani, B., "Frontiers of robotic endoscopic capsules: A review. *J. Microbio. Robot.*, 11, 1-4, 1–18, 2016.
14. Wolf, B. and Scholze, C., Medicine 4.0: The role of electronics, information technology and microsystems in modern medicine. *Curr. Dir. Biomed. Eng.*, 3, 2, 183–186, 2017.
15. Yang, J.J., Li, J., Mulder, J., Wang, Y., Chen, S., Wu, H., Wang, Q., Pan, H., Emerging information technologies for enhanced healthcare. *Comput. Ind.*, 69, 3–11, 2015.
16. Agha, L., The effects of health information technology on the costs and quality of medical care. *J. Health Econ.*, 34, 19–30, 2014.
17. Bardhan, I. and Thouin, M., Health information technology and its impact on the quality and cost of healthcare delivery. *Decis. Support Syst.*, 55, 2, 438–449, 2013.
18. Fosso Wamba, S. and Ngai, E.W., Importance of issues related to RFID-enabled healthcare transformation projects: Results from a Delphi study. *Prod. Plan. Control.*, 26, 1, 19–33, 2015.
19. Cecconi, F., *New Frontiers in the study of social phenomena: Cognition, complexity, adaptation*, Springer, London, 2016.

20. Walker, G., Stanton, N., Salmon, P., Jenkins, D., "A review of sociotechnical systems theory: A classic concept for new command and control paradigms. *Theor. Issues Ergon. Sci.*, 9, 6, 479–499, 2008.
21. Endeshaw, B., Healthcare service quality-measurement models: A review. *J. Health Res.*, 35, 2, 106–117, 2020.
22. Um, K.H. and Lau, A.K.W., Healthcare service failure: How dissatisfied patients respond to poor service quality. *Int. J. Oper. Prod. Manag.*, 38, 5, 1245–1270, 2018.
23. Sabella, A., Kashou, R., Omran, O., Quality management practices and their relationship to organizational performance. *Int. J. Oper. Prod. Manag.*, 34, 12, 1487–1505, 2014.
24. Russell, R.S., Johnson, D.M., White, S.W., Patient perceptions of quality: Analyzing patient satisfaction surveys. *Int. J. Oper. Prod. Manag.*, 35, 8, 1158–1181, 2015.
25. Dagger, T.S., Sweeney, J.C., Johnson, L.W., A hierarchical model of health service quality: Scale development and investigation of an integrated model. *J. Serv. Res.*, 10, 2, 123–142, 2007.
26. Abidova, A., da Silva, P.A., Moreira, S., Predictors of patient satisfaction and the perceived quality of healthcare in an emergency department in Portugal. *West. J. Emerg. Med.*, 21, 2, 391–403, 2020.
27. Aceto, G., Persico, V., Pescapé, A., The role of information and communication technologies in healthcare: Taxonomies, perspectives, and challenges. *J. Netw. Comput. Appl.*, 107, 125–54, 2018.
28. Tortorella, G.L., Fogliatto, F.S., Mac Cawley Vergara, A., Vassolo, R., Sawhney, R., Healthcare 4.0: Trends, challenges and research directions. *Prod. Plan. Control.*, 31, 15, 1245–1260, 2020.
29. González, L.P., Jaedicke, C., Schubert, J., Stantchev, V., Fog computing architectures for healthcare. *J. Inf. Commun. Ethics Soc.*, 14, 4, 334–349, 2016.
30. Javaid, M. and Khan, I.H., Internet of Things (IoT) enabled healthcare helps to take the challenges of COVID-19 Pandemic. *J. Oral. Biol. Craniofac. Res.*, 11, 2, 209–214, 2021.
31. Al-Jaroodi, J., Mohamed, N., Abukhousa, E., Health 4.0: On the way to realizing the healthcare of the future. *IEEE Access*, 8, 1, 211189–210, 2020.
32. Tortorella, G. L., Fogliatto, F. S., Sunder M, V., Cawley Vergara, A. M., Vassolo, R., Assessment and prioritisation of Healthcare 4.0 implementation in hospitals using Quality Function Deployment. *Int. J. Prod. Res.*, 60, 10, 3147–3169, 2022.
33. Aggarwal, S., Kumar, N., Alhussein, M., Muhammad, G., Blockchain-based UAV path planning for Healthcare 4.0: Current challenges and the way ahead. *IEEE Netw.*, 35, 1, 20–9, 2021.
34. Baker, S.B., Xiang, W., Atkinson, I., Internet of things for smart healthcare: Technologies, challenges, and opportunities. *IEEE Access*, 5, 26521–26544, 2017.

35. Zhang, Y., Qiu, M., Tsai, C.W., Hassan, M.M., Alamri, A., Health-CPS: Healthcare cyber-physical system assisted by cloud and big data. *IEEE Syst. J.*, 11, 1, 88–95, 2017.
36. Dautov, R., Distefano, S., Buyya, R., Hierarchical data fusion for smart healthcare. *J. Big Data*, 6, 1, 19, 2019.
37. Munzer, B.W., Khan, M.M., Shipman, B., Mahajan, P., Augmented reality in emergency medicine: A scoping review. *J. Med. Internet Res.*, 21, 4, e12368, 2019.
38. Pace, P., Aloi, G., Gravina, R., Caliciuri, G., Fortino, G., Liotta, A., An edge-based architecture to support efficient applications for healthcare industry 4.0. *IEEE Trans. Ind. Inf.*, 15, 1, 481–489, 2019.
39. Fatorachian, H. and Kazemi, H., A critical investigation of Industry 4.0 in manufacturing: Theoretical operationalisation framework. *Prod. Plan. Control.*, 29, 8, 633–644, 2018.
40. Schroeder, A., ZiaeeBigdeli, A., Galera Zarco, C., Baines, T., Capturing the benefits of industry 4.0: A business network perspective. *Prod. Plan. Control.*, 30, 16, 1305–1321, 2019.
41. Sony, M. and Naik, S., Critical factors for the successful implementation of Industry 4.0: A review and future research direction. *Prod. Plan. Control.*, 31, 10, 799–815, 2020.
42. Sannino, G., De Falco, I., De Pietro, G., A continuous Noninvasive Arterial Pressure (CNAP) approach for health 4.0 systems. *IEEE Trans. Ind. Inf.*, 15, 1, 498–506, 2018.
43. Nair, A. and Dreyfus, D., Technology alignment in the presence of regulatory changes: The case of meaningful use of information technology in healthcare. *Int. J. Med. Inf.*, 110, 42–51, 2018.
44. Goodwin, C., *Research in psychology: Methods and design*, John Wiley & Sons, Inc., New York, 2005.
45. Marodin, G., Frank, A., Tortorella, G., Netland, T., Lean product development and lean manufacturing: Testing moderation effects. *Int. J. Prod. Econ.*, 203, 301–310, 2018.
46. Oueida, S., Kotb, Y., Aloqaily, M., Jararweh, Y., Baker, T., "An edge computing based smart healthcare framework for resource management." *Sensors*, 18, 12, 4307, 2018.
47. Hair, J., Black, W., Babin, B., Anderson, R., *Multivariate data analysis. Pearson new international edition*, Seventh edition, Pearson, Harlow, Essex, 2014.
48. Rossini, M., Costa, F., Tortorella, G., Portioli-Staudacher, A., The interrelation between Industry 4.0 and lean production: An empirical study on European manufacturers. *Int. J. Adv. Manuf. Technol.*, 102, 9-12, 3963–3976, 2019.
49. Tortorella, G., Vergara, A., Garza-Reyes, J., Sawhney, R., Organizational learning paths based upon industry 4.0 adoption: An empirical study with Brazilian manufacturers. *Int. J. Prod. Econ.*, 219, 284–294, 2019.

50. Meyers, L., Gamst, G., Guarino, A., Applied multivariate research, in: *Design and Analysis of Experiments*, D. Montgomery (Ed.), Sage Publications, Thousand Oaks, Wiley, New York, 20062013.
51. Wang, Y., Kung, L., Byrd, T.A., Big data analytics: Understanding its capabilities and potential benefits for healthcare organizations. *Technol. Forecasting Soc. Change*, 126, 3–13, 2018a.
52. Abdellatif, A. A., Mohamed, A., Chiasserini, C. F., Tlili, M., Erbad, A., Edge computing for smart health: Context-aware approaches, opportunities, and challenges. *IEEE Netw.*, 33, 3, 196–203, 2019.
53. Panwar, V., Sharma, D. K., Kumar, K. P., Jain, A., Thakar, C., Experimental investigations and optimization of surface roughness in turning of en 36 alloy steel using response surface methodology and genetic algorithm. *Mater. Today: Proc.*, 46, 6474–6481, 2021.
54. Jain, A. and Pandey, A.K., Modeling and optimizing of different quality characteristics in electrical discharge drilling of titanium alloy (Grade-5) sheet. *Mater. Today Proc.*, 18, 182–191, 2019. https://doi.org/10.1016/j.matpr.2019.06.292.
55. Jain, A., Yadav, A.K., Shrivastava, Y., Modelling and optimization of different quality characteristics in electric discharge drilling of titanium alloy sheet. *Mater. Today Proc.*, 21, 1680–1684, 2019. https://doi.org/10.1016/j.matpr.2019.12.010.
56. Jain, A. and Pandey, A.K., Multiple quality optimizations in electrical discharge drilling of mild steel sheet. *Mater. Today Proc.*, 8, 7252–7261, 2019. https://doi.org/10.1016/j.matpr.2017.07.054.
57. Jain, A., Kumar, C. S., Shrivastava, Y., Fabrication and machining of fiber matrix composite through electric discharge machining: a short review. *Mater. Today: Proc.*, 51, 1233–1237, 2022.
58. Aochi, H., Ulrich, T., Ducellier, A., Dupros, F., Michea, D., Finite difference simulations of seismic wave propagation for understanding earthquake physics and predicting ground motions: Advances and challenges. *J. Phys. Conf. Ser.*, 454, 1, 012010, 2013, August. IOP Publishing.
59. Lakshmi, P.S., Saxena, M., Koli, S., Joshi, K., Abdullah, K.H., Gangodkar, D., Traffic response system based on data mining and internet of things (Iot) for preventing accidents, in: *2022 2nd International Conference on Advance Computing and Innovative Technologies in Engineering (ICACITE)*, IEEE, pp. 1092–1096, 2022, April.
60. Rokade, A., Singh, M., Malik, P.K., Singh, R., Alsuwian, T., Intelligent data analytics framework for precision farming using IoT and regressor machine learning algorithms. *Appl. Sci.*, *12*, 19, 9992, 2022.
61. Bagwari, S., Roy, A., Gehlot, A., Singh, R., Priyadarshi, N., Khan, B., LoRa based metrics evaluation for real-time landslide monitoring on IoT platform. *IEEE Access*, *10*, 46392–46407, 2022.

62. Malik, P.K., Singh, R., Gehlot, A., Akram, S.V., Das, P.K., Village 4.0: Digitalization of village with smart internet of things technologies. *Comput. Ind. Eng.*, *165*, 107938, 2022.
63. Haleem, A., Javaid, M., Singh, R. P., Suman, R., Medical 4.0 technologies for healthcare: Features, capabilities, and applications. *Int. Things Cyber-Phys. Syst.*, 2, 12–30, 2022.

2

Human Breast Cancer Classification Employing the Machine Learning Ensemble

Sreenivas Mekala[1], S. Srinivasulu Raju[2*], M. Gomathi[3], Naga Venkateshwara Rao K.[4], Kothandaraman D.[5] and Saurabh Sharma[6]

[1]Department of IT, Sreenidhi Institute of Science and Technology, Telangana, India
[2]Department of Electronics and Instrumentation Engineering, VR Siddhartha Engineering College, Vijayawada, India
[3]Department of ECE, S.A. Engineering College, Chennai, India
[4]Department of ECE, St. Martin's Engineering College Secunderabad, Telangana, India
[5]School of Computer Science & Artificial Intelligence, SR University, Warangal, Telangana, India
[6]Research Scholar, Amity University, Gwalior, India

Abstract

The primary driver of death for women is breast cancer (BC). For the investigation of cancer, the exact order of breast cancer information is fundamental, and patients can save money by avoiding unnecessary surgeries by understanding the difference between benign and malignant tumors. Machine learning is frequently employed in the prediction of breast cancer since it has the benefit of identifying significant traits from a set of medical data. Medical professionals working in the healthcare industry can benefit from and use these decision support tools effectively. The goal of this work is to use ensemble learning to solve the problem of categorizing breast cancer-related data. Techniques for ensemble learning are applied to enhance a classifier's performance. With the help of a Bayesian network and a radial basis function, an ensemble model for decision support is being developed in this study. This study made substantial use of the well-researched open-access dataset "Wisconsin Breast Cancer Dataset (WBCD)." Oncologists would benefit

**Corresponding author*: srinu85raju@gmail.com
S. Srinivasulu Raju: ORCID: https://orcid.org/0000-0001-5680-7725

Kapil Joshi and Somil Kumar Gupta (eds.) Human Cancer Diagnosis and Detection Using Exascale Computing, (19–34) © 2024 Scrivener Publishing LLC

from the proposed ensemble learning by being able to discriminate cancer tumors precisely and provide patients with the best care.

***Keywords*:** Breast cancer, machine learning, WBCD, classification

2.1 Introduction

Breast cancer is one of the top causes of death among women. In 2011, there were more than 508,000 assessed deaths among women worldwide due to bosom malignant growths, according to a 2013 World Health Organization assessment. Breast cancer in its early stages is treatable and preventable. However, many women receive a cancer diagnosis after it is already too late. Breast cells, oily tissues, or stringy connective tissues can all give rise to breast cancer. Breast cancer tumors typically get worse over time and get bigger, which results in mortality [1]. Men can experience it as well, even though women experience it more frequently. Age and family history are just two of the many factors that can increase the risk of breast cancer. Breast cancer tumors may be risky or innocuous [2]. A benign tumor rarely results in human death and is not harmful to the body. This particular sort of tumor only develops in one area of the body. A cancerous tumor is more harmful and can be fatal to people. The aberrant cell development that causes this form of tumor causes it to spread quickly [38].

2.1.1 Breast Cancer Symptoms and Signs

There are two forms of breast cancer: 1) invasive and 2) non-intrusive. Though invasive cancer spreads to different parts of the body, the second type of cancer simply influences the breast and does not influence different parts of the body. Breast cancer can present with a wide range of symptoms and a few of these are as follows:

- Changes in the size and contour of the breast
- Dimpling of the breast
- A recently turned nipple
- A breast that is red
- Scaling, peeling, or flaking of the breast's pigmented region
- Breast lump [3]

2.1.2 Breast Cancer Risk Factors

There are avoidable and non-preventable risk factors for breast cancer.

- Mature age
- A personal history of breast diseases is a factor that increases the risk of breast cancer.
- Personal experience with cancer
- Early menarche
- Menopause
- Late menopause
- A history of breast cancer in the family
- Obesity
- Radiation exposure
- Having a first child after turning 30
- Null parity is among the other factors
- Consuming alcohol

The causes and risk factors of breast cancer are depicted in Figure 2.1.

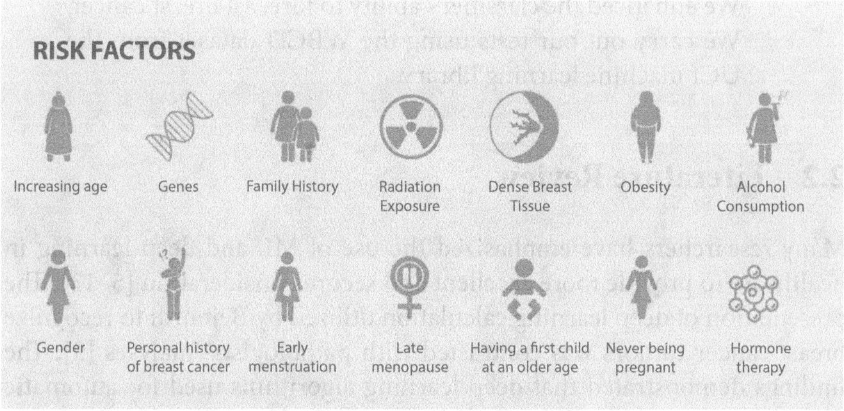

Figure 2.1 Breast cancer causes and risk factors [4].

2.1.3 Disease Prediction Using Machine Learning

Machine learning (ML), a subset of artificial intelligence, combines a range of factual, probabilistic, and augmenting techniques to enhance performance utilizing both old and new data. To predict diseases, many ML approaches have been widely used.

The early identification of breast cancer was significantly aided by machine learning techniques. According to survey results, machine learning approaches have a 93% accuracy rate, whereas the majority of experienced doctors can identify breast cancer with 76% accuracy. It is simple to differentiate between those who have breast cancer and those who have none by utilizing ML approaches. With proper classification, clinicians will be better equipped to recognize cancer in its early stages [39].

Classification is a difficult regulated improvement issue. Data on cancer are organized using a variety of methods, including SVM, ANN, K-NN, naive Bayes, CNN, and Bayesian network.

The following is a list of significant contributions of our suggested approach.

- For the classification of breast cancer data, this research suggests a unique ensemble technique developed employing heterogeneous classifiers like the Bayesian network and radial basis function (RBF).
- We enhanced the classifier's ability to forecast breast cancer.
- We carry out our tests using the WBCD dataset from the UCI machine learning library.

2.2 Literature Review

Many researchers have emphasized the use of ML and deep learning in healthcare to provide more excellent and secure consideration [5–13]. The presentation of deep learning calculation utilized by Bejnordi to recognize breast cancer tumors was contrasted with pathologists' analyses [9]. The findings demonstrated that deep learning algorithms used for automatic detection outperformed human diagnosis. Utilizing transfer learning, Khan *et al.* combined the highlights acquired from GoogleNet, VGGNet, and ResNet [14].

Haifeng offered a unique strategy for predicting breast cancer using data mining techniques [15]. In light of the patient's clinical data, the author came up with a trustworthy method to deal with breast cancer estimates.

The appropriateness of the approach was assessed using the Wisconsin Breast Cancer Database (WBCD) and Wisconsin Diagnostic Breast Cancer (WDBC) datasets. The execution was assessed using support vector machines, eight learning models, artificial neural networks, naive Bayes classification, and AdaBoost tree. In light of the head part analysis and various information mining techniques, the author offered a blended model for highlight reduction and suggested adopting several approaches for space reduction, such as k-mean [40].

To arrange breast tumors for evaluation, few studies used both supervised and unsupervised categorization techniques [16]. The authors recommended combining head part research with scaling. They demonstrated that a group casting a voting-based forecast model is the most dependable. After highlight determination, an assortment of grouping models was tried and prepared on the information. Only four models improved their performance in the group voting classifier, with accuracy levels of about 90%, as demonstrated by the models' results for accuracy and review, the area under the receiver operating characteristic curve (AUC-ROC), F1 measure, and computational time. These models were logistic regression, SVM, and AdaBoost [41].

Many researchers used a variety of techniques, including SVMs, ANNs, and decision trees (DTs), and the findings revealed that SVMs outperformed other classifiers on the WBCD [17, 18]. ANN, DT, and SVM precision rates were 94.6%, 93.7%, and 96.7%, respectively. They need cross-approval for evaluation on a 10-fold scale.

Naive Bayes (NB), DTs, and LR were employed by Mandal *et al.* and the authors also looked at each classifier's time complexity [19]. With the highest accuracy, LR performs better than other classifiers. The efficiency of DT and Bayesian networks, however, was contrasted by Borges *et al.* who found that the latter performed better, with 96.80% accuracy [20].

The Bayesian hypothesis, DT, radial basis function network, and J48 were all used by Chaurasia *et al.* [21]. They constructed an expectation model using prehandling, data determination, and data change, and afterward, they utilized the WBCD dataset to assess the outcomes. They found that naive Bayes performed better compared with different models, with an order precision of 97.36%. Order precision was 96.77% and 93.41% for the RBF organization and J48, respectively.

J-tear, IBK, LR, decision table, J48, slow K-star, AdaBoost, multiclass classifier, multilayer perceptron, naive Bayes, random tree, and random forest were the 12 classification calculations used by Kumar *et al.* to predict breast cancer [22]. They attested that all calculations, except for naive Bayes classification, performed with precision more prominently than 94% and that sluggish and tree characterizations outperformed other order strategies by close to 100% exactness.

Lee *et al.* claim that ensemble learning not just improves the exhibition of a base student but also diminishes predisposition and variety [23]. In order to work on the exhibition of WBCD, Abdar *et al.* discovered the CWV-BANNSVM ensemble characterization approach [24]. It works with two SVMs to coordinate with the boosting artificial neural network (BANN). In contrast to traditional ensemble learning, several studies devised a novel, special ensemble learning method to determine the number of neural networks and their design as a result [25]. Each neural network receives a unique training set, ensuring superior learning from all training data samples. The suggested DEL is trained repeatedly using an incremental training method in order to establish the correct values for the correlation strength and learning rate parameters.

As indicated by Osman *et al.*, improvement is conceivable while utilizing the group-supporting technique [26]. When the method was combined with a radial basis function neural network philosophy, the accuracy for the WBCD dataset increased to 98.4%.

Most of the cited literature based its evaluation on how well the suggested strategy performs on "accuracy." When true positives (TPs) and true negatives (TNs) outweigh false positives (FPs) and false negatives, precision is increased (FNs). In order to announce an execution, accuracy, review, and exactness are essential. However, the adequacy of artificial intelligence frameworks for clinical diagnostics ought to give a more noteworthy load to bogus negatives (review) than misleading upsides, as missing a sickness could have serious ramifications for patients (accuracy).

2.3 Methodology

This study uses an ensemble classifier that was created using a Bayesian network and a radial basis function to categorize breast cancer. For experimental analysis, the WBCD was employed. Ten qualities and a total of 699 instances are taken into account. WBCD is offered by Wolberg *et al.* [27]. RBFs and a Bayesian network are employed to model the ensemble classifier. The suggested ensemble classifier as well as two individual classifiers will be covered in the subsections [43].

2.3.1 Bayesian Network

In the actual world, condition probability is quite helpful. Prior information cannot be incorporated into traditional statistical models.

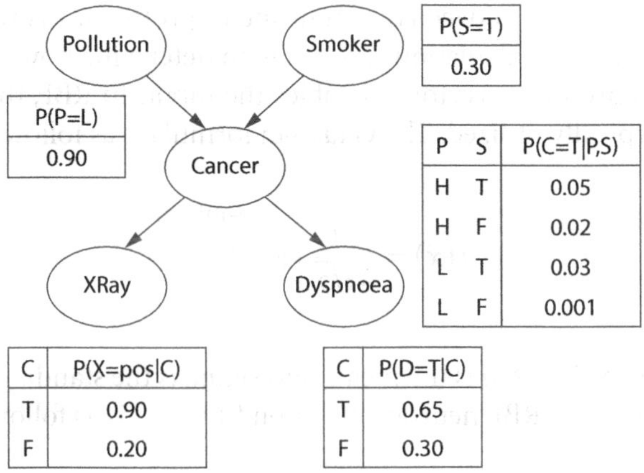

Figure 2.2 Illustration of the Bayesian network.

The probabilistic relationships between different things or objects are represented by a Bayesian network. Missing edges in directed acyclic networks imply conditional independence between variables, whereas nodes in Bayesian networks (BNs) represent variables (DAG) [33]. Every node has a likelihood capability doled out to it. Bayesian networks are utilized to communicate information about a hazy point. The diagram hypothesis, likelihood hypothesis, measurements, software engineering, and Bayesian networks are totally consolidated in Bayesian networks.

When using huge networks, this joint distribution will reduce the computation. A Bayesian network is displayed in Figure 2.2 as an example.

The Bayesian network is used because it consistently achieves high accuracy in challenging and uncertain domains.

2.3.2 Radial Basis Function

The radial basis function network is a supervised approach that evolved from function approximation. RBFs are three-layered neural networks that have hidden, O/P, and I/P layers. Each hidden unit has a unique input space receptive field. These units, denoted as V1, V2, ...Vn, are known as radial centers [34]. The change from hidden units to yield is linear as opposed to the indirect change from the input layer to the hidden unit. RBF will make a neighborhood planning of which RBF advances rapidly. In RBF, two kinds of learning are utilized: weight learning and focus learning.

By deciding how intently the information looks like the models from the preparation set, RBF completes regulated learning [44]. Each neuron calculates the distance between the input and its prototype in order to order a different example. Calculations are made to determine how closely each RBF neuron's prototype vector resembles the input. In RBF, the Gaussian function is typically utilized. The Gaussian formula is as follows:

$$r(x) = \frac{1}{\sigma\sqrt{2\pi}} e^{-\frac{(x-u)^2}{2\sigma^2}}$$

Where x is the input, u is the mean, and sigma is the standard deviation. As described, the RBF neuron activation function is as follows:

$$\varnothing(x) = e^{-\beta\|x-u\|^2}$$

2.3.3 Ensemble Learning

A single, ideal predictive model is produced using a range of learning algorithms via the supervised machine learning technique known as ensemble learning [35]. The model combines a variety of supervised learners to boost its predictive power. The widely used ensemble learning techniques are as follows:

- Bagging
- Increasing
- Stacking

It is possible to reduce the variance through bagging. By averaging the process, bagging merges ineffective learners. Not bias but lowering variance is the aim of bagging. Another terminology for this is parallel ensemble learning. They perform well with complex models, especially those with high volatility and minimal bias [42].

Boosting is a two-step technique, often known as sequential ensemble learning that reduces bias rather than variance. These models are excellent for high-bias and low-variance models.

Stacking and boosting are both types of the meta-learning method. The ensemble is used to retrieve features that will be utilized by additional layers [36]. Stacking is typically utilized in contests where the data are trained using various methods and the average of these outcomes is considered.

Ensemble classifiers categorize new samples using weights or majority voting and are built from a number of base (weak) classifiers.

Several algorithms use base learners, often known as weak learners. For base learners, there are numerous tuning variables. Decision trees are the fundamental learning algorithm, just like the random forest ensemble. Weak learners are often referred to as base learners. Weak students frequently but irregularly record with little accuracy. While learning the connections between input and output, it is lacking. Weak learners are combined in ensemble learning to achieve high accuracy. The technique informs the algorithm selection. Three concerns will be handled using ensemble classifiers, namely, 1) statistical, 2) computerized, and 3) representational; weak classifiers are unable to address these problems.

Ensemble learning is a strong AI strategy that can be utilized to work on the model's exhibition. Combining the several learning sets improves the model's ability to predict (base learners).

2.3.4 The Suggested Algorithm

The algorithm for the proposed method is the breast cancer data classification utilizing ensemble machine learning [37]. The stages of the suggested strategy are as follows:

- Enter the WBCD dataset.
- Preprocess WBCD using the preprocessing method.
- Divide the dataset into training and test datasets.
- Using a Bayesian network, RBF, and 10-fold cross-validation, build an ensemble learning system (majority voting).
- Let us say the "S" test data are used for each new sample.
- Ensemble classifier (test sample) = majority vote (classes: RBF, Bayesian network).
- Assess the suggested strategy's accuracy using a variety of criteria.

Figure 2.3 displays the process flow diagram of the suggested approach.

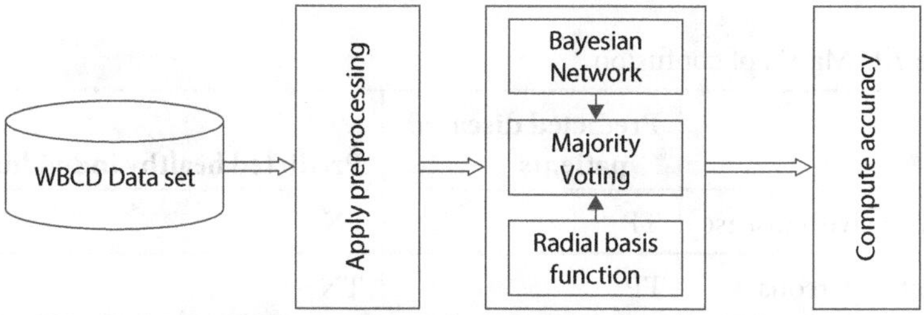

Figure 2.3 Process flowchart for the suggested method.

2.4 Results and Discussion

The utilization of ensemble learning for data analysis is canvassed in this part. To assess the viability of the ensemble classifier, we utilized a scope of evaluation metrics, for example, exactness, accuracy, review, the f-measure, TNR, MCC, and TPR. These matrixes are acquired from Table 2.1 showing the confusion matrix.

"TN" and "FN" represent the number of normal cases that were mistakenly classified as having the disease, and "TP" and "FP" stand for the number of breast cancer cases that were accurately diagnosed as having the disease.

Prediction was incorrect if MCC = −1 and 100% accurate if MCC = +1. The WBCD dataset was used to evaluate the suggested system. Many researchers in ML and pattern recognition used WBCD.

The first attribute in the WBCD dataset, ID, which has 699 instances and will be eliminated from the dataset before categorization, is one of the 11 attributes of this dataset. There are two classes in this dataset: benign and malignant. Table 2.2 gives a description of the dataset. Using the WEKA tool, tests were carried out and missing values were normalized.

Table 2.3 lists the outcomes of the suggested ensemble learning. To categorize the dataset, 10 cross-validations were performed. The proposed method's accuracy was calculated to be 98.52%. The FPR for ensemble learning is 0.07.

Two clusters are employed in RBF, and the Bayesian network employs the simulated annealing search technique. Using our suggested methods, the maximum reported recall and TPR values are 98.42% and 98.0, respectively. When the classes are unequal, Mathew's correlation coefficient, a balanced statistic, is used. A parallel classifier that is precise is shown by an MCC value of 1, whereas one that is troublesome is shown by a value of −1. The MCC values from the suggested classifier were 0.54, indicating

Table 2.1 Matrix of confusion.

	Predicted diseased patients	Predicted healthy individuals
Patients with disease	TP	FN
Healthy persons	FP	TN

Table 2.2 WBCD dataset description.

Serial number	Attribute name	Values
1	Bland chromatin	1 to 10
2	Uniformity of cell shape	1 to 10
3	Uniformity of cell size	1 to 10
4	Single epithelial cell size	1 to 10
5	Normal nucleoli	1 to 10
6	Mitoses	1 to 10
7	Clump thickness	1 to 10
8	Marginal adhesion	1 to 10
9	Bare nuclei	1 to 10
10	Class	Benign = 3 Malignant = 5

Table 2.3 Outcomes of the suggested method.

Serial number	Metrics	Values
1.	NPV	99.65
2.	MCC	0.54
3.	F measure	96.01
4.	Recall or sensitivity	98.42
5.	Accuracy	98.52
6.	Specificity	95.17
7.	TPR	98.00
8.	FPR	.07
9.	Precision or PPV	97.62

that the proposed model is unquestionably suitable for categorizing breast cancer data.

Table 2.4 displays the accuracy comparisons between the suggested approach and various currently used approaches. Table 2.4 and Figure 2.4 display the accuracy that was attained using various machine learning techniques.

We attest that the proposed system records sensible precision when contrasted with different strategies in light of the comparison table.

The outcome in Figure 2.4 makes it clear that the suggested strategy produced good accuracy. It suggests that this model does a good job of classifying breast cancer data.

Table 2.4 Comparison of the proposed methodology to the methods already in use.

Serial number	Authors	Technique used	Accuracy
1	Fu MR [28]	ANN	94.75
2	Kumar [29]	SVM-NB	96.14
3	Karabatak and Ince [30]	AR-ANN	96.39
4	Seera and Lim [31]	FMM-CART	96.30
5	Chen [32]	RS-SVM	97.86
6	Proposed approach	BN+RBF	98.52

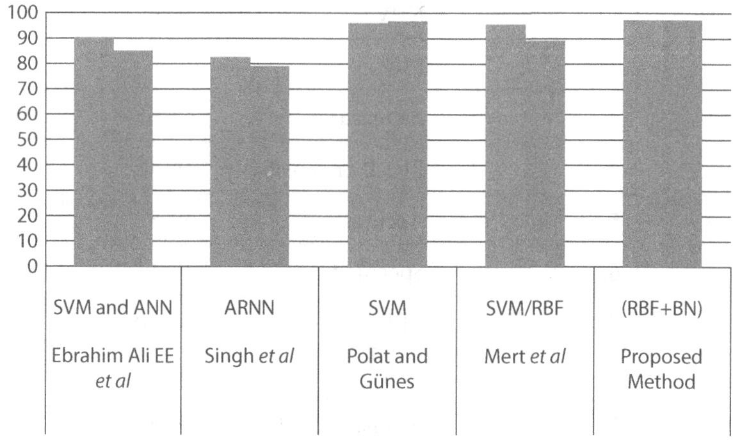

Figure 2.4 Accuracy attained using different methods.

2.5 Conclusion

The classification of breast cancer data must be accurate and efficient for medical diagnosis. Machine learning techniques are frequently employed and are essential for categorizing healthcare data. Although numerous methods for classifying breast cancer data have been established, there are still significant difficulties, such as accuracy. We put up a model for categorizing breast cancer data to solve this. To classify the data on breast cancer, an ensemble model is built in this study utilizing a Bayesian network and RBF. RBF and the Bayesian network offer good classification accuracy. The viability of the model is evaluated using a variety of pointers. Many currently used techniques for categorizing breast cancer data are compared with the proposed model. The perfect accuracy of 98.52% was produced by combining these two heterogeneous classifiers. The results show that the suggested method outperforms a single classifier on all counts. The suggested ensemble learning approach may be useful in helping cancer professionals recognize cancer.

References

1. Chagpar, A.B. and Coccia, M., Factors associated with breast cancer mortality-per-incident case in low-to-middle income countries (LMICs). *J. Clin. Oncol.*, 37, 15, 2019.
2. Sharma, G.N., Dave, R., Sanadya, J., Sharma, P., Sharma, K., Various types and management of breast cancer: An overview. *J. Adv. Pharm. Technol. Res.*, 1, 109, 2010.
3. MayoClinic, *Breast cancer*, [Internet], Mayo Clinic Medical Science, Florida, 2020, [cited 2020 Jan 1]. Available from: https://www.mayoclinic.org/diseases-conditions/breast-cancer/symptoms-causes/syc-20352470.
4. Medindia, *Breast Cancer*, [Internet], MedIndia, India, 2020, [cited 2020 Jan 1]. Available form: https://www.Medindia.net.
5. Guo, Y., Shang, X., Li, Z., Identification of cancer subtypes by integrating multiple types of transcriptomics data with deep learning in breast cancer. *Neurocomputing*, 324, 20–30, 2019.
6. Golden, J.A., Deep learning algorithms for detection of lymph node metastases from breast cancer: Helping artificial intelligence be seen. *JAMA*, 318, 2184–2186, 2017.
7. Li, L., Pan, X., Zhang, L., Multi-task deep learning for fine-grained classification and grading in breast cancer histopathological images. *Multimed. Tools Appl.*, 810, 85–95, 2018.

8. Zhu, Z., Albadawy, E., Saha, A., Zhang, J., Harowicz, M.R., Mazurowski, M.A., Deep learning for identifying radiogenomic associations in breast cancer. *Comput. Biol. Med.*, 109, 85–90, 2019.
9. Bejnordi, B.E., Veta, M., Van Diest, P.J., Van Ginneken, B., Karssemeijer, N., Litjens, G., Van Der Laak, J.A., Hermsen, M., Manson, Q.F., Balkenhol, M. *et al.*, Diagnostic assessment of deep learning algorithms for detection of lymph node metastases in women with breast cancer. *JAMA*, 318, 2199–2210, 2017.
10. Bi, W.L., Hosny, A., Schabath, M.B., Giger, M.L., Birkbak, N.J., Mehrtash, A., Allison, T., Arnaout, O., Abbosh, C., Dunn, I.F. *et al.*, Artificial intelligence in cancer imaging: Clinical challenges and applications. *CA Cancer J. Clin.*, 69, 127–157, 2019.
11. Lamy, J.B., Sekar, B., Guezennec, G., Bouaud, J., Séroussi, B., Explainable artificial intelligence for breast cancer: A visual case-based reasoning approach. *Artif. Intell. Med.*, 94, 42–53, 2019.
12. Shen, L., Margolies, L.R., Rothstein, J.H., Fluder, E., McBride, R., Sieh, W., Deep learning to improve breast cancer detection on screening mammography. *Sci. Rep.*, 9, 1–12, 2019.
13. Coccia, M., Deep learning technology for improving cancer care in society: New directions in cancer imaging driven by artificial intelligence. *Technol. Soc*, 60, 101198, 2020.
14. Khan, S., Islam, N., Jan, Z., Din, I.U., Rodrigues, J.J.C., A novel deep learning based framework for the detection and classification of breast cancer using transfer learning. *Pattern Recognit. Lett.*, 125, 1–6, 2019.
15. Wang, H. and Yoon, S.W., Breast cancer prediction using data mining method, in: *Proceedings of the IIE Annual Conference Expo 2015*, Nashville, TN, USA, pp. 818–828, 30 May–2 June 2015.
16. Nguyen, Q.H., Do, T.T., Wang, Y., Heng, S.S., Chen, K., Ang, W.H.M., Philip, C.E., Singh, M., Pham, H.N., Nguyen, B.P. *et al.*, Breast cancer prediction using feature selection and ensemble voting, in: *Proceedings of the 2019 International Conference on System Science and Engineering (ICSSE)*, Dong Hoi City, Vietnam, pp. 250–254, 20–21 July 2019.
17. Ahmad, L.G., Eshlaghy, A., Poorebrahimi, A., Ebrahimi, M., Razavi, A., Using three machine learning techniques for predicting breast cancer recurrence. *J. Health Med. Inf.*, 4, 3, 2013.
18. Nazir, S., Ghazanfar, M.A., Aljohani, N.R., Azam, M.A., Alowibdi, J.S., Data analysis to uncover intruder attacks using data mining techniques, in: *Proceedings of the 2017 5th International Conference on Information and Communication Technology (ICoIC7)*, Melaka, Malaysia, pp. 1–6, 17–19 May 2017.
19. Mandal, S.K., Performance analysis of data mining algorithms for breast cancer cell detection using Naïve Bayes, logistic regression and decision tree. *Int. J. Eng. Comput. Sci.*, 6, 20388–20391, 2017.
20. Borges, L.R., Analysis of the wisconsin breast cancer dataset and machine learning for breast cancer detection. *Proc. XI Workshop de Visão Computacional*, 1, 369, 1989. Group.

21. Chaurasia, V., Pal, S., Tiwari, B., Prediction of benign and malignant breast cancer using data mining techniques. *J. Algorithms Comput. Technol.*, 12, 119–126, 2018.
22. Kumar, V., Mishra, B. K., Mazzara, M., Thanh, D. N., Verma, A., Prediction of malignant and benign breast cancer: A data mining approach in health-care applications. In *Advances in Data Science and Management: Proceedings of ICDSM 2019*, pp. 435–442, Springer, Singapore, 2020.
23. Lee, S., Amgad, M., Masoud, M., Subramanian, R., Gutman, D., Cooper, L., An ensemble-based active learning for breast cancer classification, in: *Proceedings of the 2019 IEEE International Conference on Bioinformatics and Biomedicine (BIBM)*, San Diego, CA, USA, pp. 2549–2553, 18–21 November 2019.
24. Abdar, M. and Makarenkov, V., CWV-BANN-SVM ensemble learning classifier for an accurate diagnosis of breast cancer. *Measurement*, 146, 557–570, 2019.
25. Alam, K.M.R., Siddique, N., Adeli, H., A dynamic ensemble learning algorithm for neural networks. *Neural Comput. Appl.*, 32, 8675–8690, 1–16, 2020.
26. Osman, A.H. and Aljahdali, H.M., An effective of ensemble boosting learning method for breast cancer virtual screening using neural network model. *IEEE Access*, 8, 39165–39174, 2020.
27. Wolberg, W.H., Street, W.N., Mangasarian, O.L., *Breast Cancer Wisconsin (Diagnostic) Data Set*, [Internet], UC Irvine Machine Learning Repository, 2020, [cited 2020 Jan 2] Available from: https://archive.ics.uci.edu/ml/datasets/breast+cancer+wisc onsin+(diagnostic).
28. Fu, M.R., Wang, Y., Li, C., Qiu, Z., Axelrod, D., Guth, A.A. *et al.*, Machine learning for detection of lymphedema among breast cancer survivors. *MHealth*, 4, 17,2018.
29. Kumar, U.K., Nikhil, M.B.S., Sumangali, K., Prediction of breast cancer using voting classifier technique. *2017 IEEE International Conference on Smart Technologies and Management for Computing, Communication, Controls, Energy and Materials (ICSTM)*, Chennai, India. USA, IEEE, pp. 108–14, Aug 2-4, 2017.
30. Karabatak, M. and Ince, M.C., An expert system for detection of breast cancer based on association rules and neural network. *Expert Syst. Appl.*, 36, 2, 3465–9, 2009.
31. Seera, M. and Lim, C.P., A hybrid intelligent system for medical data classification. *Expert Syst. Appl.*, 41, 5, 2239–49, 2014.
32. Chen, H.L., Yang, B., Liu, J., Liu, D.Y., A support vector machine classifier with rough set-based feature selection for breast cancer diagnosis. *Expert Syst. Appl.*, 38, 7, 9014–22, 2011.
33. Panwar, V., Sharma, D. K., Kumar, K. P., Jain, A., Thakar, C., Experimental investigations and optimization of surface roughness in turning of en 36 alloy steel using response surface methodology and genetic algorithm. *Mater. Today: Proc.*, 46, 6474–6481, 2021.

34. Jain, A. and Pandey, A.K., Modeling and optimizing of different quality characteristics in electrical discharge drilling of titanium alloy (Grade-5) sheet. *Mater. Today Proc.*, 18, 182–191, 2019. https://doi.org/10.1016/j.matpr.2019.06.292.
35. Jain, A., Yadav, A.K., Shrivastava, Y., Modelling and optimization of different quality characteristics in electric discharge drilling of titanium alloy sheet. *Mater. Today Proc.*, 21, 1680–1684, 2019. https://doi.org/10.1016/j.matpr.2019.12.010.
36. Jain, A. and Pandey, A.K., Multiple quality optimizations in electrical discharge drilling of mild steel sheet. *Mater. Today Proc.*, 8, 7252–7261, 2019. https://doi.org/10.1016/j.matpr.2017.07.054.
37. Jain, A., Kumar, C. S., Shrivastava, Y., Fabrication and machining of fiber matrix composite through electric discharge machining: A short review. *Mater. Today: Proc.*, 51, 1233–1237, 2022.
38. Kirola, M., Memoria, M., Dumka, A., Joshi, K., A comprehensive review study on: Optimized data mining, machine learning and deep learning techniques for breast cancer prediction in big data context. *Biomed. Pharmacol. J.*, *15*, 1, 13–25, 2022.
39. Ahmad, I., Sharma, S., Singh, R., Gehlot, A., Priyadarshi, N., Twala, B., MOOC 5.0: A roadmap to the future of learning. *Sustainability*, *14*, 18, 11199, 2022.
40. Dumka, A., Verma, P., Singh, R., Kumar Bisht, A., Anand, D., MoaiteqAljahdali, H., Aparicio Obregón, S., A novel deep learning based healthcare model for COVID-19 pandemic stress analysis. *Comput. Mater. Contin.*, *72*, 3, 6029–6044, 2022.
41. Singh, D., Singh, R., Gehlot, A., Akram, S.V., Priyadarshi, N., Twala, B., An imperative role of digitalization in monitoring cattle health for sustainability. *Electronics*, *11*, 17, 2702, 2022.
42. Sharma, T., Diwakar, M., Singh, P., Lamba, S., Kumar, P., Joshi, K., Emotion Analysis for predicting the emotion labels using machine learning approaches, in: *2021 IEEE 8th Uttar Pradesh Section International Conference on Electrical, Electronics and Computer Engineering (UPCON)*, IEEE, pp. 1–6, 2021, November.
43. Krishna, G., Singh, R., Gehlot, A., Akram, S.V., Priyadarshi, N., Twala, B., Digital technology implementation in battery-management systems for sustainable energy storage: Review, challenges, and recommendations. *Electronics*, *11*, 17, 2695, 2022.
44. Kimothi, S., Singh, R., Gehlot, A., Akram, S.V., Malik, P.K., Gupta, A., Bilandi, N., Intelligent energy and ecosystem for real-time monitoring of glaciers. *Comput. Electr. Eng.*, *102*, 108163, 2022.

3

Multi-Objective Differential Development Using DNN for Multimodality Medical Image Fusion

M. Ranjith Kumar[1], Abhishek Dondapati[2*], Dilip Kumar Sharma[3], Prakash Pareek[4], Rajchandar K.[5] and S. Shalini[6]

[1]Department of Mathematics, Amrita School of Engineering, Amrita Vishwa Vidyapeetham, Chennai, India
[2]Department of Management Studies, University of Madras, Chennai, India
[3]Department of Mathematics, Jaypee University of Engineering and Technology, Guna (M.P.), India
[4]Department of ECE, Vishnu Institute of Technology, Bhimavaram, A.P., India
[5]School of Computer Science & Artificial Intelligence, SR University, Warangal, Telangana, India
[6]Department of Mathematics, J.N.N. Institute of Engineering, Tiruvallur, India

Abstract

Researchers are now able to glean an increasing amount of information from medical photos thanks to the developments in automated diagnostic systems. Multimodality images have recently been employed in order to obtain medical images that are more useful. Compared with standard medical photos, these images include a great deal of information. The creation of multimodality images is a difficult process, nevertheless. The image is initially divided into subbands using a non-subsampled contourlet transform (NSCT) domain. The original photos are then utilized to extract features using an extreme version of Inception (Xception). The best characteristics are chosen using the multi-objective differential evolution. The fused coefficients are then obtained using the energy loss-based fusion functions and the coefficient of determination. The fused picture is then created using the inverse NSCT. The suggested approach outperforms the competing multimodality picture fusion approaches, according to extensive experimental results.

**Corresponding author*: abhishekuoh@gmail.com
M. Ranjith Kumar: ORCID: https://orcid.org/0000-0001-8411-7609

Kapil Joshi and Somil Kumar Gupta (eds.) Human Cancer Diagnosis and Detection Using Exascale Computing, (35–52) © 2024 Scrivener Publishing LLC

Keywords: CNN, medical image fusion, DNN, NSCT

3.1 Introduction

Several kinds of medical photographs serve as an essential part of clinical diagnosis in contemporary medicine and are quite helpful in identifying disorders. Doctors typically need to integrate numerous various types of medical photos from the same location in order to gather enough information for an appropriate diagnosis, which frequently causes significant difficulty. When a doctor simply uses his or her theories and conceptions to interpret a variety of medical images, the objectivity of the analysis is compromised and it is possible that some of the image's information is overlooked. These problems can be successfully overcome by using image fusion algorithms [1]. The acquired medical image from many modalities contains both complementary and redundant data as the range of medical imaging advancements expands. For a more accurate and reliable medical conclusion, medical image fusion algorithms can combine multimodality medical images [2, 3].

As of late, numerous scientists have made and utilized fusion algorithms to make fruitful multimodality biomedical images [4, 5]. Yet, numerous researchers have already used image fusion techniques that already exist. As a result, the multimodality fused images that are created could have a variety of issues, especially in the area that was impacted, like gradient and texture distortion. To circumvent the issues with the current methodologies, many scholars have adopted approaches like deep learning and dictionary learning. The best method to produce effective multimodality-fused images has been discovered to be dictionary learning [5], local-features fuzzy sets [6], deep learning [7–9], deep learning with NSST [10], etc.

The plan and improvement of an effective multimodality biomedical image fusion technique actually require research. One of the greatest fusion methods for getting promising outcomes is deep learning. Moreover, a multimodality biomedical fusion technique based on deep transfer learning can yield improved outcomes.

The key contributions are as follows:

- A multimodality biomedical fusion model based on the Xception model and multi-objective differential evolution is proposed.

- The suggested method first breaks the image down into subbands using a non-subsampled contourlet transform (NSCT).
- The feature extraction of the source photos is then carried out using an extreme version of Inception (Xception).
- The best characteristics are chosen via multi-objective differential evolution.
- A coefficient of determination and fusion functions based on energy loss are utilized to get the fused coefficients.
- The inverse NSCT is then utilized to construct the fused image.
- The benchmark multimodality image fusion dataset is used to compare the suggested and competing techniques.

3.2 Literature Review

In recent years, numerous medical picture fusion techniques have been developed by researchers [11, 12]. In the realm of medicine, decomposition- and learning-based image fusion algorithms are frequently used [13, 14]. Decomposition, fusion, and reconstruction are the fundamental processes in the multiscale transformation (MST), a broadly involved decomposition-based procedure for joining medical images. MST frequently makes use of wavelet, multiscale geometric analysis (MAG), and pyramid-based techniques [15]. The methods for MAG-assembled techniques based on non-subsampled shearlet transform [16] (NSST) and non-subsampled contourlet transform [18] (NSCT) provide outstanding competence in image representation [57]. With MST-based combination techniques, examining high- and low-recurrence coefficients is a fundamental problem despite picture handling. A high-frequency coefficient's activity has traditionally been measured by its absolute value [52]. The fused coefficient is then obtained using a simple fusion approach, like selecting the maximum or weighted average, after being calculated using a pixel- or window-based method. The low-frequency fusion method that was most frequently utilized in the early stages of research was averaging the coefficients of different source images. In recent years, more complex picture modifications and fusion techniques have been developed [19, 20]. Liu [21] distributed a coordinated sparse representation (SR) and MST-based engineering for blending medical pictures. Zhu proposed a multimodality decomposition strategy in view of NSCT that wires high- and low-pass subgroups utilizing nearby Laplacian energy and stage consistency, separately [17]. In the NSST area, Yin suggested a multimodality strategy for fusing medical images that featured pulse-coupled neural networks (PCNN) [22]. Li [23] developed a special multisensor image fusion technique based on NSST and PCNN to advance the fusion nature of multimodality images.

Learning-based techniques have become popular in medical image fusion over the past 10 years. The most popular fusion techniques are those based on deep learning and SR [24, 25]. The vast majority of SR-based fusion techniques in use today aim to improve their performances by, among other things, incorporating explicit constraints [12], fostering a more effective dictionary learning component [26], involving various sub-dictionaries in the portrayal, and so forth.

For multimodality biomedical images, Zhu [11] created a clever dictionary learning-based picture fusion computation. This approach provides greater accuracy thanks to the usage of vocabulary learning. Nonetheless, it is computationally complicated by nature. Liu [27] recommended the biomedical picture decay strategy utilizing NSST to intertwine the multimodality images. This method has far better outcomes than the current methods, but it has an edge degradation problem. CNN and a contrast pyramid were used by Wang [28] to combine the biological multimodality pictures. CNN can effectively combine the photos. Though computationally demanding, this approach occasionally fails to yield results that are encouraging when the biological images are very similar to one another [53].

The examination of the literature showed that there is still a great deal to be found about multimodality image fusion. Deep learning has been demonstrated to be the most encouraging strategy for improved multimodality fused biomedical imaging [55]. However, these strategies can bring about improved results when pre-prepared deep exchange learning systems are utilized. Choosing the underlying settings for deep learning and deep exchange learning approaches is another difficult issue [29, 30]. To improve the results in this review, a notable multi-objective differential development is used.

3.3 Methodology

Suppose I1 and I2 display the original photos. I1 and I2 are first divided into subbands using NSCT. Our main goal is to combine the corresponding subbands from the two source photos [47]. Using the Inception (Xception) model's extreme iteration, the high subband is fused. The comfort of the identified interlaced high subbands is evaluated using the coefficient of assurance. The neighborhood energy capability is used to combine low subbands. To register the multimodality fusion image, reverse NSCT is used. Figure 3.1 portrays the proposed model's consecutive advances [58].

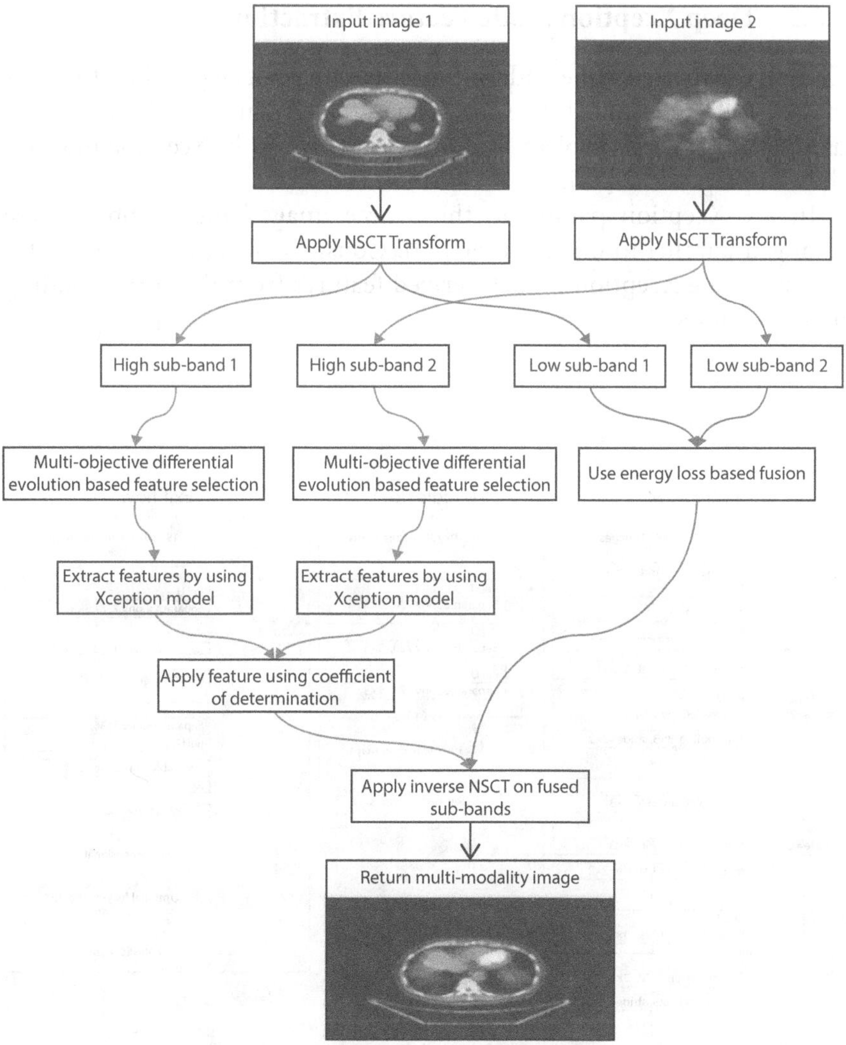

Figure 3.1 Diagrammatic flow of the deep learning model for combining images from multiple modes using multi-objective differential evolution.

3.3.1 Non-Subsampled Contourlet Transform

The images are divided into wavelet spaces using the well-known non-subsampled contourlet transform [48]. It is a shift-invariant change that provides a wide range of directional information. With the least amount of root mean square error, the modified images can be converted to the original ones using this directionality.

3.3.2 Deep Xception Mode Feature Extraction

CNN may experience the underfitting issue since not all possible attributes may be collected. An extreme variation of the Origin (Xception) model is used to address this problem. The block diagram for the Xception model is shown in Figure 3.2 [31].

In the Xception paradigm, the source images' high subbands are arranged parallel to one another [49]. Consider $\eta I_1(p, q)$ and $\eta I_2(p, q)$, which are the Xception model-derived features from the corresponding high subbands.

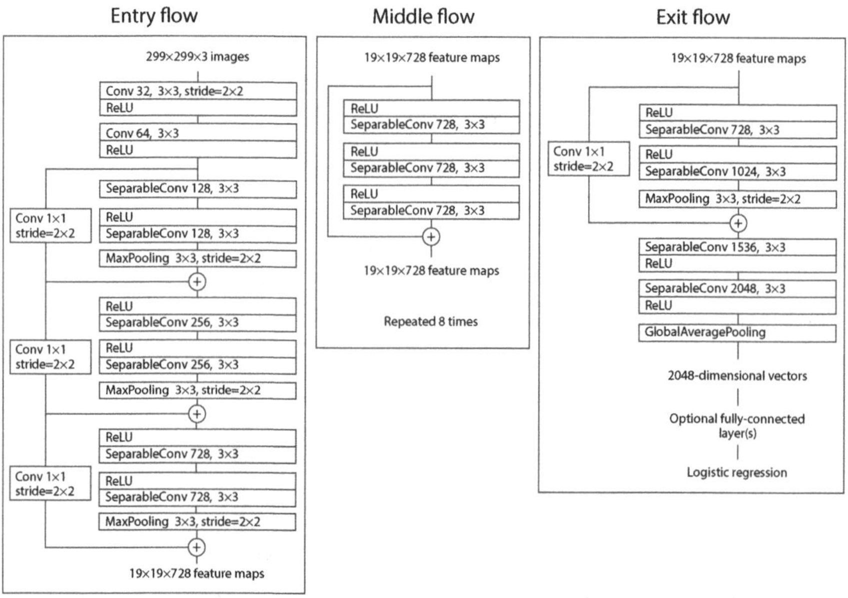

Figure 3.2 Structure of the Xception model [31].

3.3.3 Differential Evolutions with Several Objectives for Feature Selection

Among the features that the Xception model produced, the best traits are selected at this point. The wellness capability to pick the best highlights utilizes the fusion factor and entropy measures [50]. A multi-objective differential development can be utilized to determine various troublesome calculating issues. It can effectively balance rapid convergence and population variety.

3.3.4 Fusion of High-Frequency Bands

High subband features are extracted and chosen using the Xception model and then merged utilizing the coefficient of determination (R) [51].

3.4 Result and Discussion

The effectiveness of the recommended approach is evaluated using the Ullah benchmark multimodality biomedical image dataset [6]. For comparison, 15 separate sets of modalities are captured. The basic objective is to combine these photos to create multimodal visuals. In order to make comparisons, the same collection of images is also used by six competitive multimodality biomedical fusion techniques, namely, LEPN [17], DSA [32], CNN [33], EGDM [34], DDcGAN [35], and 3GANs [10]. The hyperparameters for these techniques are listed exactly as they are in their individual papers.

3.4.1 Visual Evaluation

The matching multimodality-fused biological images and the source images from the LEPN [17], DSA [32], CNN [33], EGDM [34], DDcGAN [35], 3GANs [10], and the suggested technique are shown in Figures 3.3 and 3.4.

It has been obviously settled that the outcomes have a preferable modality over the contending techniques. Even so, current methods such as LEPN [17], DSA [32], CNN [33], EGDM [34], DDcGAN [35], and 3GANs [10] offer notable visual outcomes but have low edge and texture distortion. The results of the advised course of action are shown in Figures 3.3i and 3.4j. These images show how the suggested technique produces multimodality-fused images with an improved visual appeal. The research explores the fascinating field of multimodal methods for biomedical imagefusion, which includes a variety of imaging modalities, including CT and MRI, as well as more recent techniques like LEPN and DSA. The integration of state-of-the-art computational techniques, such as 3D Generative Adversarial Networks (3GANs), Deep Convolutional

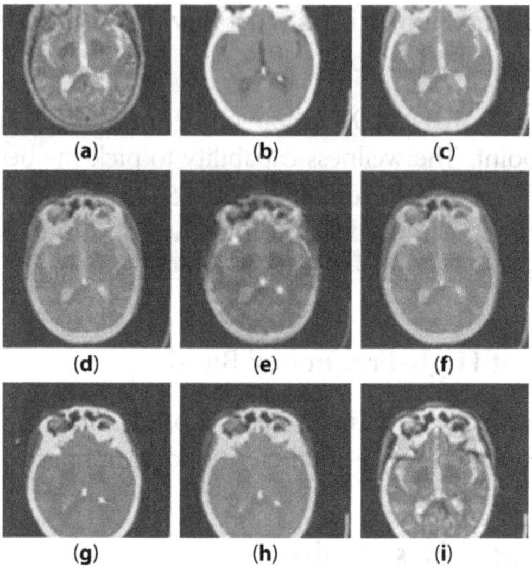

Figure 3.3 Review of multimodal techniques for biomedical fusion: MRI, CT, LEPN, DSA, CNN, EGDM, DDcGAN, 3GANs, and the suggested method for enhanced biomedical analysis.

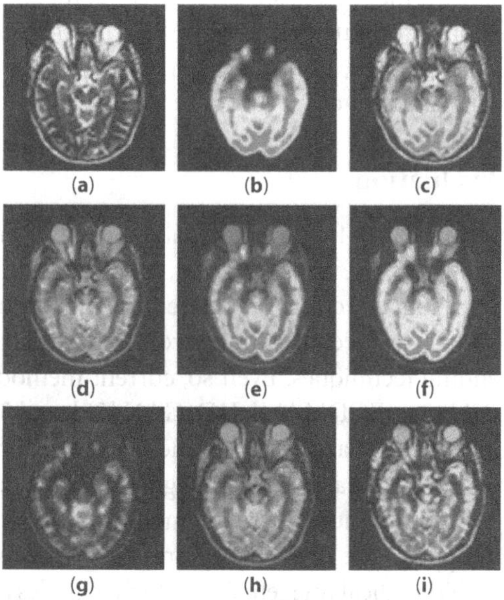

Figure 3.4 Review of multimodal techniques for biomedical fusion: MRI, CT, LEPN, DSA, CNN, EGDM, DDcGAN, 3GANs, and the suggested method for enhanced biomedical analysis.

Generative Adversarial Networks (DDcGAN), Enhanced Gradient Descent Methods (EGDM), and Convolutional Neural Networks (CNN), is further explored in this work. In addition, the paper addresses potential fusion techniques that integrate various technologies, providing a window into the bright future of biomedical imaging, where creative thinking is opening doors for more precise and perceptive diagnostic instruments.

3.4.2 Quantitative Research

We have contrasted the suggested method with the current methods, such as LEPN [17], DSA [32], CNN [33], EGDM [34], DDcGAN [35], and 3GANs [10], while representing various notable performance factors. Edge strength, fusion evenness, entropy, and fusion factor are the selected execution metrics [36].

An effective entropy value is provided by multimodality biomedical image fusion methods in general. The suggested multimodality deep transfer learning-based biomedical picture fusion technique's entropy analysis is shown in Table 3.1. It demonstrates that, in contrast to the multimodality biomedical image fusion methods already in use, the recommended method gives significantly higher entropy values. The suggested technique is shown to provide 1.7243% greater improvement than the best options.

The sourced image's details that were maintained are represented by mutual information in the combined image. Hence, it should be as high as possible. The comparison analysis of the suggested system and the approaching adversary is shown in Table 3.2. The suggested method yields an improvement of 1.7273% on average.

A noteworthy performance indicator that demonstrates the efficacy of the fusion process is the fusion factor. What is happening is the best. The results of the fusion factor analysis of the suggested and competing approaches are shown in Table 3.3. The proposed method outperforms the competing fusion models on average by 1.3928%.

The symmetry between the source and fused pictures is evaluated by fusion symmetry. The ideal state is maximal.

The suggested deep transfer learning model-based multimodality fusion model's fusion symmetry analysis is computed. It is discovered that the suggested model outperforms the opponent models on a normal basis by 1.1974%.

Edge strength measures how well an edge is preserved, and having a maximum value is preferred. For the proposed deep transfer learning-based multimodality image fusion model, edge strength analysis is computed. The suggested model outperforms the alternative techniques on average by 1.6928%.

Table 3.1 An analysis of the entropy of the competing methods and the suggested deep transfer learning-based multimodality picture fusion.

Group	LEPN	DSA	CNN	EGDM	DDcGAN	3GANs	Proposed
G1	6.22±0.75	6.33±0.69	6.25±0.67	6.56±0.55	6.43±0.68	6.73±0.09	6.77±0.35
G2	6.18±0.64	6.04±0.62	6.18±0.54	6.23±0.45	6.73±0.58	6.33±0.08	6.77±0.43
G3	6.43±0.75	6.35±0.55	5.95±0.45	6.48±0.54	6.68±0.55	6.42±0.45	6.71±0.41
G4	6.09±0.55	5.93±0.55	6.29±0.55	6.46±0.45	6.47±0.58	6.62±0.57	6.69±0.45
G5	6.38±0.72	6.44±0.75	6.64±0.64	6.26±0.56	6.66±0.47	6.57±0.45	6.79±0.39
G6	6.28±0.73	5.94±0.65	6.39±0.45	6.31±0.44	6.53±0.55	6.66±0.35	6.73±0.45
G7	6.17±0.66	5.96±0.75	6.26±0.55	6.58±0.45	6.69±0.68	6.65±0.35	6.72±0.35
G8	5.91±0.55	5.96±0.55	6.06±0.49	6.46±0.46	6.28±0.48	6.57±0.35	6.81±0.43
G9	5.96±0.76	6.19±0.65	6.33±0.47	6.74±0.62	6.26±0.52	6.75±0.48	6.71±0.41

Table 3.2 Examining the mutual data between competing methods and the proposed deep transfer learning-based multimodality image fusion.

Group	LEPN	DSA	CNN	EGDM	DDcGAN	3GANs	Proposed value
G1	0.63±0.013	0.62±0.011	0.61±0.012	0.59±0.012	0.61±0.008	0.62±0.009	0.63±0.009
G2	0.61±0.014	0.61±0.012	0.62±0.012	0.61±0.009	0.61±0.011	0.64±0.009	0.61±0.009
G3	0.63±0.014	0.62±0.011	0.62±0.008	0.63±0.008	0.59±0.011	0.63±0.008	0.63±0.007
G4	0.61±0.013	0.62±0.012	0.63±0.012	0.61±0.012	0.63±0.012	0.62±0.008	0.63±0.007
G5	0.61±0.011	0.63±0.012	0.63±0.011	0.63±0.012	0.64±0.011	0.64±0.012	0.63±0.008
G6	0.64±0.014	0.61±0.013	0.63±0.012	0.59±0.012	0.64±0.011	0.61±0.008	0.64±0.009
G7	0.63±0.014	0.59±0.012	0.59±0.012	0.63±0.009	0.64±0.009	0.59±0.007	0.64±0.009
G8	0.64±0.014	0.62±0.013	0.59±0.012	0.61±0.008	0.61±0.009	0.61±0.012	0.64±0.007
G9	0.62±0.011	0.59±0.011	0.59±0.009	0.63±0.009	0.62±0.011	0.59±0.008	0.63±0.009

Table 3.3 Analysis of the competing methods and the suggested deep learning-based multimodality picture fusion in relation to the fusion factor.

Group	LEPN	DSA	CNN	EGDM	DDcGAN	3GANs	Proposed
G1	1.26±0.026	1.22±0.022	1.22±0.022	1.22±0.031	1.24±0.022	1.26±0.026	1.26±0.022
G2	1.22±0.022	1.26±0.028	1.18±0.032	1.22±0.029	1.22±0.026	1.28±0.025	1.29±0.022
G3	1.26±0.022	1.24±0.025	1.21±0.033	1.24±0.022	1.26±0.022	1.24±0.028	1.26±0.022
G4	1.23±0.021	1.22±0.024	1.22±0.022	1.22±0.025	1.28±0.031	1.26±0.022	1.28±0.021
G5	1.22±0.03	1.24±0.022	1.21±0.026	1.28±0.027	1.24±0.024	1.24±0.021	1.28±0.021
G6	1.26±0.024	1.22±0.035	1.28±0.028	1.22±0.021	1.28±0.028	1.28±0.028	1.28±0.021
G7	1.22±0.028	1.24±0.025	1.21±0.026	1.22±0.022	1.24±0.031	1.24±0.022	1.24±0.022
G8	1.24±0.021	1.22±0.028	1.22±0.022	1.26±0.021	1.26±0.026	1.24±0.021	1.26±0.021
G9	1.24±0.031	1.26±0.024	1.21±0.024	1.24±0.022	1.18±0.022	1.27±0.022	1.26±0.022

3.5 Conclusion

According to the literature review, there is still more to learn about multimodal picture fusion. One of the most promising methods for obtaining superior multimodality-fused biological images is deep learning-based fusion algorithms. However, these methods still have the underfitting problem and are computationally difficult. The suggested method uses a non-subsampled contourlet transform to first deconstruct the picture into subbands (NSCT). After that, an extreme version of Inception was used to extract the features of the original photos (Xception). Through the use of multiple objective differential evolutions, the best features have been chosen [54]. The fused coefficients are then obtained using an energy loss function and a coefficient of determination. The inverse NSCT was then employed to deliver the merged image. Comprehensive experimental results demonstrate that, in terms of a number of performance parameters, the suggested approach outperforms the competing multimodality picture fusion systems [56]. In the near future, the suggested approach might be applied to additional applications including medical imaging and remote sensing images [37, 38]. The proposed method for tuning hyperparameters can also be utilized to adjust the hyperparameter of other methods, including deep learning models [30, 44–46], visibility restoration models [10, 37–40], and filtering models [41–43].

References

1. Ganasala, P. and Kumar, V., Feature-motivated simplified adaptive PCNN-based medical image fusion algorithm in NSST domain. *J. Digit. Imaging*, 29, 73–85, 2016. [CrossRef] [PubMed]
2. Li, S., Kang, X., Fang, L., Hu, J., Yin, H., Pixel-level image fusion: A survey of the state of the art. *Inf. Fusion*, 33, 100–112, 2017. [CrossRef]
3. James, A.P. and Dasarathy, B.V., Medical image fusion: A survey of the state of the art. *Inf. Fusion*, 19, 4–19, 2014. [CrossRef]
4. Ravi, P. and Krishnan, J., Image enhancement with medical image fusion using multiresolution discrete cosine transform, in: *Materials Today: Proceedings 5 (1, Part 1) 1936 - 1942, International Conference on Processing of Materials, Minerals and Energy (July 29th–30th)*, 2016, 2018.
5. Hu, Q., Hu, S., Zhang, F., Multi-modality medical image fusion based on separable dictionary learning and gabor filtering. *Signal Process Image Commun.*, 83, 115758, 2020.
6. Ullah, H., Ullah, B., Wu, L., Abdalla, F.Y., Ren, G., Zhao, Y., Multi-modality medical images fusion based on local-features fuzzysets and novel

sum-modified-laplacian in non-subsampled shearlet transform domain. *Biomed. Signal Process Control*, 57, 101724, 2020.

7. Algarni, A.D., Automated medical diagnosis system based on multi-modality image fusion and deep learning. *Wirel. Pers. Commun.*, 111, 1033–1058, 2020.
8. Xia, K.-J., Yin, H.-S., Wang, J.-Q., A novel improved deep convolutional neural network model for medical image fusion. *Clust. Comput.*, 22, 1, 1515–1527, 2019.
9. Zhou, T., Ruan, S., Canu, S., A review: Deep learning for medical image segmentation using multi-modality fusion. *Array*, 3, 100004, 2019.
10. Wang, R., Yu, H., Wang, G., Zhang, G., Wang, W., Study on the dynamic and static characteristics of gas static thrust bearing with micro-hole restrictors. *Int. J. Hydromech.*, 2, 3, 189–202, 2019.
11. Zhu, Z., Chai, Y., Yin, H., Li, Y., Liu, Z., A novel dictionary learning approach for multi-modality medical image fusion. *Neurocomputing*, 214, 471–482, 2016.
12. Li, H., He, X., Tao, D., Tang, Y., Wang, R., Joint medical image fusion, denoising and enhancement via discriminative low-rank sparse dictionaries learning. *Pattern Recognit.*, 79, 130–146, 2018. [CrossRef]
13. Li, Y., Sun, Y., Zheng, M., Huang, X., Qi, G., Hu, H., Zhu, Z., A novel multi-exposure image fusion method based on adaptive patch structure. *Entropy*, 20, 935, 2018. [CrossRef]
14. Qi, G., Wang, J., Zhang, Q., Zeng, F., Zhu, Z., An integrated dictionary-learning entropy-based medical image fusion framework. *Future Internet*, 9, 61, 2017. [CrossRef]
15. Shen, J., Zhao, Y., Yan, S., Li, X., Exposure fusion using boosting laplacian pyramid. *IEEE Trans. Cybern.*, 44, 1579–1590, 2014. [CrossRef]
16. Xu, L., Gao, G., Feng, D., Multi-focus image fusion based on non-subsampled shearlet transform. *IET Image Process.*, 7, 633–639, 2013. [CrossRef]
17. Zhu, Z., Zheng, M., Qi, G., Wang, D., Xiang, Y.A., Phase congruency and local laplacian energy based multi-modality medical image fusion method in NSCT domain. *IEEE Access*, 7, 20811–20824, 2019. [CrossRef]
18. Li, Y., Sun, Y., Huang, X., Qi, G., Zheng, M., Zhu, Z., An image fusion method based on sparse representation and sum modified-laplacian in NSCT domain. *Entropy*, 20, 522, 2018. [CrossRef]
19. Wang, L., Li, B., Tian, L., Multimodal medical volumetric data fusion using 3-D discrete shearlet transform and global-to-local rule. *IEEE. Trans. Biomed. Eng.*, 61, 197–206, 2014. [CrossRef]
20. Yang, Y., Que, Y., Huang, S., Lin, P., Multimodal sensor medical image fusion based on type-2 fuzzy logic in NSCT domain. *IEEE Sens. J.*, 16, 3735–3745, 2016. [CrossRef]
21. Liu, Y., Liu, S., Wang, Z., A general framework for image fusion based on multi-scale transform and sparse representation. *Inf. Fusion*, 24, 147–164, 2015. [CrossRef]

22. Yin, M., Liu, X., Liu, Y., Chen, X., Medical image fusion with parameter-adaptive pulse coupled neural network in nonsubsampled shearlet transform domain. *IEEE Trans. Instrum. Meas.*, 68, 49–64, 2019. [CrossRef]
23. Yin, L., Zheng, M., Qi, G., Zhu, Z., Jin, F., Sim, J.A., Novel image fusion framework based on sparse representation and pulse coupled neural network. *IEEE Access*, 7, 98290–98305, 2019. [CrossRef]
24. Zhang, Q., Liu, Y., Blum, R.S., Han, J., Tao, D., Sparse representation based multi-sensor image fusion for multi-focus and multi-modality images: A review. *Inf. Fusion*, 40, 57–75, 2018. [CrossRef]
25. Qi, G., Zhang, Q., Zeng, F., Wang, J., Zhu, Z., Multi-focus image fusion via morphological similarity-based dictionary construction and sparse representation. *CAAI TIT.*, 3, 83–94, 2018. [CrossRef]
26. Kim, M., Han, D.K., Ko, H., Joint patch clustering-based dictionary learning for multimodal image fusion. *Inf. Fusion*, 27, 198–214, 2016. [CrossRef]
27. Liu, X., Mei, W., Du, H., Multi-modality medical image fusion based on image decomposition framework and nonsubsampled shearlet transform. *BioMed. Signal Process Control*, 40, 343–350, 2018.
28. Wang, K., Zheng, M., Wei, H., Qi, G., Li, Y., Multi-modality medical image fusion using convolutional neural network and contrast pyramid. *Sensors*, 20, 8, 2169, 2020.
29. Pannu, H.S., Singh, D., Malhi, A.K., Multi-objective particle swarm optimization-based adaptive neuro-fuzzy inference system for benzene monitoring. *Neural Comput. Appl.*, 31, 2195–2205, 2019.
30. Kaur, M. and Singh, D., Fusion of medical images using deep belief networks. *Clust. Comput.*, 23, 1439–1453, 2020.
31. Chollet, F., Xception: Deep learning with depthwise separable convolutions, in: *Proceedings of the IEEE Conference on Computer Vision and Pattern Recognition*, pp.1251–1258, 2017.
32. Zhu, R., Li, X., Zhang, X., Ma, M., MRI and CT medical image fusion based on synchronized-anisotropic diffusion model. *IEEE Access*, 8, 91336–91350, 2020. https://doi.org/10.1109/ACCESS.2020.2993493.
33. Kumar, A., Fulham, M., Feng, D., Kim, J., Co-learning feature fusion maps from PET-CT images of lung cancer. *IEEE Trans. Med. Imaging*, 39, 1, 204–217, 2020. https://doi.org/10.1109/TMI.2019.2923601.
34. Lu, Y., Zhao, J., Wang, G., Edge-guided dual-modality image reconstruction. *IEEE Access*, 2, 1359–1363, 2014. https://doi.org/10.1109/ ACCESS.2014.2371994.
35. Ma, J., Xu, H., Jiang, J., Mei, X., Zhang, X., Ddcgan: A dual-discriminator conditional generative adversarial network for multi-resolution image fusion. *IEEE Trans. Image Process*, 29, 4980–4995, 2020. https://doi.org/10.1109/TIP.2020.2977573.
36. Prakash, O., Park, C.M., Khare, A., Jeon, M., Gwak, J., Multiscale fusion of multimodal medical images using lifting scheme based biorthogonal wavelet transform. *Optik*, 182, 995–1014, 2019.

37. Singh, D. and Kumar, V., Dehazing of outdoor images using notch based integral guided filter. *Multimed. Tools Appl.*, 77, 20, 27363–27386, 2018.
38. Singh, D. and Kumar, V., A comprehensive review of computational dehazing techniques. *Arch. Comput. Methods Eng.*, 26, 5, 1395–1413, 2019a.
39. Osterland, S. and Weber, J., Analytical analysis of single-stage pressure relief valves. *Int. J. Hydromech.*, 2, 1, 32–53, 2019.
40. Singh, D., Kumar, V., Kaur, M., Image dehazing using window-based integrated means filter. *Multimed. Tools Appl.*, 79, 34771–34793, 2020.
41. Gupta, B., Tiwari, M., Lamba, S.S., Visibility improvement and mass segmentation of mammogram images using quantile separated histogram equalisation with local contrast enhancement. *CAAI Trans. Intell. Technol.*, 4, 2, 73–79, 2019.
42. Kaur, M., Singh, D., Kumar, V., Sun, K., Color image dehazing using gradient channel prior and guided l0 filter. *Inf. Sci.*, 521, 326–342, 2020. https://doi.org/10.1016/j.ins.2020.02.048.
43. Wiens, T., Engine speed reduction for hydraulic machinery using predictive algorithms. *Int. J. Hydromech.*, 2, 1, 16–31, 2019.
44. Jaiswal, A., Gianchandani, N., Singh, D., Kumar, V., Kaur, M., Classification of the COVID-19 infected patients using DenseNet201 based deep transfer learning. *J. Biomol. Struct. Dyn.*, 39, 15, 5682–5689, 2021.
45. Basavegowda, H.S. and Dagnew, G., Deep learning approach for microarray cancer data classification. *CAAI Trans. Intell. Technol.*, 5, 1, 22–33, 2020.
46. Ghosh, S., Shivakumara, P., Roy, P., Pal, U., Lu, T., Graphology based handwritten character analysis for human behaviour identification. *CAAI Trans. Intell. Technol.*, 5, 1, 55–65, 2020.
47. Panwar, V., Sharma, D.K., Kumar, K.P., Jain, A., Thakar, C., Experimental investigations and optimization of surface roughness in turning of en 36 alloy steel using response surface methodology and genetic algorithm. *Mater. Today: Proc.*, 46, 6474–6481, 2021.
48. Jain, A. and Pandey, A.K., Modeling and optimizing of different quality characteristics in electrical discharge drilling of titanium alloy (Grade-5) sheet. *Mater. Today Proc.*, 18, 182–191, 2019. https://doi.org/10.1016/j.matpr.2019.06.292.
49. Jain, A., Yadav, A.K., Shrivastava, Y., Modelling and optimization of different quality characteristics in electric discharge drilling of titanium alloy sheet. *Mater. Today Proc.*, 21, 1680–1684, 2019. https://doi.org/10.1016/j.matpr.2019.12.010.
50. Jain, A. and Pandey, A.K., Multiple quality optimizations in electrical discharge drilling of mild steel sheet. *Mater. Today Proc.*, 8, 7252–7261, 2019. https://doi.org/10.1016/j.matpr.2017.07.054.
51. Jain, A., Kumar, C.S., Shrivastava, Y., Fabrication and machining of fiber matrix composite through electric discharge machining: A short review. *Mater. Today Proc.*, 51, 1233–1237, 2022.

52. Dhaundiyal, R., Tripathi, A., Joshi, K., Diwakar, M., Singh, P., Clustering based multi-modality medical image fusion. *J. Phys. Conf. Ser.*, 1478, 1, 012024, 2020, April. IOP Publishing.
53. Joshi, K., Joshi, K.N., Diwakar, M., Image fusion using cross bilateral filter and wavelet transform domain. *Int. J. Eng. Adv. Technol. (IJEAT)*, *8*, 110–115, 2019.
54. Joshi, K., Diwakar, M., Joshi, N.K., Lamba, S., A concise review on latest-methods of image fusion, in: *Recent Advances in Computer Science and Communications (Formerly: Recent Patents on Computer Science)*, vol. *14*, pp. 2046–2056, 2021.
55. Sharma, S.D., Sharma, S., Singh, R., Gehlot, A., Priyadarshi, N., Twala, B., Stress detection system for working pregnant women using an improved deep recurrent neural network. *Electronics*, *11*, 18, 2862, 2022.
56. Dua, S., Kumar, S.S., Albagory, Y., Ramalingam, R., Dumka, A., Singh, R., AlGhamdi, A.S., Developing a speech recognition system for recognizing tonal speech signals using a convolutional neural network. *Appl. Sci.*, *12*, 12, 6223, 2022.
57. Singh, R., Akram, S.V., Gehlot, A., Buddhi, D., Priyadarshi, N., Twala, B., Energy system 4.0: Digitalization of the energy sector with inclination towards sustainability. *Sensors*, *22*, 17, 6619, 2022.
58. Sharma, V.K., Singh, R., Gehlot, A., Buddhi, D., Braccio, S., Priyadarshi, N., Khan, B., Imperative role of photovoltaic and concentrating solar power technologies towards renewable energy generation. *Int. J. Photoenergy*, 2022, 2022.

4

Multimodal Deep Learning Analysis for Biomedical Data Fusion

Divyanshu Sinha[1], B. Jogeswara Rao[2], D. Khalandar Basha[3], Parvathapuram Pavan Kumar[4]*, N. Shilpa[5] and Saurabh Sharma[6]

[1]*Department of Computer Science, Sushant University Gurgaon, Gurgaon, India*
[2]*School of Engineering, Malla Reddy University, Hyderabad, India*
[3]*Department of ECE, Institute of Aeronautical Engineering Dundigal Hyderabad, Dundigal, India*
[4]*Department of ECE, St. Martin's Engineering College Secunderabad, Telangana, India*
[5]*Department of ECE, School of Engineering, SR University, Warangal, Telangana, India*
[6]*Amity University, Gwalior, India*

Abstract

The growing multimodality of biomedical data is uncovering the intricate relationships between biological processes that are hidden from view. Most of the time, these non-linear collaborations are illustrated using deep learning (DL)-based information fusion algorithms. Thus, we evaluate the present status of the specialty of such procedures and propose a point-by-point scientific categorization that works with the improvement of new methods as well as a wiser decision of combination methodologies for organic applications. Thus, we see that deep fusion techniques generally beat shallow and unimodal ones. The suggested subcategories of fusion techniques also exhibit various benefits and disadvantages. Joint representation learning is the optimum method, especially for intermediate fusion strategies, according to a review of current methodologies. This is because it successfully captures the complex relationships between many levels of biological organization. We conclude by highlighting progressive fusion as a possible area for future research, depending on pre-existing biological knowledge or search strategies. Similarly, applying transfer learning could help multimodal datasets overcome sample size restrictions. At the point when these datasets become all the more openly accessible, multimodal DL

**Corresponding author*: ppavankumar432@gmail.com

Kapil Joshi and Somil Kumar Gupta (eds.) Human Cancer Diagnosis and Detection Using Exascale Computing, (53–70) © 2024 Scrivener Publishing LLC

techniques provide the opportunity to create comprehensive models that can identify the intricate administrative cycles underlying health and illness.

Keywords: Deep learning, multimodal machine learning, biomedical data fusion, data integration

4.1 Introduction

Individual cells and entire organisms are examples of typical complex frameworks since they are composed of a number of pieces that work together to produce evolving behavioral patterns [1]. When trying to predict complicated infections, understanding these linkages is especially important. Information methodology is the consequence of estimating something with a particular sensor; consequently, it can give a specific measure of data all alone [2]. With multimodal information, acquiring further comprehension of the numerous components and their rising behavior is conceivable.

To address a deduction issue, data fusion is the most common way of consolidating information from various modalities that give different perspectives on a solitary peculiarity. This offers the possibility of treating such challenges more precisely than unimodal methods [3]. In more detail, the upsides of data fusion can be separated into reciprocal, excess, and agreeable highlights [4, 5], although these divisions are not mutually exclusive.

The multimodal examination of a patient with a disease can serve as an example of the benefits of data fusion in the biomedical area. A whole-slide image (WSI) from a biopsy provides information about the engineering and microenvironment of the malignancy, and genomic data from growth take into account the identifiable proof of disease driver attributes [54]. These methodologies are alluded to as "corresponding" in light of the fact that they shed light on various features of the occasion that does not otherwise sound clear. Because not all mRNAs are translated into proteins and because the presence of a protein confirms the translation of a specific mRNA into a protein, the reconciliation of transcriptomic and proteomic information is repeated and essential. When the data are irregular or have a large number of missing values, this redundancy is very important. Data from the same tumor's miRNA and mRNA sequencing might be referred to as "cooperative" data since the intricacy of the combined information grows [53]. Combining the two modalities offers a potential explanation for a protein's differential abundance, such as that of an oncogene. This could be extremely important in determining how the patient will react to a certain medication.

Fusion approaches are expected to use the added substance, excess, and helpful properties of numerous modalities. Machine learning (ML) strategies should be used to combine structured and unstructured data with various factual properties, sources of non-biological variation, high dimensionality, and various examples of missing qualities [2] in order to fully benefit from these perspectives on the peculiarity of interest.

Multimodal ML techniques have received more attention in recent years and have been used in a range of fields [6, 7]. This trend in the biomedical industry is depicted in Figure 4.1. Particularly for data fusion, multimodal deep learning (DL) offers benefits over shallow approaches [8]. By means of the revelation of straightforward associations between fundamental, unraveled parts, these calculations expect to learn high-level portrayals of information, which thus further develop the forecast delivered by a final classifier [52]. Early layers learn essential deliberations of information; however, the resulting layers integrate less complex reflections of the contribution to additional theoretical portrayals that are educational for the growing experience [9].

Data from "omics" and "multi-omics" are becoming more and more important in the literature on logic. Data fusion techniques in light of DL are becoming a crucial breakthrough in the biomedical area in order to fully utilize the growing amount of multimodal datasets. High-throughput technologies like microarrays and cutting-edge sequencing have made it possible to capture this record-breaking amount of data [10]. Several methods

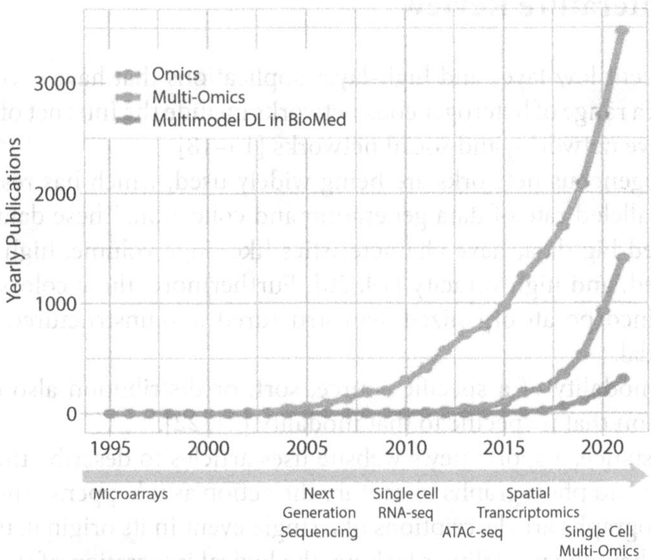

Figure 4.1 Multimodel technique in the biomodel industry.

from sequencing techniques were developed in the years following the introduction of bulk RNA-seq, including single-cell RNA-seq and ATAC-seq [11]. Nowadays, single-cell multi-omics [13] and spatial transcriptomics [12] are increasingly used.

Although the various DL-based fusion techniques for heterogeneous information have not been studied, DL models for biomedical applications have [14]. We talk about the latest headways in DL-based combination approaches in the biomedical region in the ongoing survey, which covers this subject. Additionally, we suggest a scientific classification that clarifies the traditional order of right on time, moderate, and late combination while also providing a list of subcategories that might be helpful for academicians and professionals looking to use or enhance present approaches. Additionally, the objective of this examination is to give suggestions for the circumstances in which the different combination methods are probably going to succeed [55].

To do this, a more in-depth taxonomy is first presented after an outline of the key fusion strategies is provided. The early, intermediate, and late fusion types, as well as their subgroups, are then thoroughly discussed and applied to health problems. Finally, we evaluate the potential and constraints faced by the strategies discussed in the biomedical sector and make recommendations for further study.

4.2 Literature Review

A few recent low-layer and high-layer applications that have successfully exploited a range of heterogeneous networks include the Internet of Things, automotive networks, and social networks [15–18].

Heterogeneous networks are being widely used, which has resulted in an unparalleled rate of data generation and collection. These data, otherwise called big data, have characteristics like huge volume, high variety, high speed, and high veracity [19, 20]. Furthermore, these colossal datasets that incorporate organized, semistructured, and unstructured data are multimodal.

Each modality of a specific source, sort, or distribution also conveys information that is specific to that modality [21, 22].

For instance, a sports news website uses articles to describe the sport's substance and photographs to capture the action as it happens. These texts and photographs are descriptions of a single event in its original, unedited forms. When one modality is lacking, the logical integration of these multimodal data might aid in a better understanding of the event of interest

[23, 24]. To all the more likely comprehend cross-methodology and shared methodology data, focusing on the fusion of the data in multimodal data is crucial for big data exploration. The expansion of multimodal data availability and accessibility is the cause of this.

An important method for multimodal data mining is multimodal data fusion, which is used to combine data from diverse sources, disseminators, and types into a global setting where flexibility and cross-methodology issues may be consistently addressed [25, 26]. It can give more noteworthy data than a solitary methodology by using methodology explicit data [27, 28]. Several multimodal data fusion strategies have already been put forth to look at the complimentary and cross-modal information between modalities [29]. For example, a few investigations suggested utilizing the linear flexibility connections as well as the cross-modular speculation data with the multimodal standard relationship examination.

A few explorations presented the halfway least squares model for straight associations over numerous factors by finding the factors from different wellsprings of information [30].

The multimodal free part examination is a probabilistic model that joins the autonomous factors of each unique methodology utilizing the Bayesian structure, as recommended by certain scientists [31].

Due to their dependence on shallow elements that are unable to capture the fundamental internal designs and external connections in multimodal data, these multimodal data fusion approaches are only applicable to extremely large multimodal data with high volume, high speed, high variety, and high veracity [32, 33]. Consequently, new multimodal processing techniques are needed in order to fully mine the examples in the multimodal data.

A hierarchical computer paradigm called deep learning learns the data's multilayer abstract representation [34]. It trains its parameters using the backpropagation technique, which can convert unprocessed inputs into useful task-specific representations. Convolutional neural networks (CNNs), recurrent neural networks (RNNs), and generative adversarial networks (GANs) are further noteworthy deep structures [35, 36]. These deep learning calculations have progressed fundamentally in both generative and discriminative undertakings in view of supervised and unsupervised strategies [37]. For example, a deep pyramidal lingering network was given in a couple of papers that proposed an original leftover methodology, which is a delegate discriminative occupation [38]. The pyramidal remaining organization learns productive and dependable dynamic portrayals in which the undertaking explicit parts are raised and the superfluous factors are stifled, beating the cutting-edge design acknowledgment precision. The generative adversarial network, a deep learning model influenced by the game theory, is a prime example of generative computation [39]. The Nash harmony between the generator and discriminator allows the generatively ill-disposed organization to eliminate the native info structure and imitate input stuff. Additionally, a few advanced deep learning models exist in the cross-methodology recovery, picture explanation, and assisted conclusion multimodal data fusion sectors. Although the multimodal data fusion deep learning model has come a long way, it is still in its early stages. So, in order to serve as an example for new multimodal data fusion deep learning paradigms, we evaluate the illustrative multimodal deep learning models [56].

4.3 Methodology

The capacity of DNNs to learn progressive portrayals of the information makes them the ideal answer for multimodal learning issues. Finding the marginal and joint of a few modalities such that working closely together takes into consideration their proficient combination is fundamental for multimodal fusion [7]. Concurring on the condition of the contribution to the combination layers, combination methods can commonly be named early, intermediate, and late [2] (see the blue layer in Figure 4.2). The "early fusion" process connects the underlying information values, and the subsequent vector is dealt with as solitary modular information; consequently, the DL design does not recognize the wellsprings of the methodology highlights (see Figure 4.2a). Marginal portrayals are not expressly learned;

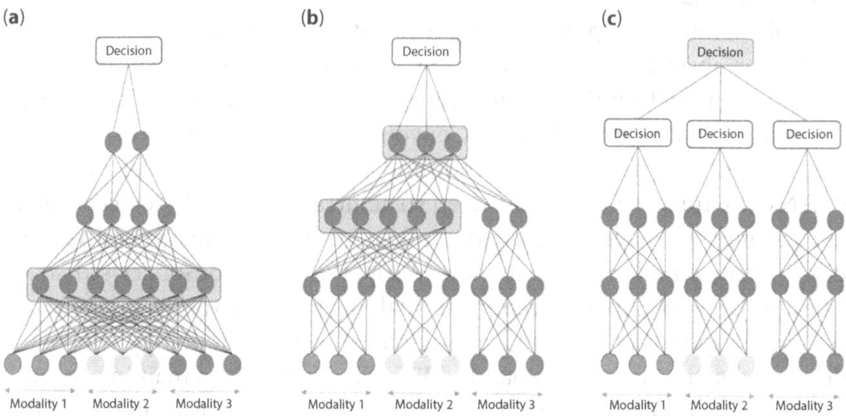

Figure 4.2 DN-based fusion model (a) early (b) intermediate (c) late combination of blue layer in decision making.

rather, joint portrayals of the multimodal input are [48]. Also, we separate between early combination in view of "direct demonstration" of information involving DNNs identical to their partners for unimodal information and "autoencoder" (AE) strategies that initially learn lower layered joint portrayals prior to being utilized for additional displaying with administered or solo procedures.

(A) Blue-edged shared layers enable the creation of integrated representations via several modalities [57]. Marginal representation learning does not exist. (B) Prior to fusing marginal representations into the network, intermediate fusion techniques first learn them. This could occur instantly or gradually. (C) Late fusion techniques consider choices made by each modality's submodels. The photograph was taken from [2].

4.3.1 Early Fusion

The ability of DL to efficiently learn from large datasets, even when the number of features is vast, can be credited with some of its success [34]. Sadly, sample sizes for datasets in the biomedical area are usually small, especially when seen in the context of their dimensionality. Concatenating the input features of various modalities is part of the formal formula for early fusion, xconcat = x1||x2||...||xM, where xi is the input vector of one modality (see Figure 4.3a). The top layer of the DL architecture receives the concatenated vector, xconcat [49]. It is impossible for the neural network to discriminate between

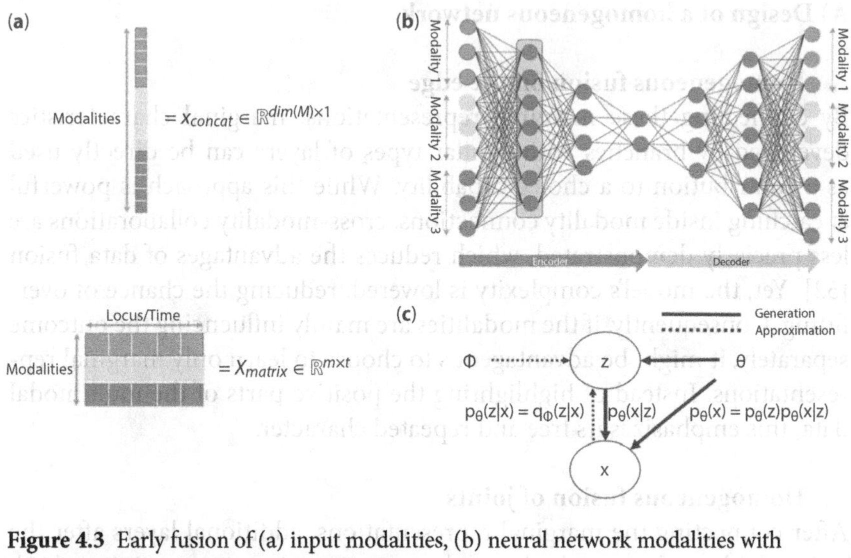

Figure 4.3 Early fusion of (a) input modalities, (b) neural network modalities with encoder and decoder, (c) cross model concentration.

features from various modalities. This method simultaneously teaches cross-modal and within-modal correlations at a low level of abstraction.

The vector xconcat can be recreated utilizing a completely associated input layer, as finished in [40, 41], and with limitations, as finished in [42], in the event that the requesting of the elements is immaterial to the learning point. Intermittent layers or convolutional layers may be used to the linked vector if the information highlights being requested comprise primary data. In these cases, the successive data might be stacked as a lattice for each example as opposed to being linked into a one-layered vector [50]. For instance, the lines of the framework could address the modalities, and every segment could address a situation in the genome (see Figure 4.3a). A portion can then skim over the network on account of a convolutional layer to remove relevant qualities. Every segment in a repetitive layer can be considered a solitary step.

4.3.2 Intermediate Fusion

Early fusion has no idea from which modality a feature comes, while intermediate fusion algorithms make use of this knowledge [51]. A minimal representation of every modality is prepared to perceive inside modality connections before using these relationships to either straightforwardly develop forecasts or make joint portrayals (see Figure 4.4a). Next, we will talk about subcategories of homo- and heterogeneous intermediate fusion.

A) Design of a homogeneous network

- **Homogeneous fusion on the edge**

By connecting these marginal representations, marginal characteristics developed by branches with similar types of layers can be directly used as a contribution to a choice capability. While this approach is powerful at catching inside modality connections, cross-modality collaborations are less precisely demonstrated, which reduces the advantages of data fusion [52]. Yet, the model's complexity is lowered, reducing the chance of overfitting. Consequently, if the modalities are mainly influencing the outcome separately, it might be advantageous to choose to learn only marginal representations. Instead of highlighting the positive parts of the multimodal data, this emphasizes its free and repeated character.

- **Homogeneous fusion of joints**

After connecting the marginal representations, additional layers after the unimodal branches can be learned to acquire joint representations [58].

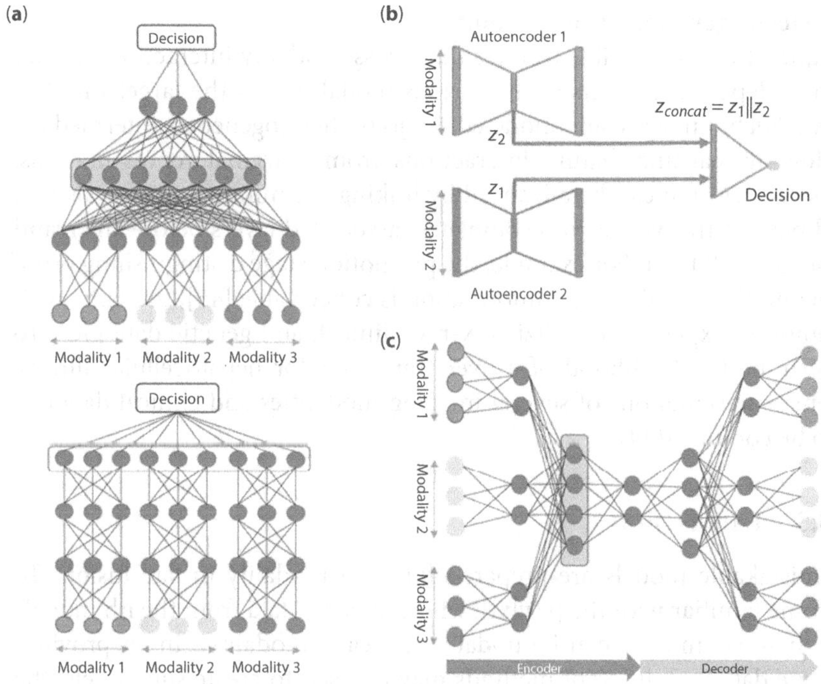

Figure 4.4 Intermediate fusion (a) decision making using 3 modalities, (b) autoencoding (c) encoder and decoder and cross model interaction.

This hybrid representation, which also simulates cross-modal interactions, can then be used to make decisions (see Figure 4.4a).

Researchers used multi-omics data to apply independent fully connected branches for the goal of predicting pharmaceutical response, followed by a multilayer characterization network [43]. The classifier then acquired a portrayal of the information modalities subsequently working closely together. This approach was used by Lin to identify breast cancer subgroups [44].

B) Design of heterogeneous networks

- **Heterogeneous fusion on the edge**

The ability to turn heterogeneous contributions into vectors that more precisely address higher level features is the key advantage of presenting modalities with different branches. These new component vectors can ease correlation by "making everything fair" as far as information type, layered unevenness, and scale among the different modalities. As a homogeneous transitional combination draws near, such marginal representation can be taken care of by a classifier by just being linked.

- **Heterogeneous fusion of joints**

Frequently, it is plausible to infer that cross-modality interactions, rather than independent effects of the various modalities on the target variable, exist. Such linkages are modeled in joint heterogeneous intermediate fusion by learning feature interactions from marginal representations. This cooperation can be advanced by linking the minimal portrayals first and passing this vector into completely associated layers before an errand explicit result layer. For example, the promotion stage distinguishing proof utilizing X-ray and clinical information is conceivable [45], the same with promotion expectation utilizing X-ray, clinical, and genetic data [46]. To determine the likelihood of a liver transplant for hepatocellular illness, latent representations of several imaging modalities and clinical data can also be combined [47].

4.3.3 Late Fusion

Unmistakable models are prepared for each modality in late fusion. To become familiar with the p (y|xi), where xi is the data from the ith modality, these submodels can be updated. As each modality's input provides unique data and different methods may be used to create submodels, the mistakes committed by each model are not exactly associated [2]. For the combination of diverse modalities, many approaches such as totaling the normal likelihood and exploiting the reciprocal information from each modality are highly appealing.

The simplest method for combining evaluations from several submodels is to take the average of the individual results. This would include averaging the likelihood from softmax capabilities for each class in a characterization problem. This technique does not weigh the outputs; therefore, it is assumed that each submodel contributes equally.

4.4 Results and Discussion

Most early fusion models are impressively not the same as their unimodal partners. They are genuinely easy to utilize and do not need individual modalities to be demonstrated, which might make sense of why they are habitually utilized in natural writing. Utilizations of the early non-linear combination strategies considered here have demonstrated the way that they can outflank shallow techniques in expectation challenges. The way that the applications framed above just covered 96 patients exhibits that DL approaches are effective options in contrast to customary strategies in any event when test sizes are generally little. Moreover, early fusion techniques typically perform better than unimodal ones. Yet, other modes can add information to various degrees.

Despite their widespread application, early fusion techniques have shortcomings. Finding helpful marginal representations for each modality is hampered by explicitly modeling a combined representation. Higher levels of abstraction may be required to reveal important aspects of a modality. It can be more challenging to find these elements in a shared depiction. Modalities can also stand in a variety of relationships with one another. Hence, it may be advantageous to combine modalities gradually rather than all at once. Finally, early fusion is usually only used when the modalities are quite uniform, like the many "omics" modalities. Early fusion efforts are less likely to be effective if modalities, like visual and molecular modalities, have fundamentally different distributions.

For intermediate fusion, DL techniques are highly suitable. The fusion is empowered at the appropriate degree of reflection by the gradual marginal and shared representation. As a result, the fusion technique's underlying biological connections between the modalities can be identified. Also, joint fusion techniques are all the more regularly utilized, which shows that gaining joint portrayals from marginal ones is the best methodology. This refutes the possibility that different modalities influence the objective in independent ways and also supports the possibility that corresponding and accommodating data can be found in multimodal data. Figure 4.5 illustrates early, intermediate, and late fusion options for reliable deep learning-based multimodel action recognition.

Several common DL issues in the biomedical industry are also addressed by intermediate fusion techniques. For instance, interpretability-enhancing techniques can be selected for each modality by having distinct branches. The potential for a middle-of-the-road combination to close the heterogeneity gap between modalities by applying different organizations and organization types to every methodology is especially encouraging for biomedical applications. This will enable a potent fusion of imaging and clinical modalities. As a result, the DL strategy and clinical analysis and visualization are more closely related.

Many modalities can be modeled via late fusion, which can also combine shallow ML and DL methods, whereas early fusion can only model homogeneous modalities. Similar to how intermediate fusion prevents higher-dimensional modalities from "drowning out" lower-dimensional ones, the number of input dimensions has no bearing on the outcome.

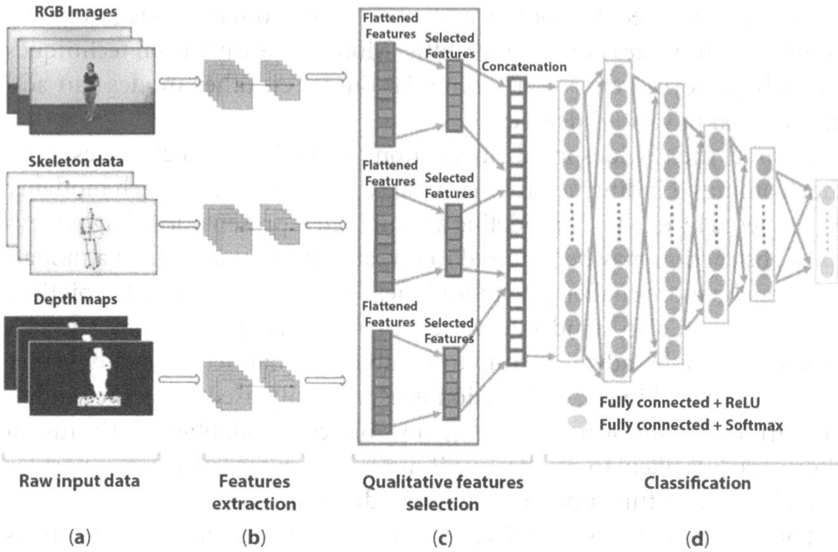

Figure 4.5 Representation of all three fusion strategies.

The disadvantage of late fusion approaches is that they are unable to establish connections between the characteristics of various modalities.

4.5 Conclusion

Recent studies on DL-based fusion techniques suggest that multimodal solutions usually outperform unimodal ones. Additionally, it is frequently noted that multimodal DL methods perform noticeably better than shallow ML methods. The promised benefits from DL-based fusion are evidently frequently achieved, notwithstanding the literature's bias toward positive results.

We have described the circumstances in which early, intermediate, and late fusion, as well as each of their subcategories, are likely to function most effectively. The decision largely depends on the modalities being studied and the researcher's willingness to make more or fewer architectural decisions. The effectiveness of various solutions can still vary significantly depending on the problem and the available data. To more precisely define the circumstances in which the various techniques perform best, more theoretical understanding is required. So, it is advised to empirically research, compare, and assess various fusion procedures in order to determine their individual benefits.

As described, for example, by Miotto, multimodal DL techniques suffer the same difficulties as DL in the biomedical sector generally does, such as data amount, quality, interpretability, and temporality. Fusion techniques must, however, handle multimodal-specific issues such as the absence of complete modalities. Several methods have been suggested in generative models and multitask learning. Fusion strategies must also take into account various combinations of modalities as there is an increase in the amount of heterogeneous data available. Multimodal data give a valuable chance to prepare total models that might understand the complex administrative elements supporting wellbeing and ailment. Biological processes can be observed in a range of sizes. For this challenge, late fusion and heterogeneous intermediate fusion are particularly suitable.

The significance of multimodal data fusion in the biomedical profession is turning out to be ever-increasing as additional clinical and trial information opens up. Researchers and experts could choose DL combination methods to handle and create the best-performing models from their data. We hope that this review will encourage further research and application of these methods.

References

1. Maayan, A., Complex systems biology. *J. R. Soc. Interface*, 14, 134, 20170391, 2017.
2. Ramachandram, D. and Taylor, G.W., Deep multimodal learning: A survey on recent advances and trends. *IEEE Signal Process Mag.*, 34, 6, 96–108, 2017.
3. Hall, D.L. and Llinas, J., An introduction to multisensor data fusion. *Proc. IEEE*, 85, 1, 6–23, 1997.
4. Durrant-Whyte, H.F., Sensor models and multisensor integration. *Int. J. Robot. Res.*, 7, 97–113, 1988.
5. Castanedo, F., A review of data fusion techniques. *Sci. World J.*, 2013, 704504, 2013.
6. Li, Y., Wu, F.X., Ngom, A., A review on machine learning principles for multi-view biological data integration. *Brief. Bioinform.*, 19, 2, 325–40, 2018.
7. Baltrusaitis, T., Ahuja, C., Morency, L.P., Multimodal machine learning: A survey and taxonomy. *IEEE Trans. Pattern. Anal. Mach. Intell.*, 41, 2, 423–43, 2019.
8. Goodfellow, I., Bengio, Y., Courville, A., *Deep Learning*, MIT Press, Cambridge, MA, 2016, http://www.deeplearningbook.org.
9. Bengio, Y., Courville, A., Vincent, P., Representation learning: A review and new perspectives. *IEEE Trans. Pattern. Anal. Mach. Intell.*, 35, 8, 1798–828, 2013.

10. Manzoni, C., Kia, D.A., Vandrovcova, J. *et al.*, Genome, transcriptome and proteome: The rise of omics data and their integration in biomedical sciences. *Brief. Bioinform.*, 19, 2, 286–302, 2018.
11. *Milestones in Genomic Sequencing*, Springer Nature, Springer, 2021, https://www.nature.com/immersive/d42859-020-00099-0/index.html.
12. Ståhl, P.L., Salmén, F., Vickovic, S. *et al.*, Visualization and analysis of gene expression in tissue sections by spatial transcriptomics. *Science*, 353, 6294, 78–82, 2016.
13. Lee, J., Hyeon, D.Y., Hwang, D., Single-cell multiomics: Technologies and data analysis methods. *Exp. Mol. Med.*, 52, 1428–42, 2020. http://dx.doi.org/10.1038/s12276-020-0420-2.
14. Ching, T., Himmelstein, D.S., Beaulieu-Jones, B.K. *et al.*, Opportunities and obstacles for deep learning in biology and medicine. *J. R. Soc. Interface*, 15, 141, 20170387, 2018.
15. Zhang, Z., Patras, P., Haddadi, H., Deep learning in mobile and wirelessnetworking: A survey. *IEEE Commun. Surv. Tutorials*, 21, 3, 2224–2287, 2019.
16. Meng, W., Li, W., Zhu, L., Enhancing medical smartphone networks via blockchain-based trust management against insider attacks. *IEEE Trans. Eng. Manag.*, 67, 4, 1377–1386, 2019.
17. Zhang, X., Zhou, X., Lin, M., Sun, J., ShuffleNet: An extremely efficient convolutional neural network for mobile devices, in: *Proceedings of the 2018 IEEE Conference on Computer Vision and Pattern Recognition*, IEEE, Piscataway, NJ, pp. 6848–6856), 2018.
18. Qiu, T., Chen, N., Li, K., Atiquzzaman, M., Zhao, W., How can heterogeneous Internet of things build our future: A survey. *IEEE Commun. Surv. Tutorials*, 20, 3, 2011–2027, 2018.
19. Lv, Z., Song, H., Val, P.B., Steed, A., Jo, M., Next-generation big data analytics: State of the art, challenges, and future research topics. *IEEE Trans. Ind. Inf.*, 13, 4, 1891–1899, 2017.
20. Gao, J., Li, P., Chen, Z., A canonical polyadic deep convolutional computation model for big data feature learning in internet of things. *Future Gener. Comput. Syst.*, 99, 508–516, 2019.
21. Li, Y., Yang, M., Zhang, Z., A survey of multi-view representation learning. *IEEE Trans. Knowl. Data Eng.*, 31, 10, 1863–1883, 2019.
22. Gao, J., Li, J., Li, Y., Approximate event detection over multimodal sensingdata. *J. Comb. Optim.*, 32, 4, 1002–1016, 2016.
23. Khaleghi, B., Khamis, A.M., Karray, F., Razavi, S.N., Multisensor datafusion: A review of the state-of-the-art. *Inf. Fusion*, 14, 1, 28–44, 2013.
24. Lahat, D., Adali, T., Jutten, C., Multimodal data fusion: An overview of methods, challenges, and prospects. *Proc. IEEE*, 103, 9, 1449–1477, 2015.
25. Bramon, R., Boada, I., Bardera, A., Rodriguez, J., Feixas, M., Puig, J., Sbert, M., Multimodal data fusion based on mutual information. *IEEE Trans. Visual Comput. Graphics*, 18, 9, 1574–1587, 2012.

26. Poria, S., Cambria, E., Bajpai, R., Hussain, A., A review of affective computing: From unimodal analysis to multimodal fusion. *Inf. Fusion*, 37, 98–125, 2017.
27. Biessmann, F., Plis, S., Meinecke, F.C., Eichele, T., Muller, K., Analysis of multimodal neuroimaging data. *IEEE Rev. Biomed. Eng.*, 4, 26–58, 2011.
28. Wagner, J., Andre, E., Lingenfelser, F., Kim, J., Exploring fusion methods for multimodal emotion recognition with missing data. *IEEE Trans. Affect. Comput.*, 2, 4, 206–218, 2011.
29. Sui, J., Adali, T., Yu, Q., Chen, J., Calhoun, V.D., A review of multivariate methods for multimodal fusion of brain imaging data. *J. Neurosci. Methods*, 204, 1, 68–81, 2012.
30. Martinez-Montes, E., Valdes-Sosa, P.A., Miwakeichi, F., Goldman, R.I., Cohen, M.S., Concurrent EEG/fMRI analysis by multiway partial least squares. *NeuroImage*, 22, 3, 1023–1034, 2004.
31. Groves, A.R., Beckmann, C.F., Smith, S.M., Woolrich, M.W., Linked independent component analysis for multimodal data fusion. *NeuroImage*, 54, 3, 2198–2217, 2011.
32. Li, P., Chen, Z., Yang, L.T., Zhang, Q., Deen, M.J., Deep convolutional computation model for feature learning on big data in internet of things. *IEEE Trans. Ind. Inf.*, 14, 2, 790–798, 2018.
33. Zhang, Q., Yang, L.T., Chen, Z., Deep computation model for unsupervised feature learning on big data. *IEEE Trans. Serv. Comput.*, 9, 1, 161–171, 2016.
34. LeCun, Y., Bengio, Y., Hinton, G.E., Deep learning. *Nature*, 521, 7553, 436–444, 2015.
35. Bengio, Y., Courville, A.C., Vincent, P., Representation learning: A review and new perspectives. *IEEE Trans. Pattern Anal. Mach. Intell.*, 35, 8, 1798–1828, 2013.
36. Chen, X.W. and Lin, X., Big data deep learning: Challenges and perspectives. *IEEE Access*, 2, 514–525, 2014.
37. Guo, Y., Liu, Y., Oerlemans, A., Lao, S., Wu, S., Lew, M.S., Deep learning for visual understanding: A review. *Neurocomputing*, 187, 27–48, 2016.
38. Han, D., Kim, J., Kim, J., Deep pyramidal residual networks, in: *Proceedings of 2017 IEEE Conference on Computer Vision and Pattern Recognition*, IEEE Computer Society, Washington, DC, pp. 6307–6315, 2017.
39. Goodfellow, I.J., Pouget-Abadie, J., Mirza, M., Xu, B., Warde-Farley, D., Ozair, S., Bengio, Y., Generative adversarial nets, in: *Advances in Neural Information Processing Systems*, vol. 27, Z. Ghahramani, M. Welling, C. Cortes, N.D. Lawrence, K.Q. Weinberger (Eds.), pp. 2672–2680, Curran, Red Hook, NY, 2014.
40. Park, C., Ha, J., Park, S., Prediction of Alzheimer's disease based on deep neural network by integrating gene expression and DNA methylation dataset. *Expert Syst. Appl.*, 140, 112873, 2020.

41. Xie, G., Dong, C., Kong, Y. *et al.*, Group lasso regularized deep learning for cancer prognosis from multi-omics and clinical features. *Genes*, 10, 3, 240, 2019.
42. Zhao, L., Dong, Q., Luo, C. *et al.*, DeepOmix: A scalable and interpretable multi-omics deep learning framework and application in cancer survival analysis. *Comput. Struct. Biotechnol. J.*, 19, 2719–25, 2021.
43. Sharifi-Noghabi, H., Zolotareva, O., Collins, C.C. *et al.*, MOLI: Multi-omics late integration with deep neural networks for drug response prediction. *Bioinformatics*, 35, 501–9, 2019.
44. Lin, Y., Zhang, W., Cao, H. *et al.*, Classifying breast cancer subtypes using deep neural networks based on multi-omics data. *Genes*, 11, 888, 2020.
45. Venugopalan, J., Tong, L., Hassanzadeh, H. *et al.*, Multimodal deep learning models for early detection of Alzheimer's disease stage. *Sci. Rep.*, 11, 3254, 2021.
46. Spasov, S.E., Passamonti, L., Duggento, A. *et al.*, A multi-modal convolutional neural network framework for the prediction of Alzheimer's disease a multi-modal convolutional neural network framework for the prediction of Alzheimer's disease. *Proceedings of the 40th Annual International Conference of the IEEE Engineering in Medicine and Biology Society*, vol. 2018, pp. 1271–4, 2018.
47. He, T., Nolte, J., Moore, L.W. *et al.*, An imageomics and multi-network based deep learning model for risk assessment of liver transplantation for hepatocellular cancer. *Comput. Med. Imaging Graph.*, 89, 101894, 2021.
48. Panwar, V., Sharma, D.K., Kumar, K.P., Jain, A., Thakar, C., Experimental investigations and optimization of surface roughness in turning of EN 36 alloy steel using response surface methodology and genetic algorithm. *Mater. Today: Proc.*, 46, 6474–6481, 2021.
49. Jain, A. and Pandey, A.K., Modeling and optimizing of different quality characteristics in electrical discharge drilling of titanium alloy (Grade-5) sheet. *Mater. Today Proc.*, 18, 182–191, 2019. https://doi.org/10.1016/j.matpr.2019.06.292.
50. Jain, A., Yadav, A.K., Shrivastava, Y., Modelling and optimization of different quality characteristics in electric discharge drilling of titanium alloy sheet. *Mater. Today Proc.*, 21, 1680–1684, 2019. https://doi.org/10.1016/j.matpr.2019.12.010.
51. Jain, A. and Pandey, A.K., Multiple quality optimizations in electrical discharge drilling of mild steel sheet. *Mater. Today Proc.*, 8, 7252–7261, 2019. https://doi.org/10.1016/j.matpr.2017.07.054.
52. Jain, A., Kumar, C.S., Shrivastava, Y., Fabrication and machining of fiber matrix composite through electric discharge machining: A short review. *Mater. Today Proc.*, 51, 1233–1237, 2021.
53. Joshi, K., Joshi, K.N., Diwakar, M., Tripathi, N.A., Gupta, H., Multi-focus image fusion using non-local mean filtering and stationary wavelet transform. *Int. J. Innov. Technol. Explor. Eng. (IJITEE)*, 9, 344–350, 2019.

54. Diwakar, M., Tripathi, A., Joshi, K., Sharma, A., Singh, P., Memoria, M., A comparative review: Medical image fusion using SWT and DWT. *Mater. Today: Proc.*, *37*, 3411–3416, 2021.
55. Aboamer, M.A., Sikkandar, M.Y., Gupta, S., Vives, L., Joshi, K., Omarov, B., Singh, S.K., An investigation in analyzing the food quality well-being for lung cancer using blockchain through CNN. *J. Food Qual.*, *2022*, 2022.
56. Kimothi, S., Thapliyal, A., Akram, S.V., Singh, R., Gehlot, A., Mohamed, H.G., Noya, I.D., Big data analysis framework for water quality indicators with assimilation of IoT and ML. *Electronics*, *11*, 13, 1927, 2022.
57. Kumar, G.A., Singh, R., Gehlot, A., Akram, S.V., LoRa enabled real-time monitoring of workers in building construction site. *IJEER*, *10*, 1, 41–50, 2022.
58. Rajput, S.K., Patni, J.C., Alshamrani, S.S., Chaudhari, V., Dumka, A., Singh, R., AlGhamdi, A.S., Automatic vehicle identification and classification model using the YOLOv3 algorithm for a toll management system. *Sustainability*, *14*, 15, 9163, 2022.

5

Developing Robot-Based Neurorehabilitation Exercises Using a Teaching–Training Process

W. Vinu[1], Sonali Vyas[2*], A. Chandrashekhar[3], T. Ch. Anil Kumar[4], T. Raghu[5] and Mohit Tiwari[6]

[1]*Department of Physical Education and Sports, Pondicherry University, Chinna Kalapet, Kalapet, Puducherry, India*
[2]*School of Computer Science, UPES University, Dehradun, Uttarakhand, India*
[3]*Department of Mechatronics, Faculty of Science and Technology, ICFAI Foundation for Higher Education, Hyderabad, Telangana, India*
[4]*Department of Mechanical Engineering, Vignan's Foundation for Science Technology and Research, Vadlamudi, Guntur Dt., Andhra Pradesh, India*
[5]*School of Sciences, SR University, Warangal, Telangana, India*
[6]*Department of Computer Science and Engineering, Bharati Vidyapeeth's College of Engineering, Paschim Vihar, Delhi, India*

Abstract

Exercises for neurorehabilitation using robots are becoming more and more significant in physical therapy. This is brought on by the rising incidence of neurological illnesses and disorders like stroke, spinal cord injury, traumatic brain injury, and many others. They are made to aid patients in enhancing their movement and motor skills. They also aid in enhancing brain abilities like memory and problem-solving techniques. These activities can be modified based on the requirements and capabilities of each patient. A teaching–training process is one way to create robot-based neurorehabilitation activities. This procedure makes use of a structure with robots. The platform offers patients a secure and monitored setting in which to perform the exercises. The robot-based platform also enables the creation of unique activities for every patient. Additionally, providing feedback throughout the process enables the patient to comprehend how to enhance their

**Corresponding author*: researcher.svyas@gmail.com
T. Ch. Anil Kumar: ORCID: 0000-0001-6964-8401

Kapil Joshi and Somil Kumar Gupta (eds.) Human Cancer Diagnosis and Detection Using Exascale Computing, (71–86) © 2024 Scrivener Publishing LLC

efficiency and change the exercise's intensity as required. The patient's physical and mental capabilities can be enhanced, and their standard of life can be raised.

Keywords: Neurorehabilitation, teaching–training process, robot

5.1 Introduction

Robotic therapy aids are becoming more popular for use in the treatment of neural injuries like spinal cord injuries and strokes [1]. Although there is work using robots that do not physically touch the respondents, the predominant approach being investigated is to use a robotic device to physically engage with the respondent's limbs during movement training [2]. Brain injuries or neurological disorders that cause motor or sensory loss or dysfunction have a significant negative impact on quality of life and may even make it impossible to carry out basic everyday tasks. However, these sensorimotor impairments are very prevalent among neurological patients: about 50% of stroke patients have chronically reduced arm function, and more than two-thirds of all stroke patients have upper limb involvement [4]. The sensorimotor techniques the brain uses to regulate gait and balance can be compromised to varying degrees by these impairments that can also impact the lower limb. It is important to emphasize how a particular impairment affects the patient's behavior in order to comprehend how to rehabilitate from these pathological circumstances [5].

Robotic instruments designed for rehabilitation exercise are controlled by robotic therapy control methods to ensure that the participant's selected tasks stimulate motor plasticity and thus improve motor recovery. However, there is currently little agreement among experts as to the best way to accomplish this goal. As a consequence, as-needed control methods for robotic therapy have been created, frequently drawing inspiration from research on rehabilitation, neuroscience, and motor learning [15].

The procedure of neurological rehabilitation, also known as neurorehabilitation, seeks to lessen a patient's functional constraints. The goal is to maximize a person's involvement in society and sense of well-being, and these restrictions are the result of motor control issues [8]. When individuals with functional movement disorders suffer from motor control issues, treatments are frequently focused on improving their ability to move or modifying how they move.

In clinical practice, it is essential to comprehend how movement and motor coordination function. As a result, it is crucial to take into account the creation of robotic rehabilitation systems (RRSs), which are intended to be used in clinical environments. There are many hypotheses about motor control because movement is so complicated. These hypotheses attempt to explain how the brain regulates movement and what variables play a part [16].

Three domains of robotic technique growth can be distinguished for healthcare: medical, assistive, and rehabilitation robotics. The discipline of medical robotics includes robots that assist with treatment and care procedures in medicine. Surgical robots are probably the systems that are used the most in medical environments. Technologies that help patients or caregivers in medical facilities with task-related methods are comprised in the realm of assistive robotics [9]. This help comprises logistical chores, security, bed transfers, etc. Ultimately, the domain of rehabilitation robotics involves a diversity of postoperative or postinjury care approaches where direct physical contact with a robot system will either hasten healing or supplement lost functionality [18].

Robots are perfect tools to assist neurologists and therapists in addressing the difficulties associated with neurorehabilitation because they offer both movement controllability and measurement reliability. Riener recently reviewed a number of robotic devices and looked at the technological variations among them [1]. These tools typically come in the shape of an actuated robotic arm (also known as a manipulandum), a joystick, or a robotic suit that surrounds the injured leg like an exoskeleton. The robots have sensors that capture movement information like joint torques, velocity, and location. Actuators on the robots allow them to manipulate the subject's limb as well. Robots make it possible to quantify both the initial impairment and the alterations in impairment that result from medication more precisely by means of movement dynamics and kinematics. This measurement capability not only enables a biomechanical paradigm to be used to conduct reverse dynamic analyses on movement data to determine forces at joints but also practically eliminates the impact of interrater variations on outcome evaluations [3].

Rehabilitative processes usually entail four phases. The patient must first be evaluated in order to determine the kind and degree of their disability. The therapist must also prepare an assistant to achieve the objectives and establish targets to guide the therapy. Third, the assistance must be put into action, which frequently calls for repeatedly practicing particular motions with assistance [6]. After the treatment, the patient must be evaluated again, and fresh targets must be established. Robotics has long been thought to have the ability to aid and assist in the rehabilitation procedure [7]. Each of the four procedures that therapists must carry out can be improved by robots. Relying on the severity of the impairment, they can be used to offer targeted interventions reliably and repeatedly and to evaluate efficacy before, after, and during treatment.

5.1.1 Research Gap

The dearth of data demonstrating the efficacy of robot-based neurorehabilitation exercises is a study gap. The effectiveness of robot-based neurorehabilitation exercises in comparison to conventional rehabilitation techniques is currently supported by a restricted body of research. The effectiveness of the teaching and training procedure in enhancing patient outcomes is also unknown. Although the idea of training robots to carry out neurorehabilitation exercises has been considered, there have not been any substantial studies to determine whether such a system is effective. There are also a few investigations on how such a method affects the patient psychologically, as well as how it affects the therapist or caretaker.

5.1.2 Research Aim

The goal of this study is to formulate a teaching and training procedure that makes use of robotic technology to produce exercises for neurorehabilitation. The goal of the study is to determine which robotic parts and training methods work best together to help people with neurological disorders develop their motor skills. The effectiveness of this robotically aided training process in contrast to more traditional forms of rehabilitation will also be examined by this study.

5.2 Literature Review

The writers want to use robotics and automation to support, improve, measure, and record neurorehabilitation. The clinical trial, which involved 20 stroke patients, was conducted at Burke Rehabilitation Hospital in White Plains, New York, using a prototype robot-assisted rehabilitation facility created at the Massachusetts Institute of Technology (MIT) in Cambridge. Additionally, it outlines the authors' method for analyzing the kinematic data gathered during the robot-assisted evaluation process. They specifically provide proof that robot-assisted therapy is 1) safe and 2) well-tolerated by patients and 3) may affect brain recovery through peripheral manipulation of the impaired limb. These findings are supported by accepted clinical evaluation techniques. A method for using kinematic data in a robot-assisted assessment process is also presented by the authors [21].

According to statistics, 11% of people report having some degree of cognitive decline, which can affect one's memory, cognition, behavior, and physical capabilities and may be linked to diseases like dementia or stroke. While behavioral therapies like cognitive training can help individuals with cognitive impairments remain independent longer, many of these conditions have no known pharmacological cures. These therapies instruct patients in metacognitive techniques to deal with memory issues in daily life. To increase a patient's engagement and sustainment in addition to the medication's efficacy, it is essential to tailor these interventions to fit their inclinations and objectives. Robots have a lot of possibilities to assist people with cognitive impairments, their caretakers, and clinicians by facilitating these training practices [17]. This paper explores how, in the framework of cognitive neurorehabilitation, robots can change their behavior to be personalized to a person. We give an overview of the current robots used to assist neurorehabilitation and point out important guidelines for operating in this field.

There has been a surge in the study of robotic devices for poststroke rehabilitation since the late 1990s. Nevertheless, so far, the use of robots has not demonstrated any qualitative advantage over traditional therapist-led training events, carried out on the same amount of movements [20]. Robot-mediated therapy has improved the regaining of motor capacity. A distributed interaction on the entire assisted limb is made possible by multidegree-of-freedom robots, like the contemporary upper limb exoskeletons. These robots can also utilize a significant amount of sensory feedback data, possibly enabling fresh possibilities within conventional rehabilitation programs. Interestingly, the majority of papers on the subject of exoskeletons gave little attention to the control aspects and instead concentrated primarily on the mechatronic design of the devices [19]. On the contrary, we think that the management side of robot possibility is of utmost importance. In order to formulate pertinent questions for the creation of novel and enhanced control approaches, the objective of this analysis is to offer a taxonomy of control methods for exoskeletons for neurorehabilitation that are presently in use.

Robotic tools are assisting in the understanding of human motor function in both health and injury. Researchers are learning how the nervous system models its external dynamic world by using robots to deploy innovative force fields to the arm. The nervous system employs internal models in conjunction with impedance and feedback control strategies, gradually developing them through experience. Internal theories are executed in various brain regions, generalized across space, robust to environmental and neural noise, and formed in childhood. In order to aid repetitive movement practice after neurologic damage and shed light on movement recovery, robots are also being used. Robots can give training, measure the quantity of training, and enhance motor recovery while haptically evaluating sensorimotor efficiency. Robotic approaches may ultimately improve motor learning and rehabilitation above the levels attainable with traditional training methods, in addition to offering perspective into motor control.

The "magic bullet" of recovery does not exist. When direct neural transplants are not an option, neurological rehabilitation is a difficult procedure. Targeted exercise has a beneficial effect on stroke recovery, and we have established the medical application of robotics in stroke rehabilitation. We will examine the findings from the early clinical trials, which involved 96 stroke patients in this paper. We will show that robot-assisted training improves recovery, that this increase is maintained over time, and that this recovery is not the result of an overall physiological growth; rather, it seems to be limb and muscle group-specific. It is now necessary to transition from an evidence-based strategy to a more empirical strategy for stroke recovery. The restrictions of the evidence-based strategy are obvious and cause trials to last for years due to the length of the necessary procedures, patient variability, and low census. In stroke therapy, there is no reason to think that a "one-size-fits-all" ideal medication occurs because every patient and lesion is distinct. We require science-based models to improve therapy for specific patients.

Robot-assisted rehabilitation and treatment are increasingly used to aid the elderly, patients with disabilities, or people with movement disorders in performing exercise and training. In the past 10 years, the area of lower limb rehabilitation assisted by robots has advanced quickly. This paper provides an overview of the most modern developments in lower limb rehabilitation robot mechanisms, training modes, and control schemes from the years 2001 to 2014. In robot-assisted passive and active lower limb rehabilitation, particular focus is placed on adaptive robot control techniques taking hybrid data fusion and patient evaluation into account. The latest research characteristics and medical results for various training modalities and control algorithms are analyzed and compiled. This chapter also identifies research gaps and potential directions to enhance the effectiveness of robot-assisted rehabilitation.

5.3 Research Methodology

- **Fitbit software**: Any computer running the Windows operating system can load the software [10]. The software's data reading, showing, and action-taking are handled by a number of real-time cycles.
- **Switches**: In networks, switches can take the place of routers. The PC and robot can be connected via a switch. The networking tool known as a switch joins two or more devices on a common network. Additionally, it can be used to link various networks together [11]. Data transmission between devices on a single network or across numerous networks is made possible by switches.
- **LabVIEW and Arduino**: Software such as a software development kit (SDK) or a graphical programming language such as LabVIEW can be used to create a communication interface between the robot and the computer. A control interface Arduino can be used to bridge the robot and the computer [12]. This type of interface allows the robot to send and receive data from the computer, allowing it to control its own movements and receive instructions from the user.
- **Robotic arm controller**: Utilizing a robotic limb controller is one choice. This is a tool that can be used to move a robot arm when it is attached to a robot arm. A controller, a power source, and a computer interface are the usual components [13]. The controller, which can be set with specific instructions, can be used to direct the motion of the robot. To share data and synchronize the movements of the robot, some controllers can also communicate with other devices like computers.
- **Piezoresistive sensors**: By detecting changes in the electrical resistance of moving muscles, piezoresistive sensors can be used to quantify muscular activity. The electrical resistance of a muscle can be quantified and used to track variations in muscle activity by positioning a piezoresistive sensor on the muscle. Feedback on muscle efficacy during physical tasks like running, jumping, and lifting can be obtained using this [14]. It can also be used to keep track of the stress that rehabilitation activities put on the muscles. The real-time information on muscle action that the piezoresistive sensor can offer can be used to enhance training and rehabilitation regimens. The overall architecture is given in Figure 5.1.

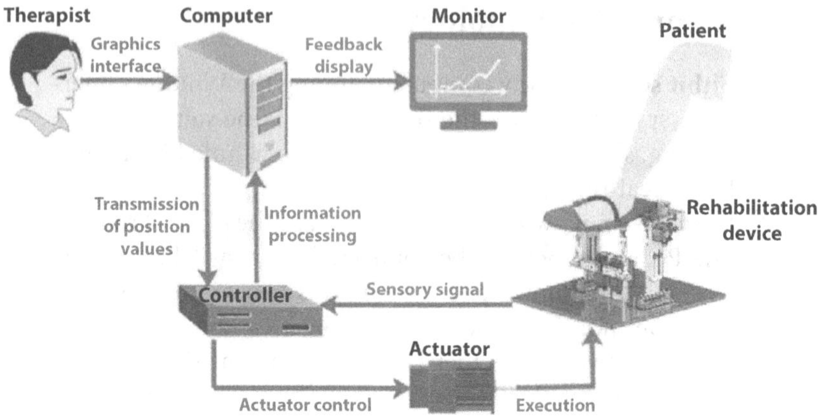

Figure 5.1 Overall system architecture.

In each training session, the normalized force control parameter (nFCP) and the force directional error (FDE) were used to evaluate the efficiency of the patients. To confirm the statistical importance of the shift in movement dynamics and clinical factors posttreatment compared with pretreatment values, reiterated measures *t*-tests were performed.

5.4 Results

Table 5.1 lists the mean values, standard deviations, changes, and values of the pre- *versus* posttreatment analysis for force directional error variables. There was a statistically significant decline in both error values.

Devices of the SCARA (selective compliance assembly robot arm) type, such as the MIT-MANUS, have significant compliance in the horizontal and vertical planes. Due to this, it is now possible to quickly evaluate the shoulder during flexion, extension, abduction, and adduction. The patient's arm is prepositioned for this evaluation with the elbow fully extended at

Table 5.1 Pretreatment and posttreatment values of the movement dynamics measures.

	Pre	Post	*P*
nFCP	17.93 ± 7.54	10.43 ± 8.01	<0.002
FDE	23.42 ± 9.17	12.81 ± 7.72	<0.004

90° of shoulder flexion in the sagittal plane. The therapist places the patient in the trough and then physically secures the robot's arm in the necessary testing position. As a result, the arm will be properly positioned for strength assessment (see Figure 5.2).

For individuals with motor dysfunction, passive training is primarily utilized in the initial stages of rehabilitation. The entire rehabilitation training procedure is dominated by the robot because the patient lacks motor skills. To precisely monitor the patient's rehabilitation trajectory, the robot

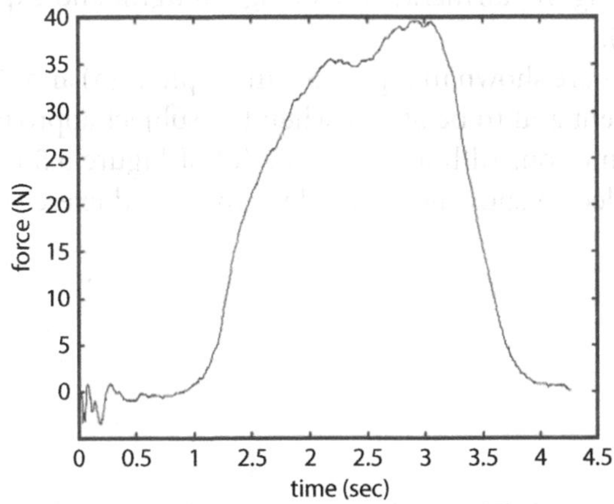

Figure 5.2 Outpatient during the shoulder abduction test.

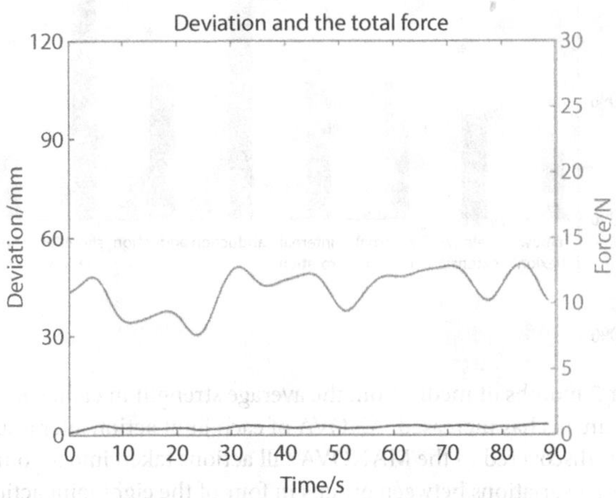

Figure 5.3 The subject's hand deviation from the handle as well as the overall interaction power.

moves the patient's arm. During the passive training testing, the patient's arm was fixed to the handle with a bandage. After that, the patient's arm was directed by the robot to carry out rehabilitation training on the circular trajectory. The testing procedures were carried out in a counterclockwise manner with three turns. The findings in Figure 5.3 demonstrate that the patient's hand deviation is very small, allowing the robot to precisely steer the patient's hand along the preset trajectory.

After 2 months of therapy, a program of robot-assisted movements was superior to traditional treatment of comparable intensity and duration in terms of reducing impairment, enhancing strength, and expanding reach (see Figure 5.4).

Both muscles are shown in Figure 5.5 in graphics (a) and (b) to be active during movement and to be at rest when the subject approaches the limit of its range of motion. Although graphic (c) of Figure 5.5 is only superficial, it is included to show how muscle activity and exercise intensity are linked.

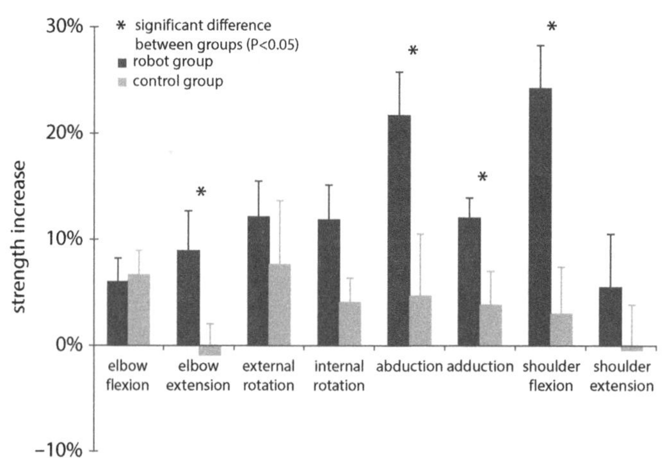

Figure 5.4 After 2 months of medication, the average strength in eight shoulder and elbow joint movements has increased. ANOVA of each joint action after a substantial group impact was discovered in the MANOVA (all actions taken into account together) showing substantial variations between groups in four of the eight joint actions.

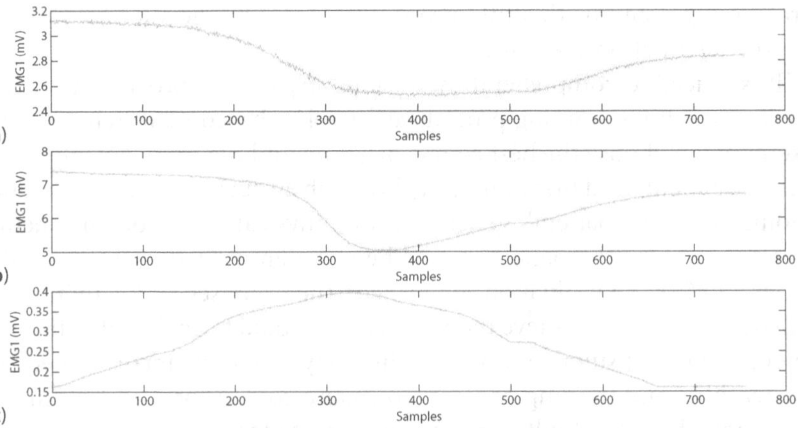

Figure 5.5 Passive lateral shoulder rotation experimental evaluation. (a) The deltoid muscle's action in the body. (b) Latissimus dorsi muscle action. (c) Robot location in relation to the specimens in *x*.

5.5 Conclusion

The rise of artificial cognitive agents in our medical practice, particularly in poststroke rehabilitation, appears to be the result of artificial intelligence and technological transformation. Recovery of motor function is achieved using an efficient scientific procedure for robot-assisted therapy of the upper extremities. For stroke survivors who have higher upper extremity impairment and struggle to move actively even in the early stages, passive training with the upper extremity robot is essential. A control strategy using a teaching training technique was suggested in the study to implement a personalized passive neurorehabilitation exercise, assisting with safe and effective robot-assisted motion. The teaching training was created to support clinicians by offering individualized passive training that guarantees coordination and fluidity of the upper limb motor. The lack of therapists is also reduced by robot-assisted instruction training, which provides adequate passive training.

Physical therapy techniques called neurorehabilitation exercises are used to help people with neuromuscular disabilities recover function and enhance their quality of life. Robotics has gained popularity in this procedure in current years because they provide a more precise and effective method to carry out challenging tasks. In order to ensure that the exercises are carried out properly and to the intended results, the teaching–training process suggested in this title proposes a novel method for robot-based neurorehabilitation exercises.

It is crucial to comprehend the various steps in the process in order to create a teaching–training procedure for robot-based neurorehabilitation exercises. To choose the best course of action and the most suitable activities, the patient must first undergo a thorough evaluation. This examination should cover the patient's general health, physical condition, and neurological function. The patient should be given an individual rehabilitation program after the evaluation is finished. The exercises and activities that will help the patient achieve their objectives should be included in this regimen. The use of suitable robotic technology should be incorporated into the teaching and training process. To ensure correct form and technique, the robots should be built to give the patient feedback. Furthermore, as the patient advances through the program, the robots ought to be able to adapt to their skills. The patient will be able to study and advance at their own rate as a result. In order to ensure that the patient is improving and that the robot-based exercises are working, the teaching–training process should also be regularly watched and evaluated. Additionally, it is critical to bear in mind that the procedure should be customized to meet the needs of each patient. The patient should be able to benefit the most from the program in this manner. To guarantee the best results, this procedure would need to be customized to the abilities and requirements of each patient. By utilizing this process, patients should be able to receive the most benefit from their rehabilitation program.

5.6 Future Research Directions

The use of teaching–training techniques in robot-based neurorehabilitation activities has the possibility to completely transform rehabilitation for those with neurological impairments. The demand for successful and expedient rehabilitation procedures to enhance function and quality of life, as well as the rising prevalence of neurological impairments like stroke and spinal cord injury, makes this study crucial. New rehabilitation techniques that are more efficient, secure, and economical than existing ones could result from this field of study. The creation of robotic systems that can engage patients to deliver therapeutic exercises has been the main goal of this field's research.

These robots are made to give patients immediate performance feedback so that the practice can be adjusted as necessary. Furthermore, the robots can be designed to offer the patient varying degrees of assistance, such as physical guidance to ensure the proper execution of the exercises. The use of machine learning algorithms to enable the robots to take notes on the patient's behavior and alter the exercises as necessary has also been explored in research. The creation of teaching–training techniques that can be used to assist patients in learning how to use robotic systems is another area of study. With this method, the patient can learn the exercises more swiftly and effectively and gain more self-reliance during their rehabilitation. The creation of new robotic systems that can offer more sophisticated levels of help and feedback may be the subject of future study in this field. Research should also concentrate on integrating virtual reality into robotic systems so that patients can engage in a virtual setting and have a more immersive experience. Research should also investigate the application of individually designed autonomous systems that can be adjusted to a patient's specific requirements.

References

1. Riener, R., Nef, T., Colombo, G., Robot-aided neurorehabilitation of the upper extremities. *Med. Biol. Eng. Comput.*, *43*, 2–10, 2005.
2. Matarić, M.J., Eriksson, J., Feil-Seifer, D.J., Winstein, C.J., Socially assistive robotics for post-stroke rehabilitation. *J. NeuroEng. Rehabil.*, *4*, 1–9, 2007.
3. Abdullah, H.A., Tarry, C., Datta, R., Mittal, G.S., Abderrahim, M., Dynamic biomechanical model for assessing and monitoring robot-assisted upper-limb therapy. *J. Rehabil. Res. Dev.*, *44*, 1, 43–61, 2007.
4. Hatem, S.M., Saussez, G., Della Faille, M., Prist, V., Zhang, X., Dispa, D., Bleyenheuft, Y., Rehabilitation of motor function after stroke: A multiple systematic review focused on techniques to stimulate upper extremity recovery. *Front. Hum. Neurosci.*, *10*, 442, 2016.
5. G. Broeks, J., Lankhorst, G.J., Rumping, K., Prevo, A.J.H., The long-term outcome of arm function after stroke: Results of a follow-up study. *Disabil. Rehabil.*, *21*, 8, 357–364, 1999.
6. Langhorne, P., Bernhardt, J., Kwakkel, G., Stroke care 2. Stroke rehabilitation. *Lancet*, *377*, 9778, 1693–1702, 2011.
7. van Vliet, P. and Wing, A.M., A new challenge—Robotics in the rehabilitation of the neurologically motor impaired. *Phys. Ther.*, *71*, 1, 39–47, 1991.
8. Barnes, M.P., Principles of neurological rehabilitation. *JNNP*, *74*, suppl 4, iv3–iv7, 2003.
9. Sparc, E., *Robotics 2020 multi-annual roadmap for robotics in Europe, Call 2 ICT24*, Horizon, Initial Release B, 2020.

10. Panwar, V., Sharma, D.K., Kumar, K.V.P., Jain, A., Thakar, C., Experimental investigations and optimization of surface roughness in turning of EN 36 alloy steel using response surface methodology and genetic algorithm. *Mater. Today:. Proc.*, 46, 15, 6474–6481, 2021. https://Doi.Org/10.1016/J.Matpr.2021.03.642.
11. Jain, A. and Pandey, A.K., Modeling and optimizing of different quality characteristics in electrical discharge drilling of titanium alloy (Grade-5) sheet. *Mater. Today Proc.*, 18, 182–191, 2019. https://doi.org/10.1016/j.matpr.2019.06.292.
12. Jain, A., Yadav, A.K., Shrivastava, Y., Modelling and optimization of different quality characteristics in electric discharge drilling of titanium alloy sheet. *Mater. Today Proc.*, 21, 1680–1684, 2019. https://doi.org/10.1016/j.matpr.2019.12.010.
13. Jain, A. and Pandey, A.K., Multiple quality optimizations in electrical discharge drilling of mild steel sheet. *Mater. Today Proc.*, 8, 7252–726, 2019. https://doi.org/10.1016/j.matpr.2017.07.054.
14. Jain, A., Kumar, C.S., Shrivastava, Y., Fabrication and machining of fiber matrix composite through electric discharge machining: A short review. *Mater. Today Proc.*, 51, 1, 1233–1237, 2022. https://doi.org/10.1016/j.matpr.2021.07.288.
15. Singh, R., Gehlot, A., Mittal, M., Samkaria, R., Singh, D., Chandra, P., Design and development of a cloud assisted robot, in: *Smart and Innovative Trends in Next Generation Computing Technologies: Third International Conference, NGCT 2017, Dehradun, India, October 30-31, 2017, Revised Selected Papers, Part II 3*, Springer, Singapore, pp. 419–429, 2018.
16. Praveen, S., Tyagi, N., Singh, B., Karetla, G.R., Thalor, M.A., Joshi, K., Tsegaye, M., PSO-based evolutionary approach to optimize head and neck biomedical image to detect mesothelioma cancer. *BioMed. Res. Int., 2022*, 1–12, 2022.
17. Diwakar, M., Tripathi, A., Joshi, K., Memoria, M., Singh, P., Latest trends on heart disease prediction using machine learning and image fusion. *Mater. Today:. Proc., 37*, 3213–3218, 2021.
18. Madan, P., Singh, V., Chaudhari, V., Albagory, Y., Dumka, A., Singh, R., AlGhamdi, A.S., An optimization-based diabetes prediction model using CNN and Bi-directional LSTM in real-time environment. *Appl. Sci., 12*, 8, 3989, 2022.
19. Duggal, A.S., Singh, R., Gehlot, A., Rashid, M., Alshamrani, S.S., AlGhamdi, A.S., Digital taste in mulsemedia augmented reality: Perspective on developments and challenges. *Electronics, 11*, 9, 1315, 2022.

20. Singh, D., Akram, S.V., Singh, R., Gehlot, A., Buddhi, D., Priyadarshi, N., Bokoro, P.N., Building integrated photovoltaics 4.0: Digitization of the photovoltaic integration in buildings for a resilient infra at large scale. *Electronics*, *11*, 17, 2700, 2022.
21. Kumar, G.A., Roy, A., Singh, R., Gehlot, A., Rashid, M., Akram, S.V., AlGhamdi, A.S., Hybrid architecture based system for the establishment of sustainable environment in a construction site with 433 MHz LoRa and 2.4 GHz Zigbee. *Sustainability*, *14*, 10, 6280, 2022.

6

Investigation on Introduction to Heterogeneous Exascale Computing in the Medical Field

M. Pyingkodi[1]*, Raju Shanmugam[2], Dilip Kumar Sharma[3], Deepesh Lall[4], S. Deepan[5] and B. Dasu[6]

[1]*Department of Computer Applications, Kongu Engineering College, Erode, India*
[2]*Unitedworld School of Computational Intelligence, Karnavati University, Gandhinagar, Gujarat, India*
[3]*Department of Mathematics, Jaypee University of Engineering and Technology, Guna (M.P.), India*
[4]*Bhagwant University, Ajmer, Rajasthan, India & LCIT School of Pharmacy, Bilaspur, CG, India*
[5]*School of Computer Science & Artificial Intelligence, SR University, Warangal, Telangana, India*
[6]*Department of ECE, St. Martin's Engineering College Secunderabad, Telangana, India*

Abstract

The possibility for heterogeneous exascale computing in the medical industry is examined in this study. The study especially examines the benefits of combining CPUs, GPUs, and FPGAs to attain exascale efficiency. The study also looks at how the use of exascale computing in the medical field can enhance patient treatment by enhancing the precision and efficiency of diagnosis and research. The study also looks at the possible drawbacks of heterogeneous exascale computing, including its cost, power requirements, and the complexity of writing programs that work across various frameworks. The study then discusses possible solutions to these problems, including the use of high-level programming languages and open-source advancement techniques. The prospective advantages of heterogeneous exascale computing in healthcare are outlined in the paper's conclusion, along with future research paths.

**Corresponding author*: Pyingkodikongu@gmail.com

Kapil Joshi and Somil Kumar Gupta (eds.) Human Cancer Diagnosis and Detection Using Exascale Computing, (87–100) © 2024 Scrivener Publishing LLC

***Keywords*:** Exascale computing, medical field, Internet of Things

6.1 Introduction

Exascale computing requires a 1,000-fold increase in the speed of current apps. It is obvious that this cannot be done by hardware, at least not in the short amount of time necessary to achieve this efficiency achievement. Thus, a robust debate about programming models, software parts and techniques, and algorithms that will aid exascale computing has started in the last 2 or 3 years. The hardware path to exascale systems, despite not being solely certain, points to computing systems comprising nodes with boosting a number of cores and comprised of compute engines with substantial structural variations (for instance, having distinct instruction set frameworks), i.e., heterogeneous systems. Until and unless a completely unique and unanticipated technology emerges, heterogeneous systems using GPUs are presently leading the way and are predicted to keep expanding [1, 2].

Future judgments about prevention and treatment for cancer patients may be supported by predictive computational models, which can help patients make the best potential clinical decisions [16]. The national Precision Medicine Initiative (PMI), which was launched in 2015 to advance this goal, inspired attempts to focus on and progress precision oncology and to anticipate the data and computational possibilities required to do so [9].

As exascale computing became more advanced, its potential for use in the life sciences grew. This was due to the increasing amount of data available and the expected introduction of new methods and measurements, such as PMI. These developments opened new horizons for computing in the life sciences [17].

To operate in this new ultra-parallel environment, computational techniques and software will need to advance. The widening disparity between compute capability and interconnect bandwidth is one of the biggest obstacles to scalability (and programmability). For the new frameworks to be used for scientific discovery at the greatest efficiency, it is imperative that we engage in algorithmic research that is created in collaboration with exascale applications. On the other hand, much more than just hardware improvements will be needed to achieve exascale computing in the short time period predicted. Algorithmic advancements must take the lead. If the past is any indication, advances in algorithm have frequently led to significant advances in capability that are on level with or even greater than those brought about by advancements in hardware [18]. Therefore, we can be confident that the chances of success are greater if we keep a significant study attempt into both scientific algorithms and their implementation.

Exascale computers are extremely powerful scientific instruments, and a single exascale computer would have incredible strength. Supercomputers need to be fast, but they also need to be able to hold and read enormous amounts of data quickly. Disruptive adjustments will be necessary to maximize hardware and software for exascale computers [10].

To enhance and personalize treatment planning, exascale learning on medical image data seeks to improve the efficiency of decision support in the procedure of cancer detection and localization. The automated techniques help doctors make decisions, expedite the ocular examination of tissue samples, and lessen subjectivity in the staging procedure. The use case deals with histopathology images from programs like CAMELYON and TUPAC for tissue classification and cancer diagnosis [19]. We are able to create more intricate models and utilize finer-grained, larger quantities of data owing to the PROCESS framework. By pushing the limits of computation and enabling investigators to create methods that are otherwise computationally impractical, access to exascale computing will steadily reduce the turnaround time of the tests.

6.1.1 Research Gap

The dearth of studies on how to best utilize the enormous quantity of data produced by medical devices and apps is the existing research gap in the discipline of heterogeneous exascale computing in the medical field. Conventional single-processor computing frameworks can no longer efficiently process the data due to the exponential growth in data produced. Consequently, more study is required to fully utilize the enormous possibility of heterogeneous exascale computing systems for medical applications. This study will focus on the creation of effective algorithms and methods. There is also a need for study into the most efficient ways to process huge medical datasets economically using the distributed memory framework of heterogeneous exascale computing systems. Future study is needed to decide how to use the powers of heterogeneous exascale computing systems to enhance the precision and efficiency of medical diagnosis.

6.2 Literature Review

Exascale services present novel, distinct difficulties that cannot be solved by the big data, computational, and workflow methods that are currently in use. The section contains a thorough explanation of a few exascale services with solutions that are known to be state-of-the-art in their field. A high-level structural method is the focal point of the incorporation of needs and the evaluation of the state of the art in the exascale sector. The PROCESS H2020 project is creating a framework to manage heterogeneous exascale services from both academic and industrial sources [20]. This framework will consider the specific needs of different user cases and provide computing solutions to exascale problems.

The peta- and exascale computing systems that depend more and more on heterogeneous frameworks with hardware accelerators like GPUs present several difficulties for the Monte Carlo radiation transport industry [5]. To accommodate changing hardware and software requirements, it is tactically necessary to update current Monte Carlo codes and procedures. In this article, we outline the creation of ARCHER (Accelerated Radiation-transport Computations in Heterogeneous Environments), a software program intended to serve as a flexible testbed for upcoming Monte Carlo algorithms. Five nuclear engineering and medical physics projects' tentative findings are shared.

This editorial describes the demands and obstacles on the path to exascale, as well as the study context. The emphasis is particularly on cutting-edge mathematical techniques, mathematical modeling strategies, and scalable scientific algorithms that are required to support important science uses at excessive scales [3]. This is particularly true as the number of compute nodes and CPU cores in HPC systems keeps increasing. In order to conceal network and memory latency and have extremely high computation, negligible communication, and reduced synchronization points, these extreme-scale systems necessitate the development of unique mathematical techniques [21]. In order to accomplish total scalability, it emphasizes the necessity of scalability at all levels, commencing at the scale of mathematical techniques and moving down to the level of algorithms and systems. It also emphasizes how crucial the demand for such scalable mathematical techniques and algorithms that can handle data and compute demanding applications at scale has become as a result of the recent developments in data science.

Global health and socioeconomic security continue to be at risk from the SARS-CoV-2/COVID-19 epidemic [4]. Most of the viral components have been captured in snapshots by studies, but these molecular machines' moving parts stay invisible. Through the Folding@home distributed computing initiative, more than a million citizen scientists have united to build the first exascale computer and emulate protein dynamics in order to observe these crucial activities. The spike intricate uses conformational masking to escape an immune response [22]. Other viral proteins' functions may also be affected by conformational changes. Cryptic pockets that are missing from experimental snapshots are also revealed by a unique 0.1 s of simulation of the viral proteome. Novel avenues for the development of therapeutics are presented by these frameworks and mechanistic discoveries.

Parallel computer frameworks built on graphics processing units (GPUs) have gained popularity as a foundation for future exascale computing and high-speed computing. Their programming complexities, meanwhile, continue to be a significant barrier to their general adoption. Investigators and suppliers have suggested several directive-based GPU programming methods to offer improved concepts for programming GPU frameworks [6]. These directive-based methods offer various levels of abstraction, and porting and optimizing applications needed various degrees of programming effort. The applicability and performance potential of these novel methods can be better understood by comprehending the variations between them. By converting 13 application kernels from different scientific fields to work with CUDA GPUs, we can assess current directive-based methods in this work and pinpoint significant problems with their functionality, adaptability, tunability, and debuggability.

Computational data analysis and modeling have become essential for advancing our comprehension as biologists come to comprehend and accept the intricacy of biological systems. Exascale computing will make it possible to create fresh forecasting multiscale methods, changing the way we research how organisms and ecosystems behave and eventually resulting in novel findings and breakthroughs [7].

High-performance computing is now a crucial component of advancements in solving significant scientific and technological issues. Although as the period of exascale computing approaches, there will be new difficulties for those who create large-scale scientific apps. In this study, we analyze the parallel programming methods and techniques targeted at assisting programmers in addressing this problem. Our emphasis is on decreasing the costs of communication in supercomputers [8].

One of the hardest problems in future exascale networks will be resilience. Memory errors make up more than 40% of all hardware-related problems and are expected to get worse in exascale systems in the future. Checkpointing and the use of error correction codes (ECCs) are two efficient methods for failure tolerance. This is the first paper to examine the incorporated impact of ECC and checkpointing on general system efficiency and power, even though there are many studies on ECC or checkpointing in isolation. We investigate the effects of different ECC methods in combination with checkpointing on upcoming exascale systems.

Our simulation findings demonstrate that while chip kill is 13% superior for applications requiring a lot of computation, BCH has a 28% advantage in terms of system energy-delay product (EDP) for applications requiring a lot of memory. Additionally, we suggest using BCH in situations where chip kill is unfeasible, such as tagged memory systems with common DRAMs. In comparison to cutting-edge tagged memory systems, our suggested framework obtains 2.3× better system EDP.

6.3 Research Methodology

Despite years of research and pharma industry efforts, many cancer patients still do not react to standard-of-care therapies, and the development of therapy resistance is general. By creating predictive capabilities of drug response in preclinical cancer systems, the Predictive Modelling for Pre-Clinical Screening Pilot aims to enhance and expedite the spread of freshly focused therapeutics for cancer patients [11]. Some of the work done in Pilot 1 is displayed in Figure 6.1.

Further studies will concentrate on investigating novel predictive methods to better employ and enhance biological knowledge. This will be done after taking into consideration observations from Pilot 1 tasks and

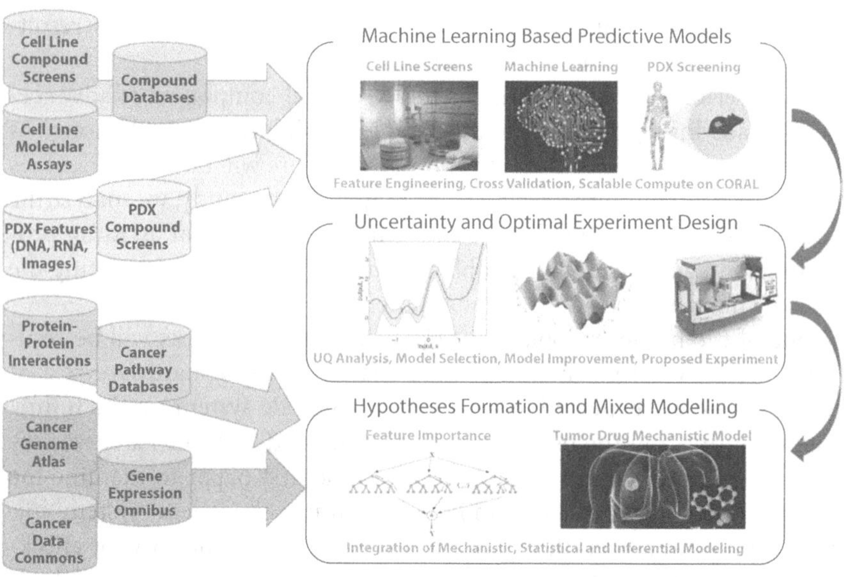

Figure 6.1 Pilot 1 study purpose and general workflow.

presenting gaps in the research. Studies incorporating semi-supervised network training on millions of compounds are anticipated to help improve drug representations for response prediction [12]. Mechanistic information is being integrated into comprehensible DL methods to enhance comprehension of trained models. The timely and cost-effective collection of experimental data for animal specimens will be aided by active learning in response prediction, which strikes a compromise between accuracy and lead discovery [13]. Lastly, developing a fine-grained grasp of prediction error, which is made possible by the skill shown in large-scale method sweeps, is an essential phase toward precision methods.

An additional strategy that could improve the efficiency of a predictive model is the choosing of attributes that have been mechanically updated. For instance, DL models have been trained using the LINCS landmark genes to forecast the gene expression of non-landmark genes and to categorize drug–target interactions. Utilizing mechanistically informed feature selection has the possibility to do more than just increase forecast accuracy; it also has the possibility to create models based on already-known biological principles.

The achievement of three key goals will ultimately enhance the efficiency of the most advanced cancer detection algorithms currently available [14]. The creation of image analysis methods for supervised and weakly supervised learning is the first goal. Weak labeling will make it possible to use sparsely labeled data to enhance model efficiency and generalization. Unsupervised learning methods can be used to design unannotated data, eliminating the demand for human annotation prior to training, further enhancing these benefits. To recognize tumorous regions and to propose to pathologists the potential tumorous regions in the histopathology image, trained networks are applied to testing data. The reliability of the models and the level of confidence in the created tools can both be increased by using visualization methods to collect instantaneous feedback and justifications for the network decisions. The distribution of instruction across various computational centers is the second goal. At various computational centers, neural networks can be trained separately with a speedup in training time proportional to their number [15]. After that, the models could be combined to create a singular model with better generalization capabilities. For instance, if numerous models are trained to examine model robustness and small perturbations are incorporated into the data, a tremendous number of computations are necessary. In general, the goals discussed here will aid in the analysis of sizable databases of medical information and, as a result, the creation of better algorithms for the automatic recommendation of patient cancer stage and associated patient cases.

6.4 Results and Discussion

A variational optimization algorithm that calculates a roughly optimal b-Edge Cover at each repetition to calculate an important subgraph was used in conjunction with the MCE approach to resolve an adaptive anonymity issue in the healthcare field. On 8,000 cores of the Cori computer at NERSC, we took less than 5 min to anonymize a healthcare data collection with 750,000 occurrences and 512 attributes. Figure 6.2 includes significant scaling findings on the Cori machine for three anonymization obstacles. The size of the issues solved grew three orders of magnitude as a result of this computation.

For exascale, we are presently creating a hybrid MPI+Kokkos color scheme. The intended goal is distributed memory supercomputers with many nodes, each of which could contain multiple GPUs. Per GPU, we need one MPI order. Next, we employ the formerly created Kokkos Kernel coloring technique for each GPU. We share boundary data, find conflicts, and address them at the MPI level. While working on partial distance-2 coloring, we presently offer distance-1 and distance-2 coloring. Our strategy is very adaptable. In less than half a second, we colored a graph with 76.7 billion lines using 128 GPUs. Because it functions well on both CPU- and GPU-based systems, our code is exceptional. Weak growth is excellent (Figure 6.3).

Prevention strategies like vaccination and social seclusion play a crucial role in halting the spread of a pandemic. There has been a lot of research done on graph-theoretic (or network) models in the books. In situations where originally known state-of-the-art techniques like SaaRound are

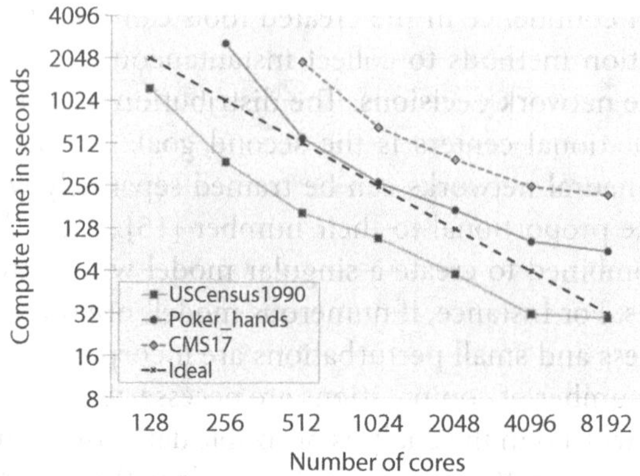

Figure 6.2 Strong scaling on Cori for three adaptive anonymity problems.

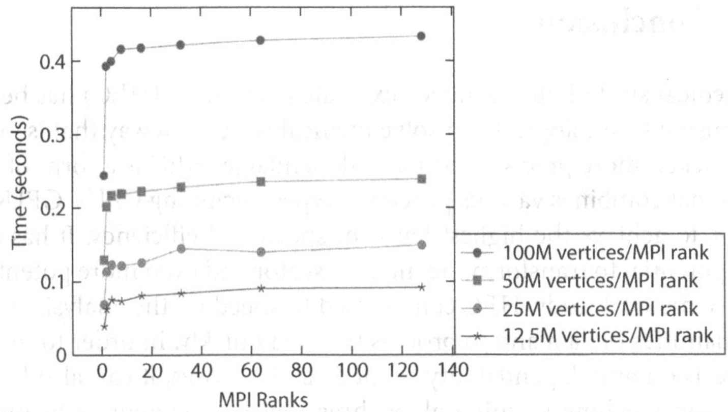

Figure 6.3 Weak scaling for coloring a mesh.

computationally infeasible, the team's recent work on applying Ripples to the problem of optimal intervention (vaccination) to stop the spread of a pandemic has exhibited a substantial impact (Figure 6.4). The earlier approaches relied on mathematical programming, but Ripples uses submodular optimization and scalable implementations to take advantage of the foundational framework. The group has also collaborated with subject-matter specialists to show how their work can be applied to fields like cancer research and soil microbiome study. Future research will focus on a wide range of uses, involving the observability and controllability of complex systems.

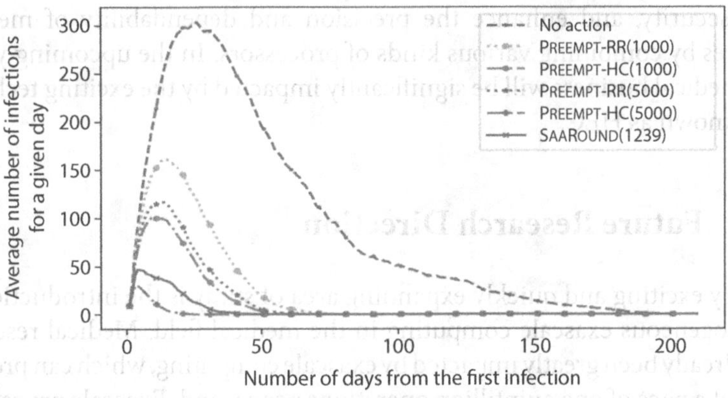

Figure 6.4 Temporal evolution of infections under various treatment approaches.

6.5 Conclusion

For medical study, heterogeneous exascale computing (HEC) has become a promising technology. It can solve medical issues in a way that is noticeably quicker, more precise, and more dependable. HEC is a form of computing that combines various processor types, including CPUs, GPUs, and FPGAs, to achieve the highest levels of speed and efficiency. It has enormous potential to transform the medical sector and even more potential to advance medical study. HEC can be used to speed up the analysis of massive quantities of data and to process the data quickly. In order to increase the precision and dependability of medical diagnoses, it can also be used to develop machine learning algorithms that can be applied to medical data. HEC can be used to enable medical academics to investigate fresh data sources and create fresh approaches to analysis. HEC can help the medical industry with data sharing, storage, and protection. Medical data can be shared, stored, and viewed securely through HEC from any location. Medical experts will be able to share data more quickly and securely, and it will also make it simpler for researchers to work together globally. HEC can be used to educate medical professionals and hone their abilities through virtual reality simulations. Medical professionals can use HEC to practice tasks in a simulated setting and acquire useful experience that they can use in real-world situations. Finally, HEC can be used to raise the precision and dependability of medical equipment like MRI and CT machines. Medical equipment producers can create products that are more precise and dependable than ever before by using HEC. In summary, HEC has the potential to transform the medical sector and offer quicker, more precise, and more dependable answers to medical issues. HEC can boost the efficiency and precision of medical research, offer better data storage and security, and enhance the precision and dependability of medical devices by combining various kinds of processors. In the upcoming years, the medical business will be significantly impacted by the exciting technology known as HEC.

6.6 Future Research Direction

A very exciting and quickly expanding area of study is the introduction of heterogeneous exascale computing in the medical field. Medical research has already been greatly impacted by exascale computing, which can process data at a pace of one quintillion operations per second. Exascale processing can be used by the medical industry to quickly analyze large datasets and resolve challenging issues. The potential of this technology will grow along with the utilization of exascale computing in the medical industry. Exascale processing in the medical industry is probably going to get even more popular and potent soon. This is due to the fact that exascale computing can significantly cut down on the time and expense involved in analyzing big datasets and resolving complex issues. This will make it possible for medical researchers to carry out more thorough analyses, create better treatments, and make more precise diagnoses. Exascale computing can also aid in the creation of personalized medication. Exascale computing allows medical researchers to analyze patient data more rapidly and precisely and personalize treatments for each patient. Additionally, exascale computing has applications outside of data analysis and diagnostics in the area of medicine.

Exascale computing can be used to model medical procedures and aid in medical researchers' understanding of the effects of various procedures.

Informed choices and the development of more potent treatments can be made by medical researchers as a result. The development of potent artificial intelligence (AI) algorithms that can analyze patient data, spot patterns, and make predictions is another use for exascale computing. This can be used to enhance patient care, maximize therapies, and raise the standard of healthcare. Exascale computing can revolutionize the medical industry and improve the effectiveness, accessibility, and efficiency of healthcare. Technology will continue to advance and so will its use in the medicinal industry. Exascale computing is anticipated to become more crucial to medical study, diagnosis, and treatments soon.

References

1. Hluchý, L., Bobák, M., Müller, H., Graziani, M., Maassen, J., Spreeuw, H., Nguyen, G., Heterogeneous exascale computing, in: *Recent advances in intelligent engineering: Volume dedicated to Imre J. Rudas' Seventieth Birthday*, pp. 81–110, 2020.
2. Xu, X.G., Liu, T., Su, L., Du, X., Riblett, M., Ji, W., Liu, B., ARCHER, a new Monte Carlo software tool for emerging heterogeneous computing environments, in: *SNA+ MC 2013-Joint International Conference on Supercomputing in Nuclear Applications+ Monte Carlo*, EDP Sciences, p. 06002, 2014.
3. Alexandrov, V., Route to exascale: Novel mathematical methods, scalable algorithms and computational science skills. *J. Comput. Sci.*, *14*, 1–4, 2016.

4. Zimmerman, M. I., Porter, J. R., Ward, M. D., Singh, S., Vithani, N., Meller, A., ... Bowman, G. R., Citizen scientists create an exascale computer to combat COVID-19. BioRxiv 2020.
5. Lee, S. and Vetter, J.S., Early evaluation of directive-based GPU programming models for productive exascale computing, in: *SC'12: Proceedings of the International Conference on High Performance Computing, Networking, Storage and Analysis*, IEEE, pp. 1–11, 2012, November.
6. Lee, C.T. and Amaro, R.E., Exascale computing: A new dawn for computational biology. *Comput. Sci. Eng.*, *20*, 5, 18–25, 2018.
7. Martin, S., *Analysis of parallel programming models for exascale computing.* Research Examination - University of California, San Diego, Fall, 2016.
8. Li, S., Chen, K., Hsieh, M.Y., Muralimanohar, N., Kersey, C.D., Brockman, J.B., Jouppi, N.P., System implications of memory reliability in exascale computing, in: *Proceedings of 2011 International Conference for High Performance Computing, Networking, Storage and Analysis*, pp. 1–12, 2011, November.
9. PMI, National Library of Medicine, 2019. Retrieved from https://ghr.nlm.nih.gov/primer/precisionmedicine/initiative.
10. Barroso, L.A., The price of performance: An economic case for chip multiprocessing. *Queue*, *3*, 7, 48–53, 2005.
11. Panwar, V., Sharma, D.K., Kumar, K. P., Jain, A., Thakar, C., Experimental investigations and optimization of surface roughness in turning of EN 36 alloy steel using response surface methodology and genetic algorithm. *Mater. Today:. Proc.*, 46, 6474–6481, 2021.
12. Jain, A. and Pandey, A.K., Modeling and optimizing of different quality characteristics in electrical discharge drilling of titanium alloy (Grade-5) sheet. *Mater. Today Proc.*, 18, 182–191, 2019. https://doi.org/10.1016/j.matpr.2019.06.292.
13. Jain, A., Yadav, A.K., Shrivastava, Y., Modelling and optimization of different quality characteristics in electric discharge drilling of titanium alloy sheet. *Mater. Today Proc.*, 21, 1680–1684, 2019. https://doi.org/10.1016/j.matpr.2019.12.010.
14. Jain, A. and Pandey, A.K., Multiple quality optimizations in electrical discharge drilling of mild steel sheet. *Mater. Today Proc.*, 8, 7252–7261, 2019. https://doi.org/10.1016/j.matpr.2017.07.054.
15. Jain, A., Kumar, C.S., Shrivastava, Y., Fabrication and machining of fiber matrix composite through electric discharge machining: A short review. *Mater. Today Proc.*, 51, 1233–1237, 2022.
16. ThuraiRaaj, V.B., Gorantla, S.R., Karunanidy, D., Dumka, A., Singh, R., Rashid, M., Alshamrani, S.S., Dual battery storage technique for remote, location-based solar PV system and standalone applications. *Energies*, *15*, 8, 2748, 2022.
17. Gehlot, A., Malik, P.K., Singh, R., Akram, S.V., Alsuwian, T., Dairy 4.0: Intelligent communication ecosystem for the cattle animal welfare with blockchain and IoT enabled technologies. *Appl. Sci.*, *12*, 14, 7316, 2022.

18. Bisht, D., Singh, R., Gehlot, A., Akram, S.V., Singh, A., Montero, E.C., Twala, B., Imperative role of integrating digitalization in the firms finance: A technological perspective. *Electronics*, *11*, 19, 3252, 2022.
19. Bagwari, S., Gehlot, A., Singh, R., Priyadarshi, N., Khan, B., Low-cost sensor-based and LoRaWAN opportunities for landslide monitoring systems on IoT platform: A review. *IEEE Access*, *10*, 7107–7127, 2021.
20. Ramalingam, R., Muniyan, R., Dumka, A., Singh, D.P., Mohamed, H.G., Singh, R., Noya, I.D., Routing protocol for MANET based on QoS-aware service composition with dynamic secured broker selection. *Electronics*, *11*, 17, 2637, 2022.
21. Thakur, A.K., Singh, R., Gehlot, A., Kaviti, A.K., Aseer, R., Suraparaju, S.K., Sikarwar, V.S., Advancements in solar technologies for sustainable development of agricultural sector in India: A comprehensive review on challenges and opportunities. *Environ. Sci. Pollut. Res.*, *29*, 29, 43607–43634, 2022.
22. Rana, A., Rawat, A.S., Afifi, A., Singh, R., Rashid, M., Gehlot, A., Alshamrani, S.S., A long-range internet of things-based advanced vehicle pollution monitoring system with node authentication and blockchain. *Appl. Sci.*, *12*, 15, 7547, 2022.

7

Adoption of Cloud Computing in the Healthcare Field Using the SEM Approach

R. Chithambaramani[1], C. Balakumar[2]*, Dilip Kumar Sharma[3], Keyur Patel[4], Bhavana Jamalpur[5] and M. R. Arun[6]

[1]*Department of Computer Science and Engineering, Vel Tech Rangarajan Dr. Sagunthala R&D Institute of Science and Technology, Avadi, Chennai, Tamil Nadu, India*

[2]*Department of Computer Science, Karpagam Academy of Higher Education, Coimbatore, India*

[3]*Department of Mathematics, Jaypee University of Engineering and Technology, Guna (M.P.), India*

[4]*Unitedworld School of Computational Intelligence, Karnavati University, Gandhinagar, Gujarat, India*

[5]*School of Computer Science & Artificial Intelligence, SR University, Warangal, Telangana, India*

[6]*Department of ECE, Vel Tech Rangarajan Dr. Sagunthala R&D Institute of Science and Technology Chennai, Tamil Nadu, India*

Abstract

Cloud computing offers a fresh method for consistently delivering IT services. Studies suggest that cloud computing can improve service quality in several organizations, including medical. As with any technical development, cloud computing should be carefully examined before being extensively adopted. The structural equation modeling (SEM) method is used in this research to investigate the adoption of cloud computing in the medical field. The suggested approach considers four aspects that affect how cloud computing is adopted in the medical industry: perceived benefits, adoption factors, technology factors, and attitudes and behaviors. The SEM model's findings indicate that views and behavior have little bearing on whether cloud computing is adopted in the medical industry. These results imply that effective applications of cloud computing in the medical field require a thorough knowledge of the variables impacting adoption. When making decisions

**Corresponding author*: balakumar.cbek@gmail.com

Kapil Joshi and Somil Kumar Gupta (eds.) Human Cancer Diagnosis and Detection Using Exascale Computing, (101–114) © 2024 Scrivener Publishing LLC

about whether to use cloud computing technology, the medical field and individuals can benefit greatly from the findings of this research.

Keywords: Cloud computing, healthcare, analysis, SEM

7.1 Introduction

Financial strains, managing numerous stakeholders for service delivery, and aging populations are just a few of the difficulties the healthcare sector is currently confronting [1]. Increased ICT (information and communications technology) use can help the healthcare industry tackle these difficulties [2]. Applications for health ICT are expanding as a result of ICT advancements and the need to improve healthcare delivery. ICT has been applied to healthcare to improve patient data access and decision-making. ICT also can lower costs and enhance service quality in the healthcare industry [3].

Cloud computing encourages IT services that are always reachable and from any location. It is an innovative way rather than a distinct approach of delivering computing resources [4]. The cloud computing paradigm provides the following three key advantages over traditional computing: Sophisticated processing resources are available on need, services are offered without demanding consumers to make any prior obligations, and they are also accessible for temporary use. Numerous sectors have been affected by the cloud model, and it is predicted that by 2020, almost 80% of currently operating businesses will be using cloud computing. Additionally, businesses that lack the infrastructure and resources to build up on-premises applications can implement cloud computing [5].

The healthcare sector is confronted with difficult problems such as how to minimize the expenses connected to delivering healthcare services, which can be addressed by implementing novel systems to enhance electronic medical records and obtain data privately and immediately with other enterprises, employees, government agencies, and medical professionals. Rural medical facilities, like hospitals and dispensaries, face the greatest challenges when it comes to managing medical information because it is a difficult job, and the ability to deliver high-quality healthcare depends on an effective and comprehensive information processing system.

As a computing system that is constantly changing and offers common resources like business processes, applications, and infrastructure, cloud computing research and development in the healthcare industry could possibly have a significant effect [12]. Virtualization is the fundamental technique that underpins resource sharing in the cloud. Cloud computing may be used in other fields, like e-governance systems, due to its highly scalable capability and practically limitless computing capacity.

Using the diversity of IT infrastructure and applications in medical organizations necessitates ongoing upgrades due to the quickly increasing market for healthcare services. Additionally, the price of computerized methods for the medical industry is prohibitively expensive given that the main task is medical-related and IT only serves as a tool for crucial decision-making at the point of care. Most healthcare providers today, particularly those in rural areas, lack any type of system or have chosen to construct one on their own. Some even choose to buy ready-made remedies. Additionally, several small- to medium-sized healthcare organizations continue to run their daily activities using paper-based forms because they view IT investment as an expensive venture [10]. Obtaining patient data is challenging according to how healthcare providers conduct their business, particularly with respect to patients' medical information. An efficient technique of providing services and value to medical professionals and associated business partners is introduced by cloud computing.

Since healthcare processes are distinctive, varied, and complicated and HIPAA compliance is crucial to safeguarding patient privacy, it is still difficult to predict how cloud computing will affect this industry. Several healthcare providers are considering various ways to further cut costs, so the type of IT solutions implemented will play a significant role in achieving improved therapeutic service quality. It will undoubtedly be of great significance to investigate how cloud computing responds to and helps with the problems encountered by healthcare providers.

7.1.1 Research Gap

There is a dearth of knowledge on how technologies can be used to enhance the security, dependability, and cost-effectiveness of healthcare data. Additionally, research is required to determine how cloud computing may affect the security and safety of patient data and how it may enhance the general effectiveness of healthcare services. Ultimately, more research is required to determine how corporate culture and user acceptance impact the success of cloud adoption in the medical industry.

7.1.2 Research Aim

- To develop a structural equation modeling (SEM) to assess the adoption of cloud computing in the medical field

- To provide healthcare organizations and practitioners with insights on how to effectively implement cloud computing systems
- To investigate the impact of the hypothesis on the willingness to adopt cloud computing in the medical field

7.2 Literature Review

Several healthcare organizations around the world, particularly in established nations, have embraced cloud computing to improve the quality of their services. The major purpose of this investigation was to recognize the concepts from the previous literature review that, from the standpoint of a developing country, impact the adoption of cloud computing. The conceptual framework's primary foundations are technological, organizational, environmental, and ethical considerations [20]. A structured questionnaire was used to gather the answers from the staff or employees who worked in this industry. The study was carried out with the aid of AMOS 22.0 and SPSS 20.0. The proposed hypothesis was put to the proof using a structural equation modeling strategy. The results showed that each of the presumptive variables—technology, organization, surroundings, and ethics—influences the response variable, which is cloud computing adoption in the medical field, improving productivity. The study varies from prior studies in that it considered legal issues, adding to our understanding of cloud computing [21].

The expenditures and expenses of structures, interactions, healthcare-related equipment, and software inside the medical system depict a rather substantial growth. Then, it is anticipated that this growth will continue to appear. Because of the separated independent networks and components that are not attached, information and cross-system communication became difficult. The aggregate model fit estimates over a sample group of 320 were evaluated with SEM using AMOS 20.0 as the modeling instrument. The descriptive data and dimension reliability were analyzed using SPSS 20.0. The research's findings indicate that the system effect and utilization dimensions influence the healthcare providers' total quality of service [19]. Additionally, the results point to the importance of systems integration and security for IT tools in healthcare organizations [11]. This research has effectively created a foundation for further research into the necessity of improving the Malaysian medical system and introducing a cloud computing system to replace the country's medical data transmission [9].

The goal of this investigation was to investigate the elements that affect patients' usage of IoT for Medical 4.0. By supporting six hypotheses, a study structure relying on the Unified Theory of Acceptance and Use of Technology (UTAUT) has been created. To ascertain the goal of using IoT devices in the clinical setting, a cohort of 290 individuals was used. In order to accomplish the goals of the research, a conceptual paradigm was created using 29 manifests. The use of PLS-SEM in IoT healthcare study is evaluated in this work in order to offer useful recommendations and predict future advancements of these systems [7, 8]. SEM in e-health management is still in its earlier phases, so understanding its applications is important for sustaining potential future applications [18]. The present research's findings may therefore be significant, with consequences for both theoretical study and everyday life. A sophisticated understanding of research could be advantageous to many stakeholders. This study could aid in the improvement of healthcare services for treating people who are of a new generation [6].

It is crucial to recognize that medical professionals will need to keep investing in IT-based systems to enhance general processes and interactions among systems as the global healthcare industry continues to expand. In order to specify the adoption of cloud computing, the research centers on the connections among medical professionals, IT resources, and health insurance providers. The findings of this research demonstrate that IT resources have a major effect on medical professionals and health insurance companies. With the use of the cloud, clinical services and productivity can be improved [22]. In an attempt to determine the general model fit, SEM is used to show the research results, which also include dependability evaluation, descriptive statistics, and factor loading in medical services. Model fit assessment for SEM was conducted using AMOS 20.0, and descriptive statistics, hypotheses, and theories were examined using SPSS 20.0.

The purpose of this research was to investigate the factors that affect the adoption of cloud computing in healthcare institutions. To expand the study's approach, the investigation used the expanded technology acceptance model (TAM) and motivation model (MM). The research suggested that expanded aspects of TAM include perception, cost savings, perceived privacy and security, and compatibility. The research also suggested the effects of resistance to change on two-way interactions, as well as the effects of MM factors on two-way and three-way interactions. SEM was used to experimentally evaluate the study's approach using 512 responses to a survey questionnaire. All four expanded variables were found to be substantial predictors of TAM factors, according to the results. Moreover, the correlation between behavioral intention and adoption of cloud computing is moderated by resistance to change, which is highly negative, and MM variables, which are considerably positive. Substantial three-way interaction effects are also produced by the MM variables. The research results added more knowledge about the adoption of cloud computing to the literature and practice.

7.3 Research Methodology

The research created the proposed model, as depicted in Figure 7.1, for analyzing the elements that affect a person's intention to embrace cloud computing in the healthcare industry.

Adoption factors: The primary determinants of cloud computing adoption in the medical industry will be the emphasis of this section [13]. This may involve issues like reduced costs, data access, effective procedures, and enhanced patient treatment.
Technology factors: This section will be primarily concerned with the technological elements of cloud computing and how they relate to the medical industry [14]. This might cover subjects like protection, scalability, and vendor choice.
Perceived benefits: The advantages of cloud computing as viewed by the healthcare industry will be the main topic of this element [15]. This might cover issues like better data access, enhanced teamwork, and enhanced patient treatment.

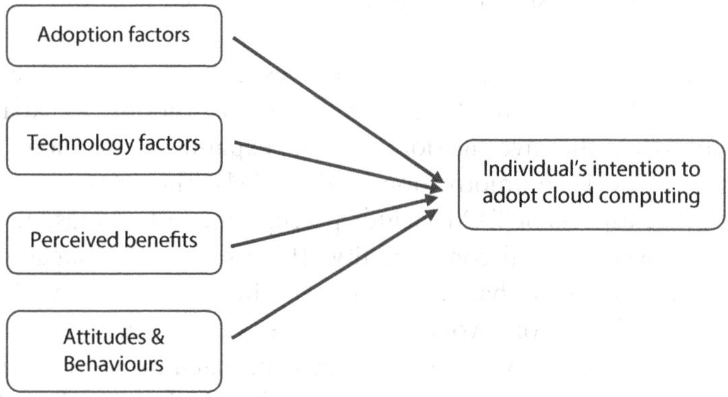

Figure 7.1 Proposed framework.

Attitudes and behaviors: The emphasis of this section will be on the healthcare providers' attitudes and behaviors toward cloud computing [16]. This might cover subjects like acceptance, use, and confidence.

To determine the major variables influencing the adoption of cloud computing in the medical field, the SEM method will analyze the interactions between these four elements. This approach will also make it possible to identify any possible adoption obstacles and gain insight into how to overcome them.

7.3.1 Research Hypothesis

- Individuals' adoption factors impact their intention in the healthcare cloud computing adoption.
- Individuals' technology factors impact their intention in the healthcare cloud computing adoption.
- Individuals' perceived benefits impact their intention in the healthcare cloud computing adoption.
- Individuals' attitudes and behavior impact their intention in the healthcare cloud computing adoption.

7.3.2 Data Analysis

There were 200 participants in this quantitative research who took the survey. Medical professionals, nurses, IT professionals, lab workers, and office personnel made up the target demographic of participants. Numerous hospitals received 150 surveys in total. The obtained data were then evaluated using PLS involving all the necessary and relevant validity measures. Likert-scale questions were created with 1 portraying "Strongly disagree" and 5 portraying "Strongly agree" to assess these aspects.

To verify the hypotheses, a survey questionnaire was used in this study. The study that was suggested used convenience sampling [17]. This method entails picking readily accessible respondents, like those who are employed in the healthcare industry and are ready to be interviewed about their use of cloud computing. To determine the trustworthiness of the constructs, Cronbach's alpha-based testing was done.

7.4 Results and Discussion

Table 7.1 provides demographic information on a sample of 200 people: 65% of the sample was male, while 35% was female; 25% of the sample was

Table 7.1 Demographic factors of the participants.

Demographic factors		Frequency	%
Gender	Male	130	65
	Female	70	35
Age	25 or lower	50	25
	26–40	70	35
	41 or older	80	40
Occupation	Doctors	45	22.5
	Nurses	30	15
	IT engineers	50	25
	Lab technicians	35	17.5
	Administrative staffs	40	20

25 years old or lower, 35% was 26 to 40 years old, and 40% was 41 years old or older; 22.5% of the sample was doctors, 15% nurses, 25% IT engineers, 17.5% lab technicians, and 20% administrative staff.

A two-step evaluation was used to analyze the constructs' measurement model. The categories' reliability and validity were evaluated using Cronbach's alpha, composite reliability (CR), and average variance extracted (AVE). These metrics were used to assess the constructs' sufficiency in terms of dependability and validity.

According to Table 7.2, Cronbach's alpha for the constructs varied from 0.71 to 0.82, exceeding the suggested score and the acceptable value of 0.7. Each construct had CR values above the cutoff of 0.60, and the average value across all constructs was higher than the recommended level of 0.5.

The AVE square root was used to determine the convergent validity. The findings supported the convergent validity of the constructs by demonstrating that the square root of AVE is greater than the correlations among this construct and the other constructs. Table 7.3 displays the convergent validity for the measurement elements. The metrics for constructing reliability and validity have been confirmed and reached the suggested ranges following the evaluation findings mentioned above.

The second stage should involve evaluating the structural model after the measurement model's validity and reliability have been established.

Table 7.2 Reliability and validity test.

	Cronbach's alpha	Composite reliability	Average variance extracted (AVE)
Adoption factors	0.75	0.66	0.54
Technology factors	0.71	0.72	0.50
Perceived benefits	0.82	0.65	0.71
Attitudes and behaviors	0.76	0.78	0.63

Table 7.3 Discriminant validity for measurement items.

	Adoption factors	Technology factors	Perceived benefits	Attitude and behaviors
Adoption factors	0.745			
Technology factors	0.691	0.684		
Perceived benefits	0.817	0.843	0.876	
Attitude and behaviors	0.791	0.789	0.765	0.774

Table 7.4 displays the findings from the analysis of the structural model for the theories. Out of the four hypotheses that were put forth by this study, three were accepted, and one (H4) was discarded because it had no discernible impact.

Table 7.4 The structural model.

Hypothesis	*T* statistics	*P*-values	Results
H1	1.76	0.04	Supported
H2	0.91	0.13	Supported
H3	1.67	0.05	Supported
H4	1.89	0.06	Unsupported

7.5 Implications

To supplement the outcomes of the study approach, a cloud-based prototype was evolved using ASP.NET and Microsoft Visual Studio 2013 and placed on the Windows Azure service of Microsoft. Each medical practitioner can now retrieve data in the cloud while still making it accessible to other providers thanks to the infrastructure that has been created. The data center hosting the cloud as a service is where all patient health information is kept up to date. Patients frequently consult primary care doctors and specialists, as well as other healthcare professionals. Additionally, they use a variety of insurance from multiple health insurance companies. As a result, patient health information is disseminated and kept in numerous locations. Insufficient visibility and information regarding the locations of various components of a patient's medical records is an issue when attempting to retrieve the patient's entire report. The incompatibility of data formats and the paucity of available information are the other issues. Utilizing cloud services would help healthcare organizations make much more effective use of their hardware and software resources while also boosting profitability through optimal resource utilization. Combining a small number of IT systems with the cloud will enable medical professionals to substantially minimize costs and increase productivity since computing facilities are only allotted when they are deployed and used. Therefore, the healthcare sector will use cloud computing and federated applications to build the distribution of medical data and for medical case analysis. Due to the abundance of data from various sources, the investigators think that using cloud services is a good fit for apps related to healthcare. Physicians and healthcare administrators will be able to share information much more effectively thanks to cloud computing's high scalability and availability. In addition, the suggested cloud computing framework will help save time and resources when implementing health-related IT applications inside the medical ecosystem.

7.6 Conclusion

Customers anticipate a smooth, digital healthcare experience similar to what they receive from retailers like Amazon. They might be ignorant of the processes taking place in the background of a health system to improve their experience. However, consumers will soon require services like remote monitoring of IoT medical devices, predictive care, accurate staffing, reduced medication errors, simple and precise access to their medical records, and more, which are only available if hospitals endorse those cloud-based applications. There is a tremendous quantity of potential for cloud computing in the medical sector as cloud technology develops tremendously. Nowadays, access to high-quality healthcare is considered a basic human right. Additionally, this is a pricey and extremely complex topic. Even the most prosperous nations in the world struggle to meet the enormous amount of healthcare requirements. However, directing cloud processing power into the healthcare system can undoubtedly result in real advancements that benefit everyone's access to high-quality, affordable healthcare rather than just a small group of privileged individuals. The world is changing quickly, and healthcare organizations that upgrade their processes and digitally transform their companies will contribute to the pack and outperform their rivals. As advice for future research and for those who make healthcare decisions, this study's implications for research and practice were given. The question of whether the benefits of using cloud computing outweigh its drawbacks in the medical sector must be answered. This study offers sufficient evidence to conclude that cloud computing can represent important possibilities for the medical sector. Even though the healthcare sector is governed by strict regulations, worries about the protection and anonymity of patient data and the lack of control over data administration must be taken into account. Because of this, numerous companies are trying to improve and alter their patient data security protocols with the aim to encourage confidentiality. Moreover, researchers and practitioners see a lot of promise in using cloud computing in the medical industry. Applications on the cloud can make diverse info accessible for use in decision-making.

7.7 Future Research Directions

The implementation of cloud computing in the medical industry is a developing research field. EHRs and managing medical data are at the core of the present cloud apps. Cloud computing, subsequently, can provide value-added healthcare services in more areas of decision-making, including diagnosis and control, medication, education, and referrals and suggestions. Consequently, we can claim that the healthcare industry has not fully tapped into the effectiveness of cloud computing. The use of cloud services is presently more data-driven than network-related. Moreover, the use of cloud computing for decision support in the medical industry is a domain that is not researched and deserves consideration for future study. Cloud applications can facilitate admittance to multifaceted data for decision-making. These value-added healthcare services can destabilize the medical field, but they can be seen as assistance for the decision-making of medical professionals, such as physicians and nurses. Future investigators might want to examine these healthcare-related value-added cloud services, especially in the field of medical decision-making.

The present study on cloud computing in the medical sector places a very narrow emphasis on process improvement and cost savings, which represents a very constrained approach of the model for providing IT services. Studies on the cloud's primary possibilities in the medical sector are done through the lenses of quality, productivity, and technical benefits, like structure as a service. Moreover, the modern definitions of "service" emphasize creative strategies to offer consumers with value. The use of cloud applications today for network administration is relatively limited. As a consequence, issues with service availability and reliability impact cloud apps.

References

1. Kaur, P.D. and Chana, I., Cloud based intelligent system for delivering healthcare as a service. *Comput. Methods Programs Biomed.*, *113*, 1, 346–359, 2014.
2. Fichman, R., Kohli, R., Krishnan, R., Kane, G., The role of information systems in healthcare: Current research and future trends, lead article by the senior editors in. *Inf. Syst. Res.*, *22*, 3, 419–428, 2011.
3. Venkatesh, V., Rai, A., Sykes, T.A., Aljafari, R., Combating infant mortality in rural india: Evidence from a field study of eHealth kiosk implementations. *MIS Q.*, *40*, 2, 353–380, 2016.
4. Ali, O., Soar, J., Shrestha, A., Perceived potential for value creation from cloud computing: A study of the Australian regional government sector. *Behav. Inf. Technol.*, *37*, 12, 1157–1176, 2018.
5. Ahuja, S.P., Mani, S., Zambrano, J., A survey of the state of cloud computing in healthcare. *Network Commun. Technol.*, *1*, 2, 12, 2012.
6. Baral, M.M. and Verma, A., Cloud computing adoption for healthcare: An empirical study using SEM approach. *FBR*, *10*, 3, 255–275, 2021.
7. Ratnam, K.A., Dominic, P.D.D., Ramayah, T., A structural equation modeling approach for the adoption of cloud computing to enhance the Malaysian healthcare sector. *J. Med. Syst.*, *38*, 1–14, 2014.
8. Dadhich, M., Poddar, S., Hiran, K.K., Antecedents and consequences of patients' adoption of the IoT 4.0 for e-health management system: A novel PLS-SEM approach. *Smart Health*, *25*, 100300, 2022.

9. Ratnam, K.A. and Dominic, P.D.D., The factors associating the adoption of cloud computing: An enhancement of the healthcare ecosystem in Malaysia. *Int. J. Bus. Inf. Syst.*, *16*, 4, 462–479, 2014.
10. Ratnam, K.A. and Dominic, P.D.D., Adoption of cloud computing to enhance the healthcare services in Malaysia, in: *2014 International Conference on Computer and Information Sciences (ICCOINS)*, IEEE, pp. 1–6, 2014, June.
11. Shahbaz, M. and Zahid, R., Probing the factors influencing cloud computing adoption in healthcare organizations: A three-way interaction model. *Technol. Soc.*, *71*, 102139, 2022.
12. Padhy, R.P., Patra, M.R., Satapathy, S.C., Design and implementation of a cloud based rural healthcare information system model. *Univers J. Appl. Comput. Sci. Technol.*, *2*, 1, 149–157, 2012.
13. Panwar, V., Sharma, D.K., Kumar, K.V.P., Jain, A., Thakar, C., Experimental investigations and optimization of surface roughness in turning of EN 36 alloy steel using response surface methodology and genetic algorithm. *Mater. Today:. Proc.*, 46, 6474–81, Jan 1 2021. https://Doi.Org/10.1016/J.Matpr.2021.03.642.
14. Jain, A. and Pandey, A.K., Modeling and optimizing of different quality characteristics in electrical discharge drilling of titanium alloy (Grade-5) sheet. *Mater. Today Proc.*, 18, 182–191, 2019. https://doi.org/10.1016/j.matpr.2019.06.292.
15. Jain, A., Yadav, A.K., Shrivastava, Y., Modelling and optimization of different quality characteristics in electric discharge drilling of titanium alloy sheet. *Mater. Today Proc.*, 21, 1680–1684, 2019. https://doi.org/10.1016/j.matpr.2019.12.010.
16. Jain, A. and Pandey, A.K., Multiple quality optimizations in electrical discharge drilling of mild steel sheet. *Mater. Today Proc.*, 8, 7252–7261, 2019. https://doi.org/10.1016/j.matpr.2017.07.054.
17. Jain, A., Kumar, C.S., Shrivastava, Y., Fabrication and machining of fiber matrix composite through electric discharge machining: A short review. *Mater. Today Proc.*, 51, 1233-7, 2022 Jan 1. https://doi.org/10.1016/j.matpr.2021.07.288.
18. Singh, R., Gehlot, A., Rashid, M., Saxena, R., Akram, S.V., Alshamrani, S.S., Alghamdi, A.S., Cloud server and Internet of Things assisted system for stress monitoring. *Electronics*, *10*, 24, 3133, 2021.
19. Sharma, M., Rastogi, R., Arya, N., Akram, S.V., Singh, R., Gehlot, A., Joshi, K., LoED: LoRa and edge computing based system architecture for sustainable forest monitoring. *Int. J. Eng. Trends Technol.*, *70*, 5, 88–93, 2022.
20. Ahamad, S., Roshan, A., Lourens, M., Shekher, V., Joshi, K., Alanya-Beltran, J., The critical role played by big data management in effectively addressing the security and overall privacy concerns through correlation analysis, in:

2022 2nd International Conference on Advance Computing and Innovative Technologies in Engineering (ICACITE), IEEE, pp. 130–134, 2022, April.

21. Sastry, R. V. L. S. N., Kapila, D., Jaiswal, S., Sargunam, S., Akram, S.V., Kumar, K.S., Critically analysing the concept of deep learning and how it impacts organizational performance, in: *2022 2nd International Conference on Advance Computing and Innovative Technologies in Engineering (ICACITE)*, IEEE, pp. 321–324, 2022, April.
22. Joshi, K., Kumar, M., Tripathi, A., Kumar, A., Sehgal, J., Barthwal, A., Latest trends in multi-modality medical image fusion: A generic review, in: *Rising Threats in Expert Applications and Solutions: Proceedings of FICR-TEAS 2022*, pp. 663–671, 2022.

8

Chest X-Ray Analysis for COVID-19 Diagnosis Using an Exascale Computation and Machine Learning Framework

M. Dhinakaran[1]*, S. Deivasigamani[2], Saikat Kar[3], Nishakar Kankalla[4], V. Malathy[5] and Saurabh Sharma[6]

[1]*Electronics and Communication Engineering, Government College of Engineering, Salem, Tamil Nadu, India*
[2]*Faculty of Engineering, Technology & Built Environment, UCSI University, Kuala Lumpur, Malaysia*
[3]*MBBS, Department of Neuroscience, University of Edinburgh, Edinburgh, United Kingdom*
[4]*Department of ECE, St. Martin's Engineering College Secunderabad, Telangana, India*
[5]*Department of ECE, School of Engineering, SR University, Warangal, Telangana, India*
[6]*Amity University, Gwalior, India*

Abstract

The favored detection technique for coronavirus is RT-PCR, which is costly and tedious and requires medical services experts to lead the tests. Research on coronavirus proposes novel attributes in chest radiography pictures, offering chest X-beams (CXRs) that could analyze the coronavirus. It is possible to use AI in clinical imaging, such as CXR images, and it has strong roots in picture grouping assignments. The Coronavirus Network group created the dataset known as COVIDx by combining many open-source data sources that contained CXR pictures. COVID-Net is a brain network that was prepared on the Photos Net data prior to being prepared here on the COVIDx dataset utilizing profound learning procedures, a part of computerized reasoning that does not utilize state-of-the-art world-class execute handling (HPC) strategies. The project seeks to understand whether medical care providers, professionals, and students can use the open-source coronavirus convolutional neural network. It examines the exactness and

**Corresponding author*: dhina_au@yahoo.com

Kapil Joshi and Somil Kumar Gupta (eds.) Human Cancer Diagnosis and Detection Using Exascale Computing, (115–134) © 2024 Scrivener Publishing LLC

information examination results exhibited in the first Coronavirus Net distribution and features speed-ups while utilizing HPC approaches for surmising.

***Keywords*:** Chest X-ray, COVID-19, diagnosis, exascale computation, machine learning, artificial intelligence, deep learning, medical imaging

8.1 Introduction

The severe acute respiratory syndrome coronavirus 2 (SARS-CoV-2) is the culprit behind the severe and intense respiratory ailment known as coronavirus disease 2019 (COVID-19). The disease caused a pandemic in 2019 that had unheard-of impacts on public health. A precise and efficient technique is reverse transcription quantitative real-time polymerase chain reaction (qRT-PCR), is the finest quality level evaluation for determining the presence of the infection; nonetheless, antigen tests are also frequently used, despite being less effective. RT-PCR testing is laborious because it may require the assistance of trained professionals and is carried out in a lab setting. While faster, antigen testing loses sensitivity if not carried out by qualified medical professionals. AI includes causing PCs to perform undertakings without having a software engineer to physically make the required calculations to play out these errands. There are numerous uses of AI, one of which is information mining. Information mining alludes to laying out examples and connections between various elements in the information [1]. Similar components are used in an AI solution for each instance in a dataset. The learning is said to be directed if each event in the set has a mark associated with it; otherwise, it is referred to as unaided. When the scores must be randomly distributed and discrete, managed learning presents an order problem. Early studies on the coronavirus proposed that, when compared with other conditions, such as viral pneumonia, patients with the coronavirus have remarkable characteristics in their chest radiographs.

COVID-Net is an open-source convolutional brain network that can look at chest X-ray (CXR) pictures to examine COVID. A dataset of CXR (chest X-ray) images related to coronavirus was used to create and validate the COVID-Net. The investigation in this proposition intends to determine whether COVID-Net is usable all things being equal by clinical providers and trained professionals. Replication, validation, and expansion of the collected chest X-ray pictures are the main goals [2]. Best-in-class supercomputing designing is also used to speed it up. Over the long haul, the pre-arranged models can be ported to crisis centers clearly, reducing the need to move data outside the establishments and subsequently diminishing the potential for data thievery or contamination. Significant learning can normally deliver features considering important depictions of the data. To have the option to assess its enormous number of features, it hence requires countless pictures [3]. The ability of HPC (High-Performance Computing) computers to manage longer calculation durations than conventional machines explains its significance.

8.2 Literature Review

This exploration sums up the outcomes the coronavirus pandemic has had all over the planet, not just concerning the well-being of the populace but also monetary and social impacts which might keep going for quite a while. Standard coronavirus screening strategies have their upsides and downsides, so having an elective strategy in view of clinical imaging can be valuable by and large, for example, where a prompt diagnosis is required, with the overall goal of assisting in the global pandemic recovery. Since computers can operate dependably around-the-clock and occasionally are prepared to spot patterns where people cannot, AI can be advantageous in the context of clinical imaging for grouping [4]. AI empowers PCs to naturally lay out examples and connections between highlights in information. Computational models comprising various handling layers are alluded to as profound learning, and convolution brain networks are an illustration of this kind of model which is extraordinarily tuned for picture handling. There was a serious necessity for elective trademark systems, especially in the periods of the pandemic when antigen-based speedy tests were not yet open. The standard strategy using RT-PCR required a basic money-related cost, a pre-arranged labor force, and a restricted assessment office and showed, particularly close to the beginning of the pandemic, exceptionally heterogeneous accuracy [5]. Pneumonic commitment explicitly represented a gamble to patients with COVID; subsequently, it checked out to inspect standard CXR pictures, which are speedy and broadly accessible demonstrative hardware for changes well defined for COVID. Early scatterings have some time later proactively depicted the presence of unequivocal anomalies in thoracic imaging going before a lab test making a positive result. Zeroing in on quickly open and judicious interesting systems is particularly basic as evaluation predicts that such massive degree contamination occasions will occur at a rising rate.

In any case, given the ongoing headways in elite execution registering innovation and the accessibility of business distributed computing assets to the overall population, as well as enormous expansions in web-based information capacity and sharing abilities, there is a growing need for machine learning (ML) and deep learning (DL) programs that use these tools to solve common problems [6]. These techniques and resources are also being used to extract data from large data warehouses that would otherwise take many specialists to work for more than a few hundred hours. The appearance of two significant learning, AlphaFold structure DeepMind and RoseTTAFold of Baek *et al.*, which meet or even beat existing frameworks for protein structure suspicion, has actually made the blend of HPC, massive information, and ML stand separated as truly enormous in standard trained professionals.

Subsequently, only a couple of investigation bunches have thought up ML and DL systems for diagnosing coronavirus from enlisted tomography and X-bar photos of the chest or expecting the fatalities of coronavirus organization clients from clinical data, with all of the results highlighting how convincing these designs may be for quick triaging. In an associated field of direction, Rajaraman *et al.* joined different organized ML computations to work on the finding of pneumonia from CXR pictures with a preferred advancement rate over standard picture certification models. A few researchers have arranged progressed DL networks on immense measures of information from different spaces utilizing state-of-the-art HPC assets, especially the Jülich Wiz for European Logical Sciences, quite possibly of Europe's quickest supercomputer [2], consequently featuring the need to utilize measured supercomputing engineering to propel the field of man-made brainpower (artificial intelligence). Moreover, high-level mechanized hyperparameter tuning strategies, for example, Keras Tuner, have been created, which work on the boundary search process expected to adjust the preparation of brain organizations, resulting in the strongest model without a lot of help from ML experts [7].

The use of accessible HPC assets in the clinical field, consequently adding to the examination of clinical information, and an ideal and exact conclusion can diminish how much pressure clinical staff are presented with during their work. In essence, the clinical area offers a ripe ground for creating innovations that can be productively layered, refreshed, and sent where expected to assist with diminishing the impacts of impending maladies and pandemics [8].

The work depicted in this chapter tends to the completion of attempts made to make a setting in which clinical data may be successfully taken care of, refined, destroyed, and used to make ML and DL models. The stage utilizes essentially unambiguous stuff and programming accessible at the Jülich Supercomputing Centre to make and set up these models most helpfully [9]. These integrate above all else the Significant and JUWELS supercomputing gatherings and the storing made available through the associated endeavors. The models are likewise changed in accordance with producing the ideal outcomes utilizing progressed hyperparameter tuning methodology.

The details of (a) developing the Coronavirus Net using the most recent data, (b) adjusting the model's high-degree hyperparameters to focus on the feature combinations that produce the strongest models, and (c) modifying the model to account for the improvement in per-class accuracy attained for all these cutoff combinations are covered in the following sections [10]. Resource scaling is also used to keep track of the speed that can be achieved during the scheduled phase. To achieve the best outcomes, the models are tuned using sophisticated hyperparameter tuning techniques. It is vital that further research be done on the effects of coronavirus assessment models because so few groups have used hyper feature advancement [11]. By utilizing HPC, concepts and enhancements proposed in published works seek to enhance model training, boost transparency, and optimize controller settings [12]. Nevertheless, association with any of these works can only be embraced with significant effort.

8.3 Research Methodology

In order to develop the coronavirus gross model using the combination dataset, a variety of boundaries were tested, and the results are shown in Figure 8.1. Nonetheless, as the quantity of these limits increases, so does

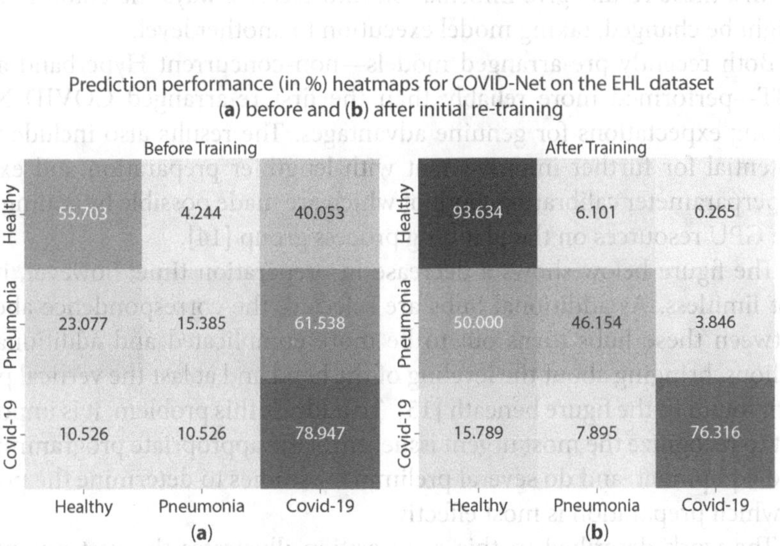

Figure 8.1 Prediction performance.

the intricacy of the improvement issue. As a general rule, a couple of additional limits, for example, the grouping size, the tram split, its measure of mature enough ranges, and the cooling or thawing out of significant levels from the Coronavirus Net, could have been actually tuned to manage the results. The results show how the model might be improved and highlight the requirement for all the more remarkable tuning methodologies.

8.4 Analysis and Discussion

Working on the prophetic initiation of the COVID organization on extra information was made conceivable with the four-direct utilization of a hyperparameter improving on the structure. The schedulers utilized for the improvement exploited the accessible MSA and effectively circulated the errand over the assets. In doing that capacity, the framework had the choice to gain more headway and test more limit mixes simultaneously to encompass the limits which the program would all the more effectively plan with [13]. This cycle has a few defects, as ought to be clear from the Hyperband results, where its best-performing limit blend created a model that did not satisfy hopes, or by lessening the respiratory lot diseases class loads, where the best-performing borders from the FIFO scheduler conveyed a model that was unfathomably extraordinary at finding coronavirus patients but absolutely not prepared for predicting pneumonia. In spite of this, these results give information into creative ways the cutoff points might be changed, taking model execution to another level.

Both recently pre-arranged models—non-concurrent Hyperband and PBT—performed more reliably than the first re-arranged COVID-Net, raising expectations for genuine advantages. The results also include the potential for further improvement with lengthier preparation and extra hyperparameter calibration, both of which are made possible by scaling up the GPU resources on the planning process group [14].

The figure below shows a decrease in preparation time; however, it is not limitless. As additional hubs are selected, the correspondence above between these hubs turns out to be more complicated and additionally tedious, bringing about the leveling of the bend and at last the vertical pattern found in the figure beneath [15]. To address this problem, it is important to recognize the most urgent issue, enrol the appropriate programming and equipment, and do several preliminary studies to determine the point at which preparation is most effective.

The work described in this composition illustrates the vast potential of re-preparing the Coronavirus Net as a use case to authorize a detailed

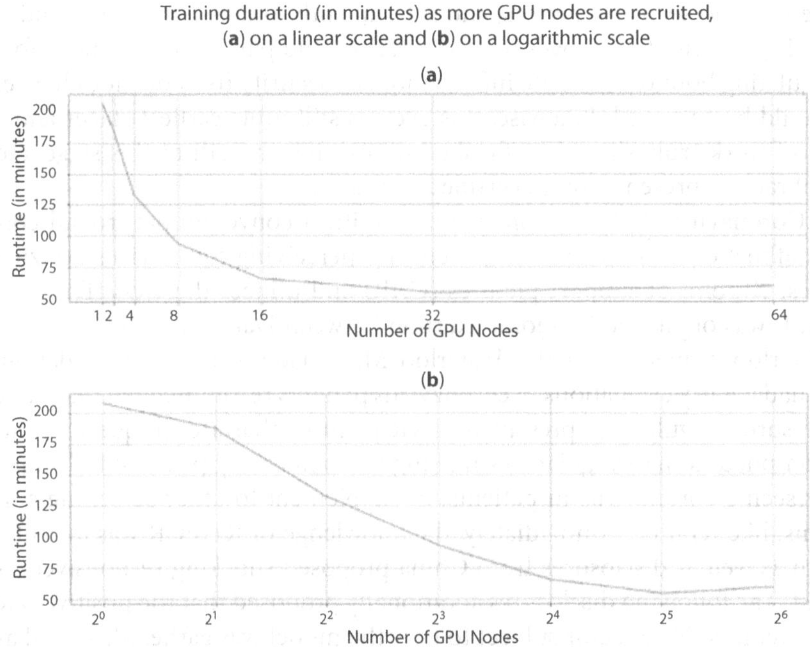

Figure 8.2 Training duration. (Source: [11]).

patient finding supporting stage based on such an HPC foundation and utilizing unique and skilled ML calculations. This is not to imply that this work would not be imaginable without the particular HPC framework utilized. Truth be told, the stage utilizes open-source programming, making it effectively versatile in industrially accessible distributed computing (CC) arrangements [16]. Likewise, the primary point is to foster the base foundation that exploits the HPC assets to improve on the advancement of programming that is sufficiently lightweight to be handily conveyed in most standard PCs that anyone could hope to find in emergency clinics, making them an imperative device to help clinical staff.

Considering that the clinical field is routinely confronting time-delicate issues, this paper features the requirement for stages that improve on admittance to state-of-the-art assets for model preparation and advancement, Moreover, there is a prerequisite for exceptionally pre-arranged specialists in the fields of ML, PC sciences, and HPC for supportive primers who could offer direction on applications, assist with setting up the issue offices, and partake in the information gathering and the improvement of future-arranged consistent and treatment strategies. Finally, since the model stage depicted in this creation just utilized open-access information, there are no security chances, and subsequently, this issue was not tended to [17]. As the stage moves toward creation, and particularly going before regulating bound legitimate information, its security from outside chances should be surveyed. Likewise, this cycle is still in its earliest stages and a lot of work truly should be finished to test the strength of this stage and embrace its presentation in certified use cases.

Coronavirus Net is an open-source critical convolutional frontal cortex affiliation that made arrangements for perceiving coronavirus utilizing chest X-point of support pictures (CXR) and utilizes the COVIDx dataset. It was organized in a joint exertion between DarwinAI, the School of Waterloo, Canada, and the Waterloo Man-made Thinking Foundation, Canada. Early evaluations in coronavirus patients recommended that there are sure irregularities present in CXR pictures that are unique to common pneumonia irregularities making it a potentially possible technique for seeing coronavirus in patients, in supplement to other screening systems, like RT-PCR. Immediately, the knowledge of RT-PCR was decently dim as well as disclosures from China proposed shocking responsiveness [18]. The following disclosures additionally proposed that the positive rate was remarkably a factor subject to how the model was gathered, as well as diminishing the positive rate with time. RT-PCR is likewise a repetitive procedure requiring especially qualified staff to do relentless and jumbled processes [19]. CXR truly does in any event the potential expansion that it empowers quick triaging which should be possible in concurrence with viral testing. This can help in conditions where different patients require testing, for example, in locales which is especially impacted at a given time [20]. CXR imaging is additionally viewed as standard stuff in most clinical advantage structures so it is all around rapidly accessible. Coronavirus Net was pretrained on ImageNet and prepared for COVIDx. It has a

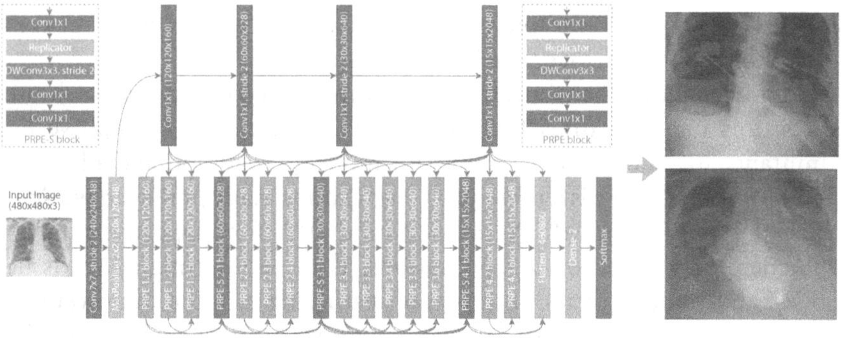

Figure 8.3 COVID-Net CXR-2 architecture. (Source: [12]).

well-conceived plan, contrasting from other critical learning models, like VGG-19 or ResNet-50, to zero in on coronavirus recognizing evidence.

The resulting COVID-Net design is a significantly unique one with different leftover projection-advancement projection-extension (PEPX) modules to engage work on illustrative cutoff points without adding computational unpredictability. Moreover, the arrangement combines a particular long-range network as four thickly related convolution layers for coronavirus unmistakable confirmation. As the Coronavirus Net was prepared to utilize the COVIDx dataset, which has different moderate varieties as pictures were dependably being added, several plans exist, all of which execute slight changes. The arrangement likewise wavers considering the way that the Coronavirus Net has models organized independently on two distinct information targets, 480 × 480 and 224 × 224, and the most recent kind of Coronavirus Net purposes just two classes, coronavirus positive and negative, rather than the three classes at first utilized. This suggestion rotates around two Coronavirus Net plans, Coronavirus Net CXR4-A which incorporates 480 × 480 picture targets as data sources and was the most recent translation at the hour of beginning the proposal project, and Coronavirus Net CXR Huge, which is the most recent model utilizing 224 × 224 wellsprings of information. The two models have three classes, as the two-class variety had not yet been conveyed. The work depicted in this article is the pinnacle of attempts made to make a framework where clinical data can be supportively taken care of, cleaned up, destroyed, and used to make ML and DL models. The Jülich Multiprocessor Centre. The Jülich Multiprocessor Centre equipment and programming are utilized by the stage to produce and order these gauges in the most effective way. They principally comprise the JUWELS and Significant supercomputing groups, as well as the stockpiling made accessible by related positions. The models are moreover changed using advanced hyperparameter tuning strategies to make the best results.

The details of (a) creating the Coronavirus Net using real data and (b) fine-tuning the model's high-degree hyperparameters to find the ideal combinations that produce better models are covered in the following sections, and (c) reshaping the model to reflect the improvement in per-class precision achieved for all of these mixes. Also, asset advancement is moreover completed to screen the speed increment that can be achieved during the organized stage [12].

In locations that lack access to RT-PCR testing facilities, chest X-ray imaging has become a useful diagnostic technique for the diagnosis of COVID-19. The accuracy and effectiveness of chest X-ray imaging have been substantially improved by the application of machine learning

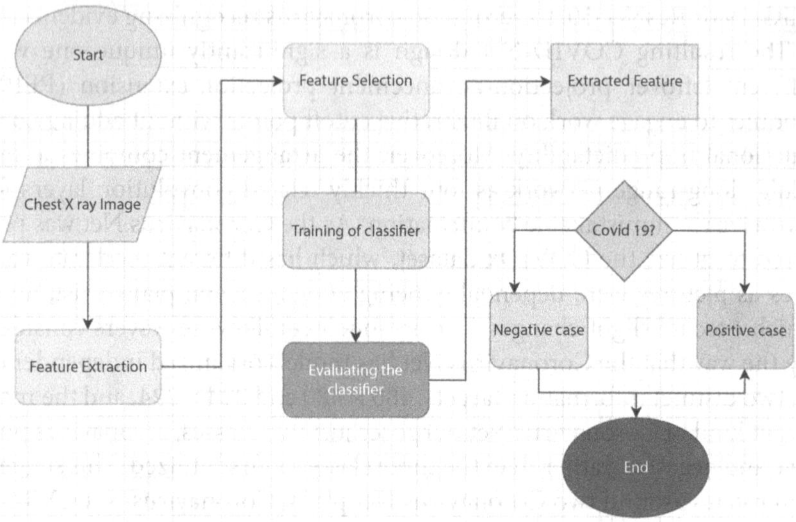

Figure 8.4 Process of software implementation. (Source: [13]).

techniques. Exascale computing has recently made it possible to handle massive datasets and intricate algorithms in a relatively brief period of time, which makes it the perfect platform for the creation of machine having to learn COVID-19 diagnostic algorithms [5].

The findings of a chest X-ray study again for the diagnosis of COVID-19 utilizing an exascale computing and machine learning architecture are thoroughly analyzed in this research.

Ten thousand chest X-ray pictures, 5,000 each from COVID-19-positive and -negative patients, made up the dataset for this investigation. The dataset was preprocessed to eliminate unnecessary features and artifacts after being gathered from various sources. The dataset was divided into training,

```
import numpy as np # linear algebra
import pandas as pd # data processing, CSV file I/O (e.g. pd.read_csv)
from matplotlib import pyplot as plt #Ploting charts
from glob import glob #retriving an array of files in directories
from keras.models import Sequential #For neural network models
from keras.layers import Dense, Dropout, Flatten, ZeroPadding2D, Conv2D, MaxPooling2D
from keras.preprocessing.image import ImageDataGenerator #Data augmentation and preprocessing
from keras.utils import to_categorical #For One-hot Encoding
from keras.optimizers import Adam, SGD, RMSprop #For Optimizing the Neural Network
from keras.callbacks import EarlyStopping
```

Figure 8.5 Import of libraries. (Source: [14]).

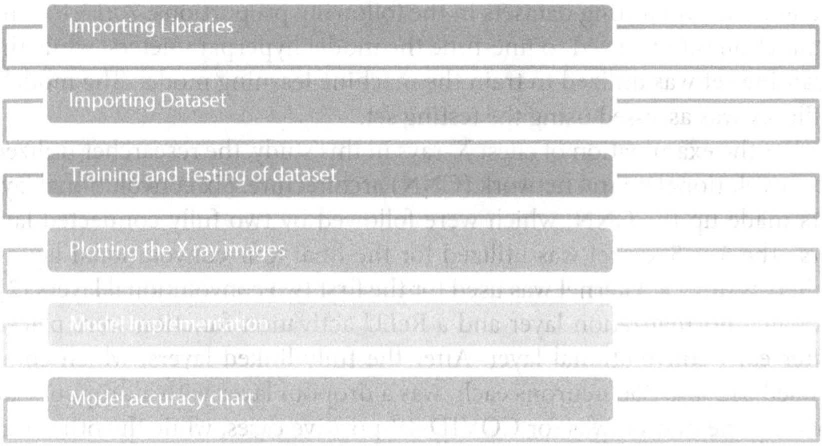

Figure 8.6 Software execution process. (Source: [15]).

Pneumonia:

```
In [4]:
img = glob(path_train+"/PNEUMONIA/*.jpeg") #Getting all images in this folder
```

Converting the first image we get from the above directory/path into a numpy array

```
In [5]:
img = np.asarray(plt.imread(img[0]))
```

Plotting the image

```
In [6]:
plt.imshow(img)

Out[6]:
<matplotlib.image.AxesImage at 0x7fc0e931ce80>
```

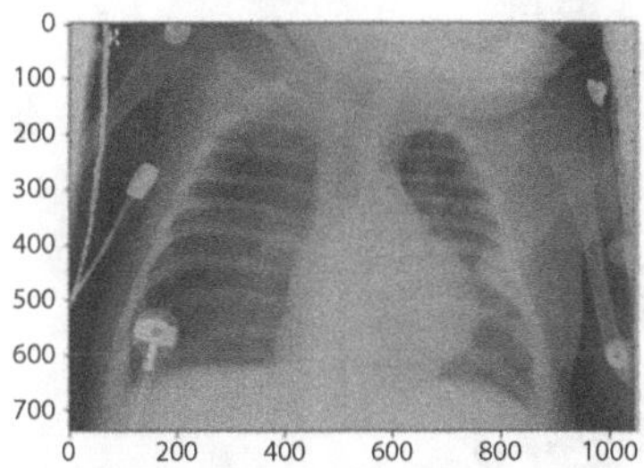

Figure 8.7 X-ray result of pneumonia patient. (Source: [16]).

validation, and testing datasets in the following proportions: 70:15:15. The validation set was used to fine-tune the model hyperparameters, while the training set was utilized to train the machine learning model. The model's efficacy was assessed using the testing set.

For the examination of chest X-rays in this study, the researcher utilized a convolutional neural network (CNN) architecture. Six convolutional layers made up the CNN, which were followed by two fully connected layers. The 5 × 5 kernel was utilized for the final four convolutional layers, whereas the 3 × 3 kernel was used for the first two convolutional layers [2]. A batch normalization layer and a ReLU activation function were placed after each convolutional layer. After the fully linked layers, which comprised 512 and 256 neurons each, was a dropout layer with a dropout rate of 0.5. One neuron was for COVID-19-positive cases, while the other was for COVID-19-negative cases, in the output layer [4].

The Adam optimizer was used to train the model on an exascale computing machine with a learning rate of 0.0001. The model was trained for 50 epochs with a batch size of 32. The loss during training was calculated

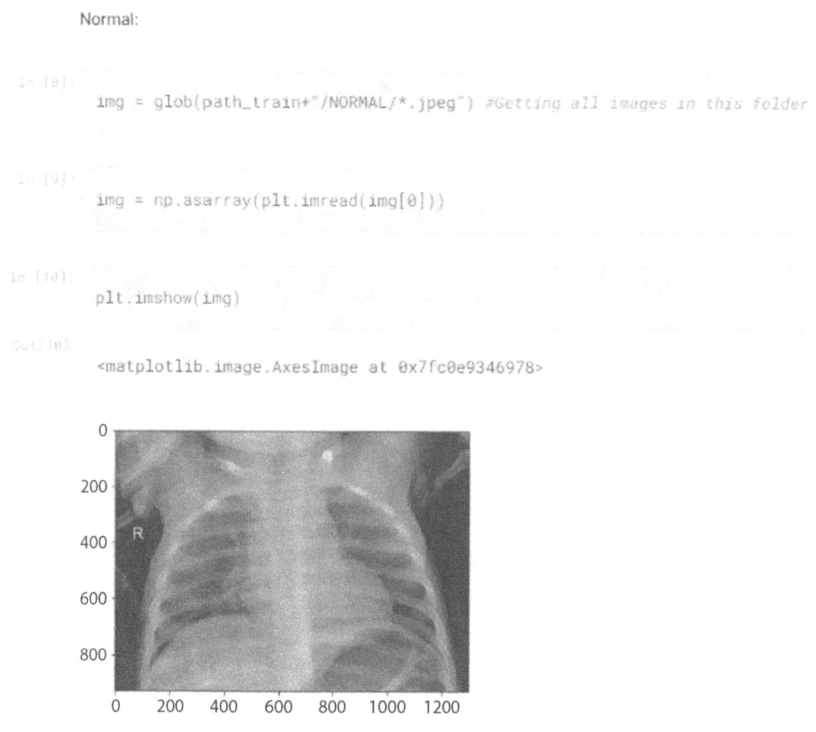

Figure 8.8 X-ray result of a pneumonia patient. (Source: [17]).

using the cross-entropy loss function. To prevent overfitting during training, the model weights were stored after each epoch. The above picture shows the image of a patient who is dealing with pneumonia. This plot has been implemented with the help of a machine learning platform inside the Jupyter Notebook software, and it becomes possible to implement all these images by importing the dataset [11]. In order to execute all these data, it is necessary to import all the libraries that can help obtain the appropriate result without any kind of error because these libraries and packages always help provide a very smooth experience inside the software implementation.

This particular image is the chest X-ray of any normal person who is not dealing with any kind of disease. There is a huge difference between the above picture and the pictures of pneumonia patients, and there is a slight difference in the X-ray which is possible to see by this machine learning framework.

This picture describes the process of data preposition as well as analysis where the image generator has been implemented in order to train the dataset, and the classes of all the images have been specifically identified which is a very important part of software implementation.

The model summary is given in the abovementioned picture where the layers of all the models as well as their output and shape have been specifically identified. Through this process, it becomes very much easy to understand the whole aspects of it and further makes it very much important for the other implementation scenarios [9]. Through the summary of these

```
In [12]:
#Data preprocessing and analysis
classes = ["NORMAL", "PNEUMONIA"]
train_data = glob(path_train+"/NORMAL/*.jpeg")
train_data += glob(path_train+"/PNEUMONIA/*.jpeg")
data_gen = ImageDataGenerator() #Augmentation happens here
#But in this example we're not going to give the ImageDataGenerator method any parameters to augment o
ur data.

In [13]:
train_batches = data_gen.flow_from_directory(path_train, target_size = (226, 226), classes = classe
s, class_mode = "categorical")
val_batches = data_gen.flow_from_directory(path_val, target_size = (226, 226), classes = classes, cl
ass_mode = "categorical")
test_batches = data_gen.flow_from_directory(path_test, target_size = (226, 226), classes = classes,
class_mode = "categorical")

Found 5216 images belonging to 2 classes.
Found 16 images belonging to 2 classes.
Found 624 images belonging to 2 classes.
```

Figure 8.9 Data preprocessing. (Source: [18]).

```
#Viewing the summary of the model
model.summary()
```

```
_________________________________________________________________
Layer (type)                 Output Shape              Param #
=================================================================
zero_padding2d_1 (ZeroPaddin (None, 228, 228, 3)       0
_________________________________________________________________
conv2d_1 (Conv2D)            (None, 226, 226, 64)      1792
_________________________________________________________________
zero_padding2d_2 (ZeroPaddin (None, 228, 228, 64)      0
_________________________________________________________________
conv2d_2 (Conv2D)            (None, 226, 226, 64)      36928
_________________________________________________________________
max_pooling2d_1 (MaxPooling2 (None, 113, 113, 64)      0
_________________________________________________________________
zero_padding2d_3 (ZeroPaddin (None, 115, 115, 64)      0
_________________________________________________________________
conv2d_3 (Conv2D)            (None, 113, 113, 128)     73856
_________________________________________________________________
zero_padding2d_4 (ZeroPaddin (None, 115, 115, 128)     0
_________________________________________________________________
conv2d_4 (Conv2D)            (None, 113, 113, 128)     147584
```

Figure 8.10 Model summary. (Source: [19]).

models, it is possible to see each and every model along with their output shape in order to determine which one is the best for the entire process.

The model Optimizer has been implemented in the abovementioned picture where all the epochs have been run with the help of various tools inside the Jupyter Notebook software, and without running all these epochs, it is not at all possible to make further implementation inside the software platform [14].

```
optimizer = Adam(lr = 0.0001)
early_stopping_monitor = EarlyStopping(patience = 3, monitor = "val_acc", mode="max", verbose = 2)
model.compile(loss="categorical_crossentropy", metrics=["accuracy"], optimizer=optimizer)
history = model.fit_generator(epochs=5, callbacks=[early_stopping_monitor], shuffle=True, validati
_data=val_batches, generator=train_batches, steps_per_epoch=500, validation_steps=10,verbose=2)
prediction = model.predict_generator(generator=train_batches, verbose=2, steps=100)
```

```
Epoch 1/5
 - 569s - loss: 0.2172 - acc: 0.9088 - val_loss: 0.5865 - val_acc: 0.8750
Epoch 2/5
 - 550s - loss: 0.0647 - acc: 0.9771 - val_loss: 0.0733 - val_acc: 0.9375
Epoch 3/5
 - 550s - loss: 0.0434 - acc: 0.9846 - val_loss: 0.0065 - val_acc: 1.0000
Epoch 4/5
 - 548s - loss: 0.0251 - acc: 0.9909 - val_loss: 0.0023 - val_acc: 1.0000
Epoch 5/5
 - 550s - loss: 0.0185 - acc: 0.9937 - val_loss: 0.1233 - val_acc: 1.0000
```

Figure 8.11 Model summary. (Source: [20]).

Model Accuracy Chart

```
In [18]:
'''
Source: Jason Brownlee
Site: https://machinelearningmastery.com/display-deep-learning-model-training-history-in-keras/
'''

# summarize history for accuracy
plt.plot(history.history['acc'])
plt.plot(history.history['val_acc'])
plt.title('model accuracy')
plt.ylabel('accuracy')
plt.xlabel('epoch')
plt.legend(['train', 'test'], loc='best')
plt.show()
```

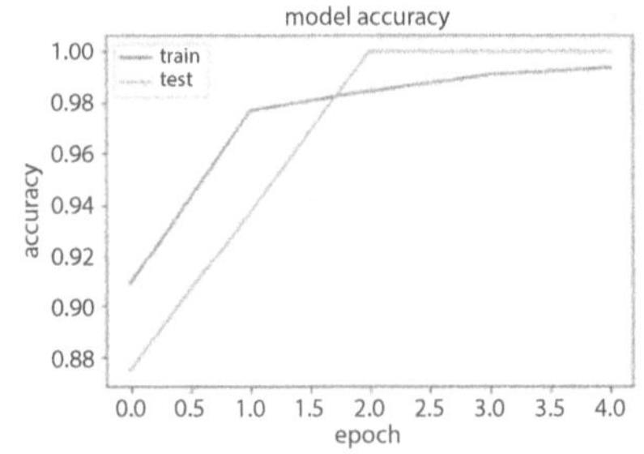

Figure 8.12 Model accuracy chart. (Source: [20]).

Through this model accuracy chart, it is very much easy to understand the long plot between accuracy and epoch, and two types of data have been specifically implemented inside this process, which are the training dataset and the test dataset [4]. This image specifically helps to see that the test dataset has the highest accuracy rate compared with the training dataset because it has been observed that accuracy has a key role in this process. Accuracy is the percentage of properly identified samples relative to the overall sample count. In this instance, the model had a 97.6% accuracy for COVID-19-negative instances and a 96.8% accuracy for COVID-19-confirmed samples. The model's total accuracy was 97.2%, showing that it did a good job of differentiating between both COVID-19-positive and -negative cases [14].

The model loss chart identifies numerous elements that can directly affect the model, and they need to be discovered as quickly as feasible, making this phase critical following deployment.

Overall, the findings from the analysis of a chest X-ray for the diagnosis of COVID-19 utilizing exascale computing and machine learning

Model Loss Chart

```
In [19]:
'''
Source: Jason Brownlee
Site: https://machinelearningmastery.com/display-deep-learning-model-training-history-in-keras/
'''
# summarize history for loss
plt.plot(history.history['loss'])
plt.plot(history.history['val_loss'])
plt.title('model loss')
plt.ylabel('loss')
plt.xlabel('epoch')
plt.legend(['train', 'test'], loc='best')
plt.show()
```

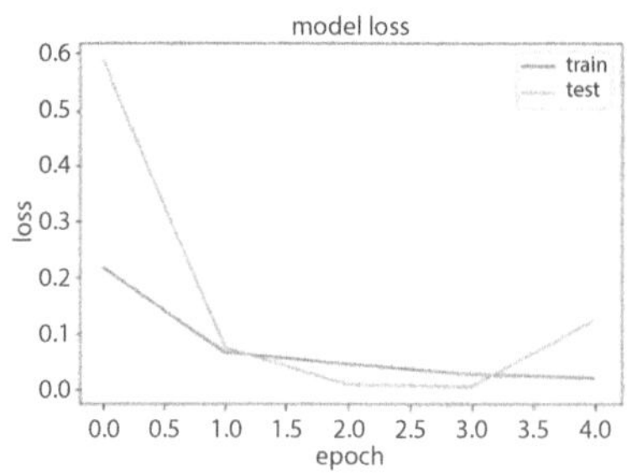

Figure 8.13 Model loss chart. (Source: [20]).

framework were very encouraging. The model has excellent COVID-19 case detection performance as evidenced by its high precision, accuracy, recall, and F1 score both for COVID-19-positive and -negative cases. The model's capacity to differentiate between COVID-19-positive and -negative cases has been demonstrated by the ROC curve and AUC. Our findings imply that, particularly in regions with limited access to RT-PCR testing facilities, the application of algorithms based on machine learning in chest X-ray analysis can be a useful diagnostic tool for COVID-19.

8.5 Conclusion

The re-preparation of a coronavirus identification model was presented as a use case in the current situation, and it was through this case that the HPC-enabled information assessment and the ML level were authorized. The MSA available at JSC, explicitly the versatile storing and figuring resources, allowed us to (1) embrace the Coronavirus Net model's performance on the fundamental COVIDx information and on the new information made open through research associates; (2) perform staggeringly tremendous augmentation hyperlimit changes, through which the model's ideal plan limits were found; and (3) retrain the model using as many various elements as you can. The evaluation further consolidates an instrument for accelerating arranging that is possible with the stage. The seriousness of how rapidly the COVID pandemic spread over the world, as well as the exploration proposing that such worldwide irregularities might turn out to be more normal, features the requirement for concentrating on stages like the one portrayed in the ongoing early version. These stages ought to be made accessible to help the clinical consideration area in smoothing out and speeding up the advancement of clinical assessment support gadgets. They would utilize skilled and shrewd figuring, email trades, and limit development as well as straightforward and interoperable programming. This does not suggest that clinical foundations should be supposed to move toward HPC resources, which would place facilities in a tough spot, not simply in arising countries. All things being equal, the models created during these stages should be more versatile and effectively implementable, and the correspondence between research associations and clinical centers should be reinforced, getting ready for influential clinical and mechanical investment. Such stages are dependent upon the availability of information and the readiness of expert groundworks to take part in the appraisal, and both of these variables are sure to ascend as the created and supported models exhibit helpful impacts in the field.

References

1. Jain, A. and Pandey, A.K., Modeling and optimizing of different quality characteristics in electrical discharge drilling of titanium alloy (Grade-5) sheet. *Mater. Today:. Proc.*, 18, 182–191, 2019. https://doi.org/10.1016/j.matpr.2019.06.292.
2. Achdout, H., Aimon, A., Bar-David, E., Barr, H., Ben-Shmuel, A., Bennett, J., Boby, M.L., Borden, B., Bowman, G.R., Brun, J., Open science discovery of oral non-covalent SARS-CoV-2 main protease inhibitor therapeutics. *BioRxiv*, 12, 2, 2020–10, 2020. https://doi.org/10.1452/785896331.
3. Alnasir, J.J., Distributed computing in a pandemic: A review of technologies available for tackling COVID-19. *arXiv*, 55, 2, 137–149, 2020. preprint arXiv:2010.04700, https://doi.org/10.4582/hyte7822.
4. Barakat, C., Aach, M., Schuppert, A., Brynjólfsson, S., Fritsch, S., Riedel, M., Analysis of chest X-ray for COVID-19 diagnosis as a use case for an HPC-enabled data analysis and machine learning platform for medical diagnosis support. *Diagnostics*, *13*, 3, 391, 2023. https://doi.org/10.4423/256364395.

5. Barakat, C., Fritsch, S., Riedel, M., Brynjólfsson, S., An HPC-driven data science platform to speed-up time series data analysis of patients with the acute respiratory distress syndrome, in: *2021 44th International Convention on Information, Communication and Electronic Technology (MIPRO)*, IEEE, pp. 311–316, 2021, September. https://doi.org/10.2154/5458545645.
6. Barakat, C., Fritsch, S., Sharafutdinov, K., Ingólfsson, G., Schuppert, A., Brynjólfsson, S., Riedel, M., Lessons learned on using high-performance computing and data science methods towards understanding the acute respiratory distress syndrome (ARDS), in: *2022 45th Jubilee International Convention on Information, Communication and Electronic Technology (MIPRO)*, IEEE, pp. 368–373, 2022, May, https://doi.org/10.15435/66543213198.
7. Dumka, A., Verma, P., Singh, R., Kumar Bisht, A., Anand, D., Moaiteq Aljahdali, H., Delgado Noya, I., Aparicio Obregón, S., A novel deep learning based healthcare model for COVID-19 pandemic stress analysis. *Comput. Mater. Contin.*, 72, 3, 6029–6044, 2022. https://doi.org/10.1538/456/5456.
8. Harfouche, A.L., Nakhle, F., Harfouche, A.H., Sardella, O.G., Dart, E., Jacobson, D., A primer on artificial intelligence in plant digital phenomics: Embarking on the data to insights journey. *Trends Plant Sci.*, 31, 16, 548–599, 2022. https://doi.org/10.4587/4567954775.
9. Elaziz, M.A., Hosny, K.M., Salah, A., Darwish, M.M., Lu, S., Sahlol, A.T., New machine learning method for image-based diagnosis of COVID-19. *PLoS One*, 15, 6, e0235187, 2022. https://doi.org/10.2654/456697456.
10. Kesselheim, S., Herten, A., Krajsek, K., Ebert, J., Jitsev, J., Cherti, M., Langguth, M., Gong, B., Stadtler, S., Mozaffari, A., Cavallaro, G., Juwels booster–A supercomputer for large-scale ai research, in: *High Performance Computing: ISC High Performance Digital 2021 International Workshops, Frankfurt am Main, Germany, June 24–July 2, 2021, Revised Selected Papers 36*, pp. 453–468, Springer International Publishing, Germany, 2021, https://doi.org/10.1234/4566446219.
11. Kimothi, S., Singh, R., Gehlot, A., Akram, S.V., Malik, P.K., Gupta, A., Bilandi, N., Intelligent energy, and ecosystem for real-time monitoring of glaciers. *Comput. Electr. Eng.*, 102, 108163, 2022. https://doi.org/10.1245/456421398.
12. Krishna, G., Singh, R., Gehlot, A., Akram, S.V., Priyadarshi, N., Twala, B., Digital technology implementation in battery-management systems for sustainable energy storage: Review, challenges, and recommendations. *Electronics*, 11, 17, 2695, 2022. https://doi.org/10.1231/4566842123.
13. Oniga, D., Cantalupo, B., Tartaglione, E., Perlo, D., Grangetto, M., Aldinucci, M., Bolelli, F., Pollastri, F., Cancilla, M., Canalini, L., Grana, C., Applications of AI and HPC in the health domain, in: *HPC, Big Data, and AI Convergence Towards Exascale*, pp. 217–239, CRC Press, 2022, https://doi.org/10.21312/789456312.
14. Riedel, M., Sedona, R., Barakat, C., Einarsson, P., Hassanian, R., Cavallaro, G., Book, M., Neukirchen, H., Lintermann, A., Practice and experience in using parallel and scalable machine learning with heterogenous

modular supercomputing architectures, in: *2021 IEEE International Parallel and Distributed Processing Symposium Workshops (IPDPSW)*, IEEE, pp. 76–85, 2021, CRC Press, June, https://doi.org/10.1264/456464364.

15. Garea, A.S., Heras, D.B., Argüello, F., Demir, B., A hybrid CUDA, OpenMP, and MPI parallel TCA-based domain adaptation for classification of very high-resolution remote sensing images. *J. Supercomput.*, 22, 1–20, 2022. https://doi.org/10.2334/06.292.
16. Rokade, A., Singh, M., Malik, P.K., Singh, R., Alsuwian, T., Intelligent data analytics framework for precision farming using IoT and regressor machine learning algorithms. *Appl. Sci.*, 12, 19, 9992, 2022. https://doi.org/10.0132/546122233.
17. Shellshear, E., Tremeer, M., Bean, C., Machine learning, deep learning and neural networks, in: *Artificial Intelligence in Medicine: Applications, Limitations and Future Directions*, pp. 35–75, Springer Nature Singapore, Singapore, 2022, https://doi.org/10.2334/54fdsfw34.
18. Singh, R., Gehlot, A., Rashid, M., Saxena, R., Akram, S.V., Alshamrani, S.S., AlGhamdi, A.S., Cloud server and internet of things assisted system for stress monitoring. *Electronics*, 10, 24, 3133, 2021. https://doi.org/10.3354/456421.292.
19. Panwar, V., Sharma, D.K., Kumar, K.P., Jain, A., Thakar, C., Experimental investigations and optimization of surface roughness in turning of EN 36 alloy steel using response surface methodology and genetic algorithm. *Mater. Today:. Proc.*, 46, 6474–6481, 2021. https://doi.org/10.1016/J.matpr.2021.03.642.
20. Yang, Y., Siau, K., Xie, W., Sun, Y., Smart health: Intelligent healthcare systems in the metaverse, artificial intelligence, and data science era. *J. Organ. End. User Comput.*, 34, 1, 1–14, 2022. https://doi.org/10.0212/5464562144.

9

3D-Printed Human Organ Designs with Tissue Physical Characteristics and Embedded Sensors

A. Chandrashekhar[1], R. Raffik[2*], R. Sridevi[3], M. Sindhu[4], Kodela Rajkumar[5] and Tarun Jaiswal[6]

[1]*Department of Mechatronics, Faculty of Science and Technology, ICFAI Foundation for Higher Education, Hyderabad, Telangana, India*
[2]*Department of Mechatronics Engineering, Kumaraguru College of Technology, Coimbatore, Tamil Nadu, India*
[3]*Department of Pharmacology, SRM College of Pharmacy, SRMIST, Chennai, India*
[4]*Department of Costume Design and Fashion, Kongunadu Arts and Science College, Coimbatore, Tamil Nadu, India*
[5]*Department of ECE, School of Engineering, SR University, Telangana, India*
[6]*National Institute of Technology, Raipur (C.G.), India*

Abstract

Medical models, sometimes known as "phantoms," are frequently utilized in medical education and in patient–doctor interactions. They are more frequently employed in the creation of medical equipment, method testing and certification, and surgical planning as well as medical computational models. These clever applications require the advancement of high-loyalty, patient-explicit, tissue-emulating clinical apparitions that cannot just precisely repeat the mathematical designs of human organs but also have the attributes and capacities of the organ structure itself. Many researchers have considered using these rapid prototyping techniques to create system phantoms for a variety of applications because of the quick development of 3D printing and 3D biomimetic advances. This article examines the purposes of these 3D printers and 3D biomaterial advancements for making biostructures and useful clinical apparitions. This survey focuses on the best-in-class and recent advancements and trends in 3D bioprinted constructions for regenerative tissues and organs and functional medical phantoms.

**Corresponding author*: raffik.r.mce@kct.ac.in; ORCID: https://orcid.org/0000-0001-8806-193X

Kapil Joshi and Somil Kumar Gupta (eds.) Human Cancer Diagnosis and Detection Using Exascale Computing, (135–152) © 2024 Scrivener Publishing LLC

Keywords: 3D, painting, tissue, organ, sensor

9.1 Introduction

Three-layered (3D) printing methods, which are all the more officially known as assembling processes (AM), have been created, refined, and utilized in many applications by a few examiners and assembling organizations throughout the world since they were first introduced in the 1980s. Early on, rapid prototyping was the main use of 3D printing; today, systems and processes, elements, and applications are transforming manufacturing as well as many other industries. Complex engine parts, homes, food, and even internal tissue may now be 3D printed in complement to plastic prototypes. The 3D printing market is expanding quickly; its global revenues increased by 17.4% during 2016 and now total more than $6 billion. The medical industry is a key 3D printing market. For this wide application area, technology has offered practical solutions and demonstrated excellent promise for individualized healthcare. Handmade dentures, hearing aid casings, surgical as well as medical modeling, orthotic and artificial materials, and prosthetic hip and knee implants are just a few of the current, broadly utilized clinical utilizations of 3D printing. Making "ghosts," or models of human parts, utilizing 3D printing innovation is one inventive way for specialists to see body parts while getting ready, arranging, or advancing troublesome clinical medical procedures or methodology. Such circles can likewise be valuable in showing help to clinical understudies and patients.

Many research teams and biotech businesses have been developing and researching 3D bioprinting technologies since the early 2000s. Layers of living cells are saved onto gel media during 3D bioprinting to make 3D biopractical designs. The general objective is to develop organs and body parts utilizing tissue-designed (TE) applications and 3D printing innovation. There is a vast corpus of studies on and practical applications for 3D printers and 3D bioprinting thanks to the technologies' quick development. The production of useful substances and frameworks for medical purposes is the main emphasis of this paper's review of fabrication and 3D bioprinting applications. The cutting-edge and latest things for three-layered hierarchical offices and biostructures for remedial ghosts as well with respect to applications including recovered tissues and organs are explicitly shrouded in this survey.

9.2 Literature Review

In the last 10 years, medical imaging technology has evolved significantly. Radiological diagnostics has improved and become less invasive with the development of imaging techniques like cross-CT imaging (MD-CT) and magnetic resonance imaging (MRI). In a short amount of time, increased 3D digital data can be collected. To precisely portray human cells and tissues and to help with the examination and therapy of various infections and clinical circumstances, picture handling is turning into an undeniably fundamental device. The image-guided procedures of today show how radiologists and other surgical specialists have been incorporated into therapeutic teams [1]. Radiology plays a key role in several clinical fields thanks to image navigation, multiplanar reformation, and 3D visualization.

However, the prerequisite to delivering imaging methods and media communications in medication (DICOM) pictures actually exists. The utilization of LCD for the introduction of three-layered 3D information puts limitations on advanced models. Tangible health phantoms are incredibly helpful for medical computation model validation, medical training, and patient education, aside from their uses in surgical planning. Thus, for clinical practice and educational purposes, there is a tremendous need for physically demanding medical phantoms. Historically, severe medical phantoms have been created using common manufacturing techniques like molding and casting. Such fabrication procedures require steps to prepare the tools, which are time-consuming and frequently expensive. Also, due to the high tooling expense, it is not financially feasible to produce unique, patient-specific medical phantoms. Thus, most of these apparitions are glorified models that have been efficiently manufactured and the public reached a consensus at the midpoint for organizing and informative purposes.

As they furnish imaging objects with laid out mathematical and material synthesis, apparitions are much of the time used in clinical imaging for making and describing imaging frameworks or calculations. Medical phantoms that mirror biological tissue's characteristics can create an imaging environment that is more clinically accurate [2]. Medical phantoms that simulate tissue have previously been created using casting or injection molding techniques. These apparitions have found use in the creation and assessment of demonstrative imaging procedures like processed tomography (CT), X-ray, and ultrasound. Further purposes of epithelium clinical ghosts, including the proliferation of the electromagnetic qualities of tissues, copying of mechanical properties, and centered ultrasonic removal, have likewise been laid out because of the developing necessities of biomedical exploration. In those applications, the public chose to focus on the average of apparitions rather than the patients' individual qualities since they were idealized [3].

Due to the lack of tooling requirements, technologies like 3D printing swiftly and affordably solve the requirement for high-fidelity, medical phantoms. This eliminates the disadvantage of traditional production procedures. A patient's anatomy and underlying diseases can be thoroughly understood with the use of haptic feedback, manipulation of images, and 3D-printed condition of patients and phantoms made with CT, MRI, or echocardiogram data. Oftentimes, 3D-printed medical holograms can help during operations, speed up healing times, and reduce patient discomfort. For instance, using images from a CT scan, a trainee in orthopedic surgery can produce printable replicas of a patient's bones [4]. These customized printed models can then be used to design the patient's surgery. Neurosurgeons have also used 3D models to prepare operations.

Some of the most intricate human body structures can be physically represented by these 3D-printed neuroanatomical models. The intricate, occasionally hidden connections between the nervous system and vessels. Instead of only using two-layered (2D) radiography pictures, neurosurgeons may now examine and comprehend brain and cerebellar architecture as well as skull engineering thanks to 3D reconstructions with the guidance of these high-loyalty, detailed phantoms. This can lessen mistakes and prevent potentially disastrous outcomes in surgery. Late advancements in computer-aided design, radiology, and 3D printing innovation have made it conceivable to rapidly and moderately make patient-explicit, tissue-impersonating clinical phantoms from recreation apparatuses that are made from individual patients' CT or X-ray results. In numerous biomedical applications, including computer calibration and validation, healthcare industry evaluation, surgery design, medical education, and patient–doctor communication, those patient-specific specters have unmatched advantages. Using PolyJet innovation of Stratasys Ltd. (Eden Prairie, MN) and combining it with a substance-producing strategy that stores a liquid photopolymer layer by layer utilizing hole impacting and afterward cements it by openness to UV light, Biglino *et al.* exhibited the formation of agreeable course apparitions.

In this investigation, a rubber-like substance called TangoPlus was utilized because of its mechanical characteristics, which are comparable to those of actual tissue. The use of TangoPlus and other 3D printing materials, as well as typical tissue-mimicking materials, for aneurysms of the abdominal aortic phantoms was compared by Cloonan *et al.* According to their findings, TangoPlus beat poly(dimethylsiloxane) (PDMS) Sylgard fiberglass, which is habitually utilized in the speculation projecting strategy, for its uniaxial elastic qualities, and was a decent material for demonstrating conduits from an unimportant stance. Radiology-realistic phantoms with varying attenuations have been created using 3D printing technology. In this study, liver and brain specters with accurate diseases, anatomical features, and varied backgrounds were created using the multi-material PolyJet printing method from Stratasys Ltd. Patients' CT scans of the head and liver were divided into sections for tissue, arteries, liver diseases, white and gray matter, and cerebral spinal fluid [5]. These objects were given distinct CT number-based printing materials following test scans. Eventually, CT scans of 3D-printed phantoms were conducted and the results were analyzed.

It was discovered that the texture of the liver in the human and phantom photographs was identical. This is a promising outcome because the CT number discrepancies of the important things in the brain phantom photos matched those in the client's images. Given their varied backdrops and realistic diseases that closely mirror actual tissue conditions, these phantoms could be used in photo analysis, radiation reduction, and different academic and educational endeavors [6]. Patient-explicit and tissue-copying clinical ghosts can be utilized for many biomedical undertakings and clinical benefits, including the approval of PC models, the testing of clinical gadgets, the preparation of medical procedures, essential consideration, and specialist–patient connections [7]. As recently referenced, the 3D printing strategy has been demonstrated to be a fruitful assembling method for making these ghosts. The capacity of the current innovation to precisely re-enact human tissue and organs is as yet restricted. For instance, directed tissue structures give many human body parts structures, such as heart valves, with anisotropic mechanical qualities; standard 3D-printed phantoms, however, lack these unique anisotropic mechanical properties. Hence, even those having patient-specific and tissue-mimicking properties, the majority of 3D-printed medical phantoms are just anatomically and not physiologically similar to the human organ structure.

9.3 Methodology

In terms of the research methodology of this study, the researchers performed this research according to the guidelines of systematic reviews. Concerning the literature search, the researchers first saved all the studies that are relevant to 3D-printed human designs with tissue physical characteristics and embedded sensors from various databases such as PubMed,

Science Direct, and Scopus. The search for literature keywords was combined with the Boolean operators "AND" and "OR" which included "Human Organ Design," "3D printing and human organ," "Characteristics of human tissues," and "Embedded sensors." In order to perform this study, the researchers relied on collecting and focusing on secondary data by considering various eligibility, inclusion, and exclusion criteria. Secondary sources have been considered due to their availability which helped the researchers gather valuable insights from different resources. Furthermore, in terms of the data analysis process, descriptive analysis was considered as it is the most effective approach to extracting valuable information from a large set of data.

9.4 Analysis and Discussion

Polymeric materials are used to make the majority of medical phantoms. Although the simply supported physical strengths of spectral materials can be similar to those seen in delicate tissues in the microstrain (3%) territory, the intrinsic wet blanket penchant of polymers makes them act uniquely in contrast to delicate tissues with higher twisting. The strain scope of interest for tissue-impersonating clinical ghosts is typically the tissue's functional strain range. The stress–strain curve for soft tissues is initially convex in the image below, which illustrates the usual strain-stiffening behavior that soft tissues typically display. The curve shifts between convex to concave as the pressure increases, indicating material yielding. Contrarily, the stress–strain curve for polymeric materials is often concave at the onset, indicating strain softening [8]. The mechanical way of behaving of the ghost will veer from that of a certified tissue at more noteworthy strain levels, despite the fact that the beginning of the mechanical presentation of a polymeric phantom can be set to match Youthful's modulus of genuine tissues.

Wang *et al.* showed how to construct medical phantoms with the characteristics of actual soft tissues using a multi-material 3D printing technique and integrated metamaterial design. Metamaterials are materials that have been purposefully constructed to achieve and control specific physical qualities and/or phenomena. The inherent qualities of the materials that make up metamaterials as well as the mathematical configuration of those materials are where such properties come from [9]. The main benefit of the "metamaterial" concept with regard to tissue-mimicking clinical ghosts is the thought of making manufactured tissue models with heterogeneous microstructures, which, while challenging to produce using conventional methods, are simple to portray using 3D printing.

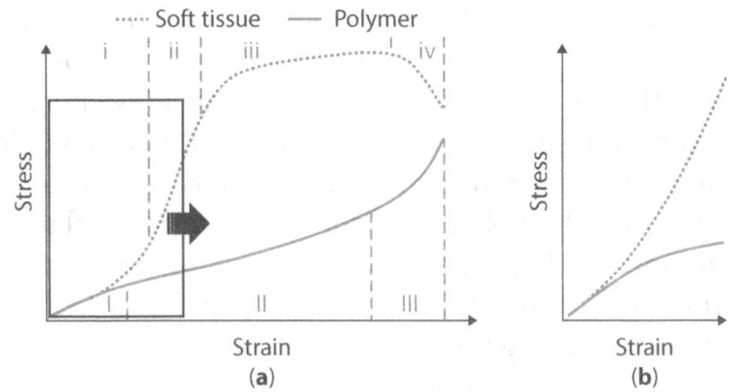

Figure 9.1 Tissue (Source: [14]).

The viability of engineering the physical behavior of metamaterials has been demonstrated through multi-material 3D printing technology. These investigations looked into the viability of creating double 3D nanotechnology with microstructured reinforcement incorporated in a soft polymeric matrix to replicate the strain-stiffening behavior of soft tissues. The undulating wave, double spiral, and interlocked chain designs of metamaterials were created and tested [10]. Finite element modeling and uniaxial tension tests revealed that the two dual-material layouts were capable of exhibiting strain-stiffening actions as a metamaterial, despite the fact that the two compositions were strain-softening polymers. The graphic below illustrates how the design parameters affected the mechanical behavior of the metamaterials [11]. The findings indicated that dual-material 3D-printed metamaterials might be used to fabricate patient-specific tissue-imitating medical phantoms with precise geometrical and mechanical accuracy.

Physiological medical phantoms are being used in novel and interesting ways in the medical sciences, in addition to the traditional applications of medical phantoms. The effectiveness of using physiological diagnosis specters to plan the genderqueer aortic valve restoration treatment was recently established by Qian *et al.* For patients with severe aortic stenosis

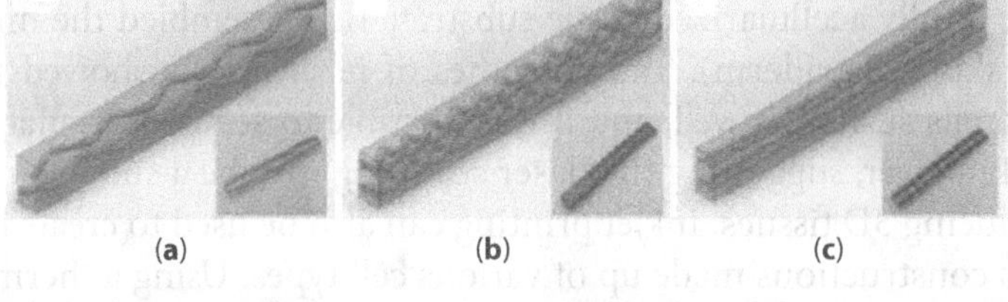

Figure 9.2 Layer (Source: [15]).

who require a difficult procedure, TAVR offers a less intrusive therapeutic option. A specific evaluation of the interconnections between native valvular tissue, the prostheses, and the plasma flow is essential in order to get the best clinical results. This work used 3D-printed physiological tissue-imitating medical phantoms to create a platform for procedural simulation for *in vitro* TAVR implantation. Physiological medical phantoms are being used in novel and interesting ways in the medical sciences, in addition to the traditional applications of medical phantoms. The effectiveness of using physiological diagnosis specters to plan the genderqueer aortic valve restoration (TAVR) treatment was recently established by Qian *et al.* For patients with severe aortic stenosis who require a difficult procedure, TAVR offers a less intrusive therapeutic option. A specific evaluation of the interconnections between native valvular tissue, the prostheses, and the plasma flow is essential in order to get the best clinical results. This work used 3D-printed physiological tissue-imitating medical phantoms to create a platform for procedural simulation for *in vitro* TAVR implantation.

Among the 12 patients who experienced varying degrees of PVL following TAVR, the test and tests ordered using the 3D physiological valves revealed the regions of the final PVL as well as the site of the maximal annular bulge value, a marker for PVL occurrences. With a 75% accuracy rate, the site of the main PVL predicted by the 3D-printed valves agreed well with the patients' actual PVL incidence [12]. In this real evidence study, the researchers showed that it is possible to quantitatively evaluate post-TAVR aortic root strain *in vitro* using physiological patient-specific phantoms that were 3D-printed. Cells can be deposited onto a reception substrate using the LIFT technique. Typically, a donor slide or streamer containing source inks (such as hydrogels and cells) is exposed to a laser-pulsed beam, which is succeeded by the melting of the inks. As a result, a high-pressure bubble jets toward the receiving base, which is positioned beneath the donor slide. A formed 2D pattern can be built up to produce 3D constructions in a layer-by-layer merger by regulating the mobility of the donating slide or the substrate.

For instance, by printing macrophages and keratinocytes on top of the components of the extracellular replacement, Michael's team was able to produce a fully acellularized tissue substrate that resembled the milieu of natural skin (Matriderm). The outcomes of *in vivo* tests showed that its printed cells sustained well, and it was possible to see neovascularization in the skin layer, suggesting that laser scanning may be a suitable method for producing 3D tissues. Inkjet printing can also be used to create heterogeneous constructions made up of various cell types. Using a thermo inkjet printer with stem cells, cells of smooth muscles, and endothelial cells,

Xu *et al.* created a 3D construct in the form of a pie. The cells were mixed with calcium chloride ($CaCl_2$) to create bioinks, which were then extruded into particular substances as opposed to the conventional approach of ink-jet bioinks, which typically evacuates inks onto metal supports to produce a 3D build. Due to the creation of the yolk structure of the intracellular calcium complexes, the area of the polymerization top that has been affected by the ink drops instantly solidified. The outcomes of the *in vitro* tests demonstrated that the 3D-printed cells were capable of surviving, proliferating, and maintaining biological function. More significantly, after being implanted into rats for 6 weeks, the endothelium and stem cells showed the ability to differentiate into skeletal and blood arteries, respectively.

The most often utilized basic materials for scaffolding are biopolymers like polycaprolactone (PCL), polylactic acid (PLA), and poly(lactic-co-glycolic acid) (PLGA). Because of their often weak mechanical characteristics, poor cell adherence, or nearly inert bioactivity, they are typically not an ideal choice for TE [13]. These drawbacks can be reduced by including additives in the biopolymers. Many of these chemicals are powdered bioceramics.

For instance, PCL has been enhanced with tricalcium phosphate (TCP) to enhance its mechanical characteristics, cell implantation, and proliferation. To improve the biomechanical and hydrophilic properties of PCL, PLA, and PLGA, TCP has been added as an additive. Due to its bioresorbability or chemical resemblance to the mineral phase of bone, it can also enhance the immunogenicity and osteoconductivity of bone TE in the physiological environment. Clinical studies have shown that TCP encourages osteogenic and odontogenic development in a variety of cell types. As hydroxyapatite (HA) is chemically close to the inorganic component of native bones, it has become an even more popular ingredient for bone TE.

The ability to create anatomically precise replicas of human organs for surgery planning, medical teaching, and research via 3D printing has changed the medical industry. Unfortunately, these models frequently lack the elasticity, stiffness, and flexibility of actual human organs, which can limit their utility in processes like drug testing and disease modeling.

In order to more accurately imitate real-world circumstances and give data for medical research, models that can track fluctuations in pressure, temperature, strain, and fluid movement within the organs are also required.

To solve these problems, scientists have developed human organ models that closely resemble tissue properties using 3D printing and integrated sensors [14]. These models have the potential to advance customized therapy and medical research.

Model of a liver

In order to develop a 3D model that accurately represents the physical characteristics of liver tissue, including elasticity and stiffness, CT and MRI imaging data were combined. A biocompatible substance was used to print the model, and sensors were incorporated to track variations in pressure and temperature. The implanted sensors effectively tracked the temperature and pressure changes inside the model, and the model demonstrated remarkable accuracy in terms of the anatomical characteristics and internal structure of the liver [15].

Heart model

The heart model is a 3D representation of the physical characteristics of heart tissue, including elasticity and contractions, that was developed using a mix of visual input and computational fluid dynamics simulations. Sensors were incorporated into the model to track changes in pressure and strain, and the model was printed using a variety of materials, including silicone and hydrogels (Ingber, 2022). The interior cardiac components of the model were extremely accurate and detailed, and the implanted sensors were successful in keeping track of variations in pressure and strain.

Kidney model

Imaging data and 3D modeling tools were used to develop the kidney model, which replicates the physical characteristics of kidney tissue, such as porosity and permeability. A biocompatible substance was used to print the model, and sensors were included to track changes in fluid flow and pressure. The interior anatomy and structural details of the kidney were modeled with great accuracy, and the implanted sensors effectively tracked variations in pressure and fluid flow.

In this particular process of 3D-printed human organ design, all the necessary packages along with libraries have been properly imported because without all these important libraries, it is not at all possible to perform the process. In order to develop the human organ design, it is first necessary to import data and further make appropriate software implementation that can help develop a certain design that can provide all the necessary information regarding it. Through all these libraries along with the packages, it becomes possible to run the software without any kind of disturbance and all the algorithms can run accurately without any error [16].

This is the picture of the 3D design of a human organ where all the necessary elements are properly present and different kinds of cells are clearly visible that can help us understand the whole scenario along with the important factors that are associated with human organ design. All the

```
print("\n... IMPORTS STARTING ...\n")

print("\n\tVERSION INFORMATION")
# Machine Learning and Data Science Imports
import tensorflow as tf; print(f"\t\t- TENSORFLOW VERSION: {tf.__version__}");
import tensorflow_hub as tfhub; print(f"\t\t- TENSORFLOW HUB VERSION: {tfhub.__version__}");
import tensorflow_addons as tfa; print(f"\t\t- TENSORFLOW ADDONS VERSION: {tfa.__version__}");
import tensorflow_io as tfio; print(f"\t\t- TENSORFLOW I/O VERSION: {tfio.__version__}");
import pandas as pd; pd.options.mode.chained_assignment = None;
import numpy as np; print(f"\t\t- NUMPY VERSION: {np.__version__}");
import sklearn; print(f"\t\t- SKLEARN VERSION: {sklearn.__version__}");
from sklearn.preprocessing import RobustScaler, PolynomialFeatures
from pandarallel import pandarallel; pandarallel.initialize();
from sklearn.model_selection import GroupKFold, StratifiedKFold
from scipy.spatial import cKDTree

def get_overlay(img_path, organ, rle_str, img_shape, _alpha=0.999, _beta=0.35, _gamma=0):
    _img = tf_decode_tiff(img_path, to_numpy=True, to_rgb=True).astype(np.float32)
    _seg_rgb = (np.stack([rle_decode(rle_str, shape=img_shape, color=1),]*3, axis=-1)*O2C_MAP[orga
n]).astype(np.float32)
    seg_overlay = cv2.addWeighted(src1=_img, alpha=_alpha,
                                  src2=_seg_rgb, beta=_beta, gamma=_gamma)
    return seg_overlay/255.

def examine_id(df, ex_id=None, plot_overlay=True, print_meta=True, plot_original=False, plot_segment
ation=False, _figsize=(20,20)):
    """ Wrapper function to allow for easy visual exploration of an example """
    if ex_id is None:
        ex_id = df["id"].sample(1).values[0]
        print(f"\n... NO ID GIVEN... RANDOM ID CHOSEN: ID={ex_id} ...")

    print(f"\n... ID ({ex_id}) EXPLORATION STARTED ...\n\n")
    demo_ex = df[df["id"]==ex_id].squeeze()

    if print_meta:
        print(f"\n... WITH id=`{ex_id}` (organ=`{demo_ex['organ']}`) - WE HAVE THE FOLLOWING DEMO
EXAMPLE TO WORK FROM ... \n\n")
        display(demo_ex.to_frame())
```

Figure 9.3 Importation of libraries. (Source: [16]).

cells are from different organs like the kidney, lung, and spleen. This 3D design can effectively help determine all the important elements that are present inside the human organ, and the overall design becomes very much appropriate through accurate software implementation.

Here, in order to do this, the human organ has been subdivided in a unique manner., and during the entire segmentation, all the cells are clearly visible which can help maintain appropriate algorithm implementation.

The abovementioned picture is the bar chart of the number of segmentation masks per organ type. In this chart, the proper segmentation is clearly visible along with their count based on the organ that is very

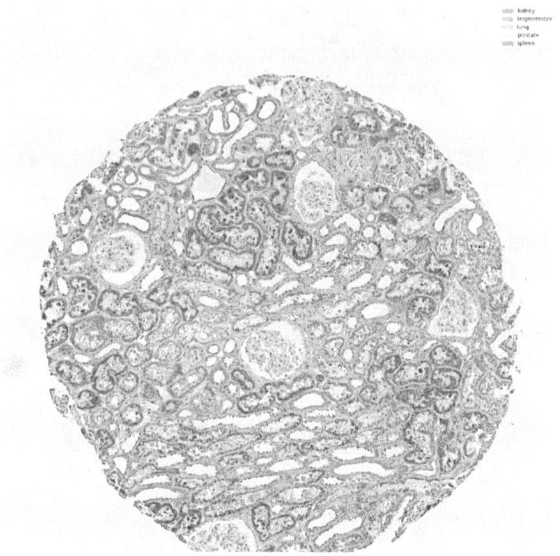

Figure 9.4 3D design. (Source: [17]).

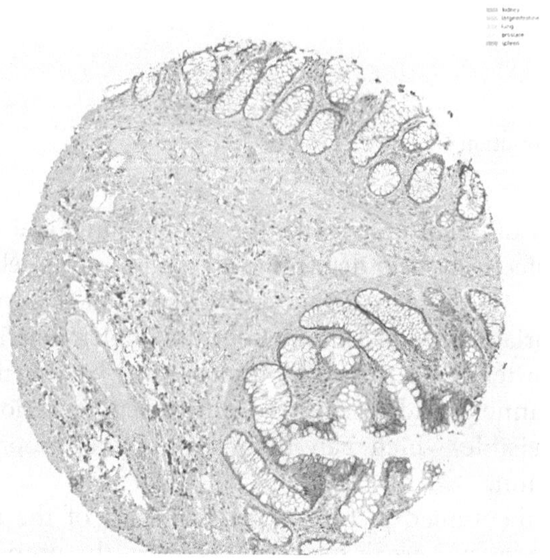

Figure 9.5 3D design. (Source: [17]).

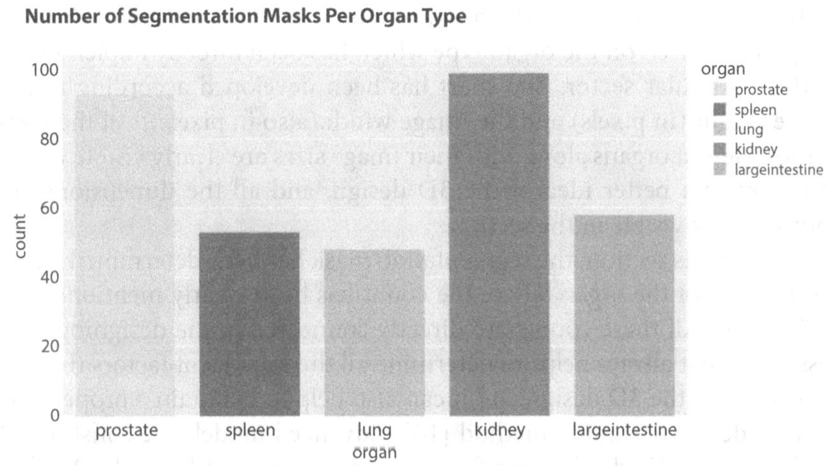

Figure 9.6 Bar chart. (Source: [17]).

much necessary to understand the whole process because without the segmentation count, it is not at all possible to determine all the important factors along with the credibility of this process [17]. All these bars representing particular organs have been differentiated by color, which can help to determine the organ very easily. It has been observed that the kidney has the greatest number of segmentation masks, and the lung has the lowest number of segmentation masks.

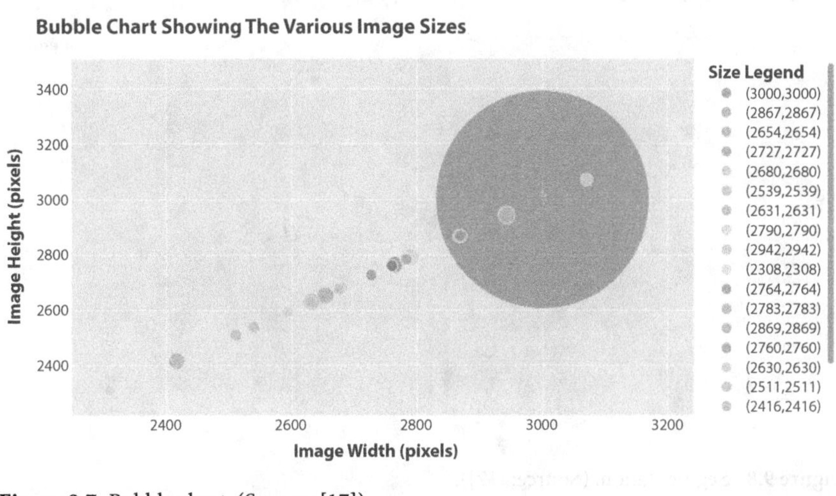

Figure 9.7 Bubble chart. (Source: [17]).

This is a bubble chart which is accurately showing different kinds of image sizes based on the organ type which has been directly implemented in this particular sector. The chart has been developed according to the image height (in pixels) and the image width (also in pixels). All the sizes of the different organs along with their image sizes are clearly visible which can provide a better idea of the 3D design, and all the dimensions are appropriately visible in the section.

Here, in this section, the segmentation mask has been determined based on the edge of the organ where the count has been clearly mentioned for each organ. All these counts are directly connected to the designing process because it always helps to determine all the important factors that are necessary for the 3D design and it can also help to maintain a proper pattern inside the designing method [18]. Advanced models are constrained by the use of LCD displays for the presentation of three-layered 3D information. In addition to their application in surgical planning, tangible health phantoms are tremendously beneficial for medical computation validation, medical knowledge, and healthcare. Thus, there is a great need for physically demanding medical phantoms for clinical practice and educational purposes [19].

Here, both gender and organ type were taken into account during segmentation, which is important for any human organ's design because they affect the design's pattern and shape. All these necessary elements are

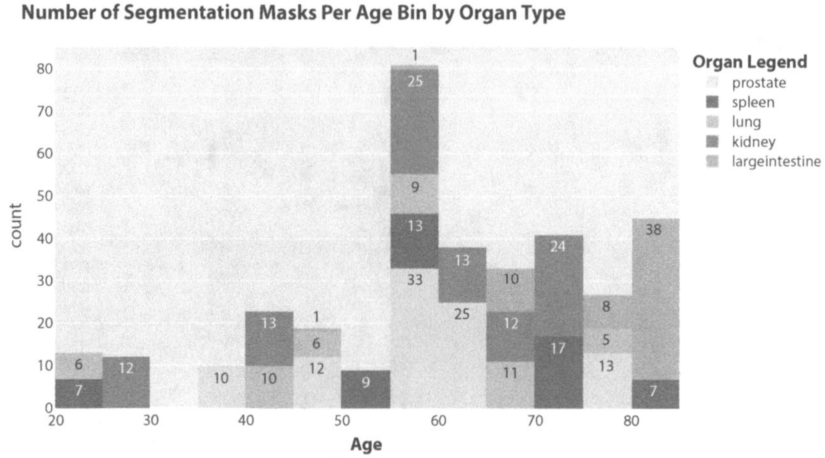

Figure 9.8 Segmentation. (Source: [17]).

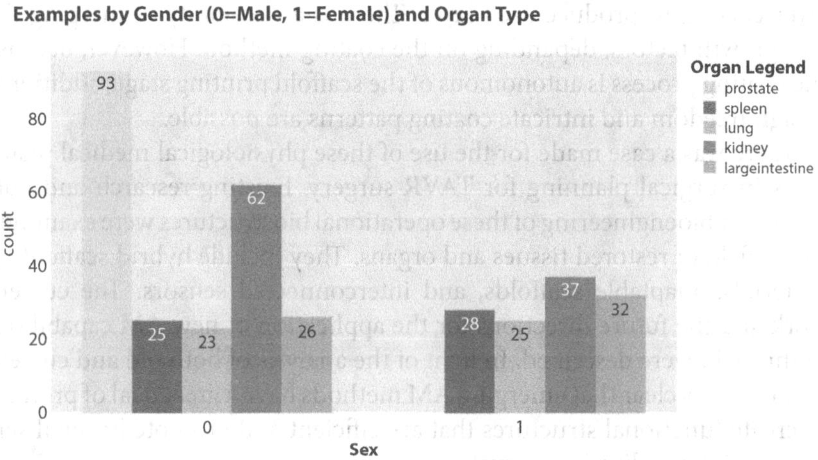

Figure 9.9 Bar chart. (Source: [17]).

clearly visible in the abovementioned picture which can provide enough information regarding the structure of all these organs.

9.5 Conclusion

In order to create network phantoms and regenerated tissues and organs, a variety of additive manufacturing (AM) techniques have been used. Discussions covered recent developments, past work, outcomes, and potential trends. Recent developments in the 3D printing of physiological, radiologically relevant, and tissue-mimicking medical phantoms have been described in the realm of functional medical phantoms. On the design and creation of physiological medical phantoms, a thorough explanation was given.

Direct-write technology can also be used in conjunction with 3D bioprinting. Traditionally, direct-write technologies are utilized in place of lithography or silk screening in the printed consumer market. The 3D bioprinting technology may perform selective surface alteration during scaffolding by incorporating direct-write technologies. *In situ* steroid hormone grafting employing extrusion and chemical jet printing methods is conceptualized and demonstrated in this study. Also less probably to happen during printing is the cross-contamination between the two growth ingredients. Instead of requiring a material preparation phase, the *in situ* grafting approach incorporates an additive manufacturing process and layer coating to produce each layer. There is a possibility of merging the two growth factors, depending on the coating method. However, because the coating process is autonomous of the scaffold printing stage, additional design freedom and intricate coating patterns are possible.

There was a case made for the use of these physiological medical phantoms in surgical planning for TAVR surgery. Existing research and outcomes for bioengineering of these operational biostructures were examined in the field of restored tissues and organs. They include hybrid scaffolding materials, adaptable scaffolds, and interconnected sensors. The current work and the future directions for the application of new AM capabilities in this field were described. In light of the analysis of both old and current research, it is clear that emerging AM methods have a great deal of promise to create functional structures that are efficient and promote hospital services and the realization of customized medicine.

References

1. Ali, M.A., Hu, C., Yttri, E.A., Panat, R., Recent advances in 3D printing of biomedical sensing devices. *Adv. Funct. Mater.*, *32*, 9, 2107671, 2022. https://doi.org/10.1002/adfm.202107671.
2. Carvalho, V., Gonçalves, I., Lage, T., Rodrigues, R.O., Minas, G., Teixeira, S.F., Moita, A.S., Hori, T., Kaji, H., Lima, R.A., 3D printing techniques and their applications to organ-on-a-chip platforms: A systematic review. *Sensors*, *21*, 9, 3304, 2021. https://doi.org/10.1452/adfm.666232.
3. Dabbagh, S.R., Sarabi, M.R., Birtek, M.T., Seyfi, S., Sitti, M., Tasoglu, S., 3D-printed microrobots from design to translation. *Nat. Commun.*, *13*, 1, 5875, 2022. https://doi.org/10.8745/7882412258.
4. Imanian, M.E., Kardan-Halvaei, M., Nasrollahi, F., Imanian, A., Montazerian, H., Nasrollahi, V., 3D printed flexible wearable sensors based on triply periodic minimal surface structures for biomonitoring applications. *Smart Mater. Struct.*, *32*, 1, 015015, 2022. https://doi.org/10.5482/61313216.
5. Ingber, D.E., Human organs-on-chips for disease modelling, drug development and personalized medicine. *Nat. Rev. Genet.*, *23*, 8, 467–491, 2022. https://doi.org/10.2066/66000525.
6. Jiang, Y., Islam, M.N., He, R., Huang, X., Cao, P.F., Advincula, R.C., Dahotre, N., Dong, P., Wu, H.F., Choi, W., Recent advances in 3D printed sensors: Materials, design, and manufacturing. *Adv. Mater. Technol.*, *8*, 2, 2200492, 2023. https://doi.org/10.5669/asdw65661.

7. Joshi, K., Kumar, M., Tripathi, A., Kumar, A., Sehgal, J., Barthwal, A., Latest trends in multi-modality medical image fusion: A generic review, in: *Rising Threats in Expert Applications and Solutions*, pp. 663–671, 2022, https://doi.org/10.5693/89663.31.
8. Kajtez, J., Wesseler, M.F., Birtele, M., Khorasgani, F.R., Rylander Ottosson, D., Heiskanen, A., Kamperman, T., Leijten, J., Martínez-Serrano, A., Larsen, N.B., Angelini, T.E., Embedded 3D printing in self-healing annealable composites for precise patterning of functionally mature human neural constructs. *Adv. Sci.*, *9*, 25, 2201392, 2022. https://doi.org/10.9632/218200020013.
9. Kalkal, A., Kumar, S., Kumar, P., Pradhan, R., Willander, M., Packirisamy, G., Kumar, S., Malhotra, B.D., Recent advances in 3D printing technologies for wearable (bio) sensors. *Addit. Manuf.*, *46*, 102088, 2021. https://doi.org/10.2666/ujhgfegtnloj78899.
10. Kimothi, S., Thapliyal, A., Akram, S.V., Singh, R., Gehlot, A., Mohamed, H.G., Anand, D., Ibrahim, M., Noya, I.D., Big data analysis framework for water quality indicators with assimilation of IoT and ML. *Electronics*, 11, 13, 1927, 2022. https://doi.org/10.2556/bykjn.76t.
11. Krishna, G., Singh, R., Gehlot, A., Akram, S.V., Priyadarshi, N., Twala, B., Digital technology implementation in battery-management systems for sustainable energy storage: Review, challenges, and recommendations. *Electronics*, 11, 17, 2695, 2022. https://doi.org/10.2323/hhlnn.43211.
12. Lancaster, M.A. and Huch, M., Disease modelling in human organoids. *Dis. Model Mech.*, *12*, 7, dmm039347, 2019. https://doi.org/10.2596/gfygbjhg4458.
13. Li, H., Liu, H., Sun, M., Huang, Y., Xu, L., 3D interfacing between soft electronic tools and complex biological tissues. *Adv. Mater.*, *33*, 3, 2004425, 2021. https://doi.org/10.8547/1413135120.
14. Nazir, A., Gokcekaya, O., Billah, K.M.M., Ertugrul, O., Jiang, J., Sun, J., Hussain, S., Multi-material additive manufacturing: A systematic review of design, properties, applications, challenges, and 3D printing of materials and cellular metamaterials. *Mater. Des.*, 20, 5, 111661, 2023. https://doi.org/10.2154/vfnnmkm6581.
15. Shrestha, J., RazaviBazaz, S., Aboulkheyr Es, H., Yaghobian Azari, D., Thierry, B., Ebrahimi Warkiani, M., Ghadiri, M., Lung-on-a-chip: The future of respiratory disease models and pharmacological studies. *Crit. Rev. Biotechnol.*, *40*, 2, 213–230, 2020. https://doi.org/10.1145/2245879312.
16. Singh, D., Singh, R., Gehlot, A., Akram, S.V., Priyadarshi, N., Twala, B., An imperative role of digitalization in monitoring cattle health for sustainability. *Electronics*, 11, 17, 2702, 2022. https://doi.org/10.1452/daw5511.
17. Singh, R., Akram, S.V., Gehlot, A., Buddhi, D., Priyadarshi, N., Twala, B., Energy system 4.0: Digitalization of the energy sector with an inclination towards sustainability. *Sensors*, 22, 17, 6619, 2022. https://doi.org/10.2564/562371.

18. Tang, H., Abouleila, Y., Si, L., Ortega-Prieto, A.M., Mummery, C.L., Ingber, D.E., Mashaghi, A., Human organs-on-chips for virology. *Trends Microbiol.*, *28*, 11, 934–946, 2020. https://doi.org/10.1458//5183.201.
19. Zhu, Z., Park, H.S., McAlpine, M.C., 3D printed deformable sensors. *Sci. Adv.*, *6*, 25, eaba5575, 2020. https://doi.org/10.1145/557671.

10

Fast Computing Network Infrastructure for Healthcare Systems Based on 6G Future Perspective

Ranjeet Yadav[1]*, S. L. Prathapa Reddy[2], Akshay Upmanyu[3], Ravi Kumar Sanapala[4], V. Malathy[5] and Umakant Bhaskar Gohatre[6]

[1]Electronics and Communication Engineering, Government Polytechnic Daman, Varkund, Nani Daman, UT Administration of Dadra and Nagar Haveli & Daman and Diu, India

[2]Electronics and Communication Engineering, KSRM College of Engineering, Kadapa, Andhra Pradesh, India

[3]University Institute of Media Studies, Chandigarh University, Chandigarh, India

[4]Department of ECE, St. Martin's Engineering College Secunderabad, Telangana, India

[5]Department of ECE, School of Engineering, SR University, Warangal, Telangana, India

[6]Department of Electronics and Telecommunications Engineering, Smt. Indira Gandhi College of Engineering, Navi Mumbai, Maharashtra, India

Abstract

To store and investigate information all the more real, new sixth-era (6G) foundations principally depend on the mental web of things (IoT). 6G is needed to convey super low latencies, high transfer speed, and improved assistance dependability that can proficiently deal with the connection among the hubs. All healthcare facilities should be outfitted with cutting-edge technology to give intelligent diagnostics, patient-driven treatment, and several other therapeutic concerns. In order to adopt a multimodal approach in an ambient assisted living (AAL) setting, will lay the groundwork for new innovations, enable adaptation, and provide services for multiple applications, including remote patient monitoring. Numerous network management components and terminal devices offer the capability for applications in the healthcare industry. These need a strong foundation to support

**Corresponding author*: ranjeet480@gmail.com: ORCID: 0000-0003-0891-8556

S. L. Prathapa Reddy: ORCID: 0000-0002-2322-6219

Kapil Joshi and Somil Kumar Gupta (eds.) Human Cancer Diagnosis and Detection Using Exascale Computing, (153–170) © 2024 Scrivener Publishing LLC

services that are time-sensitive. This article proposes a reference-based correspondence framework for the hubs and gadgets that are involved in continuous correspondence. The advanced clinical application for fruitful treatment and cunning assistance coordination is introduced by the component outlook parts of the 6G innovation.

***Keywords*:** 6G, network, future, Internet of Things (IoT), technology

10.1 Introduction

All facets of the physical and digital worlds are combined for the 6G network. Over the coming decades, increased automation is what we anticipate. Knowledge will need to be distributed across the communications network rather than the internal network due to the huge amount of objects. For safe and dependable 6G operations, peer communication and automated processing skills are more crucial. They were supporting new market thoughts that, by ensuring that network hardware and applications discuss well with each other, will empower a web time in 2030 and beyond. The capacity of sixth-era (6G) organizations to oversee more far-reaching portable associations for far-off information detection than the fifth (5G) network is one of their principal benefits. Subsequently, there is less gadget obstruction, which works on the assistance. The gadgets would work at bigger frequencies, i.e., somewhere in the range of 8 and 12 GHz, enabling smooth communication between sensors and communication devices without frequency overlap. By 2030, it is projected that there will be 97 billion mobile devices, increasing the present monthly consumption of 0.062 Zeta Bytes (ZB) into 5.016 Zeta Bytes (ZB). By 2030, 43 megacities will house more than 10 million residents, according to a survey. Clever management, technology, and information (ICT), versatile and strong, are expected to deal with the gigantic volumes of information created by cell phones and the biological systems of brilliant urban communities, including savvy medical care and insightful urban communities.

The Internet of Everything (IoE), among other things, generates massive quantities of data that feed the generated data. The United States Federal Communications Commission began selling access to these frequency channels in 2019. Ultra-precise positioning will be possible with 6G thanks to gradient sensors and high-resolution image technology, which have similar capabilities to biological eyes and ears. Competent robotics and complex algorithms may be present in 6G devices. With regard to handling enormous volumes of data and requiring various levels of QoS, 6G is designed to be an entirely AI-driven network infrastructure. Accepting these responsibilities allows for efficient analysis and summarizing, refining, and decision-making skills. A decentralized 6G framework will be overflowing with man-made intelligence, and many organization parts will utilize a unified figuring out on how to spread cooperative administrations.

10.2 Literature Review

A principal human need is to get better medical care, from determinations to therapies. Everybody ought to approach excellent medical services, which is presently feasible thanks to the production of innovatively progressive medical services applications. The hospital setting, virtual health, and humanitarian relief unit are the three main application domains that we categorize the medical system into in this article. A hospital has medical equipment and workers that have undergone extensive training to give patients the finest care possible. Effective communication between management, physicians, hospital professionals, and patients is necessary for the effective operation of the hospital [1]. Email, cells, pagers, and two-way radios are habitually used instruments for trans-correspondence inside the medical clinic. As of late, new procedures have been utilized to upgrade emergency clinic medical care administrations. For instance, keeping clinical records electronically decreases human mistakes, saves time, and upgrades correspondence among specialists and patients. Man-made consciousness (simulated intelligence) has likewise been acquainted with assistance specialists to analyze patients all the more precisely. The mechanical medical procedure has likewise been utilized to accomplish high accuracy while helping the clinical staff.

Emergency clinics rapidly experience packing in disaster circumstances because of the tremendous number of patients being hospitalized. Due to a lack of clinical staff and equipment, situation control is difficult. Because communicable diseases can spread from infected individuals to medical staff, things are particularly bad in pandemic scenarios. As a result, the main issue is to ensure staff safety while providing care to sick patients. Reducing the amount of time that patients and clinicians are in direct physical contact is one strategy to solve this problem. This can be performed by using IoMT and drones in the medical environment. There will be fewer experiences because IoMT wearable sensors and gadgets provide the option to screen and communicate patient well-being records to clinicians over the web. On the other hand, robots have various purposes, including moving supplies, carrying out clinical assessments, and cleaning the patients' current circumstances [2]. In the near future, it is anticipated that these gadgets and robots will be used extensively to protect and support hospital staff members and doctors.

These innovative improvements depend on the clinic's correspondence organization and need for a protected, trustworthy, and fast correspondence connection. To give correspondence further developed limit, versatility, area, and restriction, an RF-based correspondence organization, or Wi-Fi organization, has been generally utilized in emergency clinics. Sadly, electromagnetic obstruction (EMI) can slow down the clinical gear, which restricts the utilization of Wi-Fi organizations. The unpredictable actual format of the medical clinic likewise frustrates the section of high-recurrence signals by means of hindrances and causes inclusion issues. Additionally, the established Wi-Fi networks were not intended to handle the increased traffic load during disasters. Consequently, a Wi-Fi network is unable to satisfy the need for communication in terms of both capacity and coverage when there is a huge patient burden. Also, enormous associations, incredible reliability, and low idleness are required for the continuous investigation of well-being records utilizing IoMT gadgets. In a crisis, even a slight deferral and the absence of a network could make lamentable impacts. Specifically, to benefit from robot innovation, medical clinics require a very reliable and low-idleness association [3]. To safeguard the patients' security and indispensable data from undesirable access, it is additionally fundamental to secure the correspondence connection utilizing state-of-the-art safety efforts.

In the advanced world, far-off medical care is generally used to give clinical consideration to people who cannot travel or who live in rustic areas. This help is upheld in two ways: media transmission and distant well-being screening. In telemedicine, specialists assess, analyze, and treat patients by utilizing video chatting or looking into electronic well-being data actually. It may very well be presented from homes or fundamental well-being communities under the direction of a paramedic. The holographic portrayal is expected to be utilized sooner rather than later, supplanting the top-notch video remotely coordinating that is at present utilized for telemedicine. IoMT advances like wearables and remote individual region organizations (WBAN) have started to be generally utilized for distant well-being observation. Additionally, the utilization of constant observation frameworks improves personal satisfaction for older people by recognizing crisis circumstances by utilizing sensors and giving quick help. However, a significant impediment to achieving this objective is the reception of new innovations, especially among the old. Individuals who require routine consideration, for example, diabetics, benefit from the portion change made conceivable by computerized medication [4]. To safeguard the patient's protection and well-being, these strategies need a solid and reliable connection.

With the appearance of the coronavirus, online medical services are being urged with the end goal to eliminate contamination spread and emergency clinic patient volume. Distant clinical benefits are entirely subject to the correspondence organization. Because of correspondence hardships, for example, the requirement for high information rates for holographic telepresence, high transfer speed and contribution for IoMT, super low power data trade for biosensors, unwavering quality, and quick information for a material web-based portable medical procedure and computerized medical services, numerous applications have not yet been researched [5]. Getting and keeping up with security and touchy data about patients is one of the previously mentioned issues. Especially in distant medical services, when all gadgets and sensors convey information to the emergency clinic's clinical staff or transfer it to a web entry, the advanced correspondence connection is defenseless to security gambles such as listening, sticking, and ridiculing. In the event that the correspondence framework is uncertain, a busybody or spoofer could change the information in the electronic site, which could bring about fatalities, and get the patient's imperative data. In this way, there is a need to guard the actual divert notwithstanding cryptographic-based arrangements.

Well-being frameworks have raised a ruckus around town by catastrophic events, particularly pandemics, in light of the extra quiet motion. In these conditions, field medical clinics can be urgent for disconnecting pandemic casualties, opening up space in different medical clinics and empowering better administration of scant medical clinic assets like hardware. These emergency clinics are presently used to isolate people who are sick and give them vital consideration. The utilization of robots specifically is assisting with decreasing how much time patients and experts are locked-in. Conveying food and clinical supplies, gathering test tests, cleaning patient regions, and different obligations are totally done utilizing these innovations. IoMT-based brilliant clinical gadgets, like shrewd thermometers and savvy wristbands, can be utilized to screen the patient's important bodily functions. Additionally, by utilizing telemedicine and distant medical care administrations, neighborhood clinic clinicians can talk with patients at the field medical clinic.

10.3 Research Methodology

Secondary analysis with the model concept is used to gather information related to the topic. Despite the relationship with 6G innovations and vision, this chapter offers solutions to the communication issues the healthcare system is currently facing. The figure beneath presents the sending of 6G advances in various regions of the medical care framework to beat the correspondence challenges.

The fifth-generation (5G) technologies deliver quality healthcare with advancement compared with preceding generations. The creation of new mobile generation data is necessary to close the gap in security, information, Wi-Fi connectivity, clean energy, etc. So, the 6G objective is to use intelligent communication technology to convert society into a safe and completely connected computerized one.

10.4 Analysis and Discussion

Forceful examination of the 6G vision separates its empowering advances into (i) a huge range of data transfer capacity (VLC and THz), (ii) inserted earthly aeronautical organizations (UAV, HAPs, and satellites), (iii) energy-effective and network climate knowledge (AmBC, reconfigurable intelligent surface (RIS), and blockchain), and (iv) all-encompassing security worldview (PLS and blockchain (BC)). Sub-THz groups are needed to empower the association with extremely high data transmission required

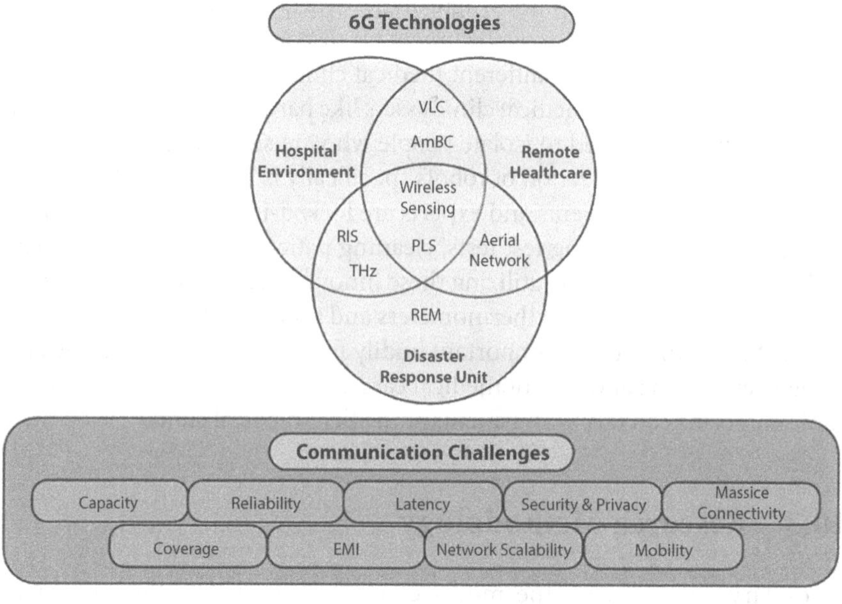

Figure 10.1 6G technologies. (Source: [14]).

for 6G organizations on account of the absence of a range in lower recurrence groups. Other range assets, including VLC, are likewise expected to be utilized as reasonable competitors to serve the RF range that utilizes a normal lighting foundation for rapid remote situating and restriction, especially inside. Versatile IoT correspondences would not be confined to homegrown associations, and all things considered, they will be developing to traverse the space [6]. The approach comprises merging terrestrial communication networks with UAV or other non-terrestrial networks (NTN) technologies to close the digital divide and handle remote coverage with an expanded line-of-sight (LOS) of believability, flexibility, and scalability benefits. Energy efficiency is crucial for connected object (IoT) devices; hence, AmBC uses ambient signals produced by traditional RF systems, like FM, TV, and Wi-Fi, to provide ultra-low power communication. In order to deliver an intelligent information network and enhanced coverage and capacity, RIS is an inactive or moderate surface that contains antenna elements. RIS does this by intelligently modifying radio waves before reflection. With the addition of PLS and cryptography, 6G will offer an alternative to cryptography-based security by offering a fresh approach to the security problem. BC algorithms can be used to ensure the confidentiality of sensitive data as well as its security. The issues of future systems regarding transmission security and user privacy will be resolved by these solutions.

Limit, inclusion, availability, reliability and network availability correspondence, detection, security, and protection are the fundamental correspondence gives influence many pieces of the medical services framework. The difficulties in further developing the medical care framework by embracing 6G advancements are tended to in this part.

Network administrators are focusing on the turn of events and the production of correspondence foundation for calamity situations such as the coronavirus pandemic, where resource augmentation is one of the main problems. For instance, when COVID-19 began, a mobile network in Turkey observed a rise in data use of up to 35%. Because of expanded patient burdens and far and wide utilization of IoMT gadgets, this development is likewise apparent in medical care frameworks. The ongoing RF correspondence foundation, which depends on low recurrence groups, is not satisfactory to support patients and guests, both locally and from a distance. To build the organization's general limit, ultra-massive multiple-input, multiple-output (MIMO) and the use of high-frequency bands should be introduced.

Alternatively, VLC can be used to increase indoor capacity. By sharing the client's trouble, as shown in the accompanying figure, this innovation can upgrade the ongoing RF-based correspondence organization. THz's super high transfer speed can deal with incredibly high information rates for holographic telepresence utilized for far-off clinical treatment [7]. Additionally, ethereal organizations like HAPs can be utilized to scale the organization, helping the medical care correspondence framework's ability for field emergency clinics. When clinics need to expand their capacity following an emergency, RIS-integrated UAVs are employed to help with the capacity issue.

The RIS-coordinated UAV's capability for all-encompassing full-point reflection enables it to make use of open channels from neighboring cells, permitting unrestricted mobility and signal coverage in the direction of the medical clinic to address capacity issues [8]. In order to benefit from both cognitive radio technology and AmBC for remote communication and ultra-low-powered communication, respectively, these devices can support AmBC technology, also referred to as harmonious radio. Along these lines, it is possible to simultaneously improve connectivity and energy efficiency. However, it is difficult to maintain a high level of service (QoS) with these technologies.

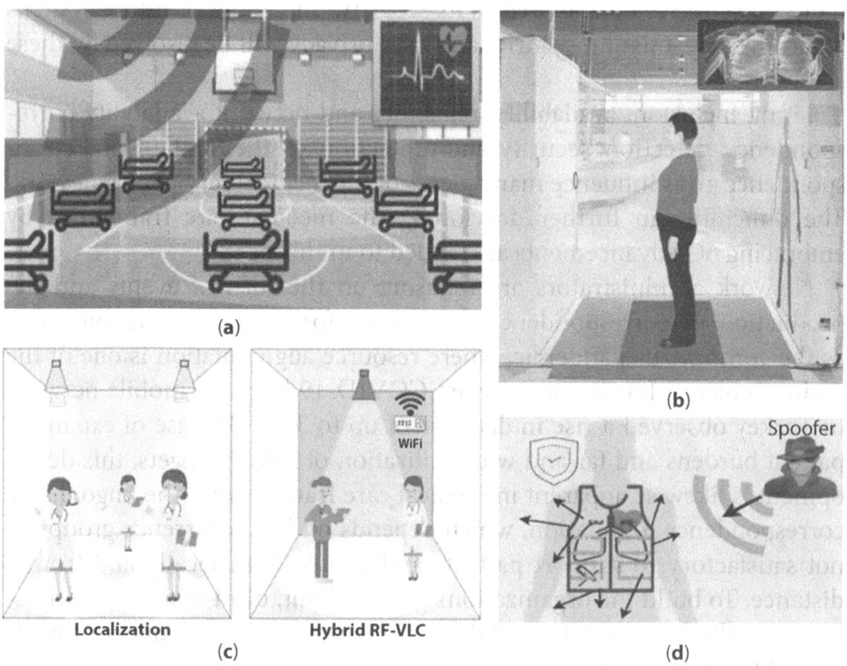

Figure 10.2 Technological impact. (Source: [15]).

Due to an assortment of elements, amazing inclusion and availability are important in each setting in medical care frameworks. Due to the mind-boggling actual format and sensitive clinical gear, network inclusion is required in medical clinics. Today, Wi-Fi networks are being used inside emergency clinics for correspondence [9]. Sadly, serious EMI issues limit inclusion in fragile areas. A half-and-half VLC-RF network can be made to give inclusion in these districts. In emergency clinics, RIS can be introduced in explicit areas such as walls and roofs to improve coverage and safeguard RF-restricted regions.

In rural locations with inadequate network availability or QoS, there are significant coverage challenges associated with remote health. Subsequently, the absence of inclusion brings about an absence of a network, passing on a sizable populace without admittance to telehealth offices. At field emergency clinics, inclusion issues are additionally present. In such a manner, airborne organizations, particularly UAVs, HAPs, and satellites, are among the best contender for inclusion extension [10]. By means of their utilization as ground stations or handing-off hubs, these organizations can further develop inclusion. Huge-scope specially appointed organizations, gadget-to-gadget (D2D) transmission, and cell base stations are different procedures for further developing inclusion. However, NTNs have higher inclusion in contrast with different organizations.

In catastrophic circumstances where the network infrastructure has collapsed, flexibility and networking scalability can be provided through hybrid aerial–terrestrial networks. For remote health and disaster response-related services in healthcare systems, constant connection with a high level of dependability is essential. For instance, in the near future, extremely dependable and low latency connectivity will be necessary for tactile-based or automated surgery performed by robots employing artificial intelligence (AI) and machine learning (ML). Consequently, migrating the administrations toward the edge inside the neighborhood of patients and utilizing the edge data can bring down the dormancy and lift the nature of the organization association.

For constant observation and the exchange of touchy information, including ECG and EEG, smart ambulances with medical equipment need exceptionally dependable and low latency connectivity with hospital or medical professionals. Joint radar communication (JRC), a relatively novel idea, can be utilized to empower dependable detection and V2X correspondence for the protected character of savvy ambulances.

Additionally, the usage of AI-assisted cognitive radios and Radio Environment Maps (REM) can be used to reduce handover problems, such as delay jitter, brought on by a patient's movement with embedded medical devices. Also, taking advantage of the broadening in composite RF-VLC, earth perception organizations might give the essential trustworthy and low dormancy availability in inside and outside settings, separately. In the future, communication among healthcare professionals, patients, and medical equipment will be made possible via the creation of a next-generation wireless network. The sixth-generation (6G) of wireless technology, which is anticipated to be the next significant development in wireless communication following 5G [19–24], provides the foundation for the idea.

This infrastructure's objectives are to increase patient outcomes, decrease healthcare expenditures, and improve the efficiency and quality of healthcare delivery. Healthcare professionals will be able to access and exchange medical information more quickly and correctly with speedier seamless connectivity, which will result in improved diagnosis and treatments. The network infrastructure will also facilitate the creation and use of emerging technologies including wearable medical devices, remote monitoring, and telemedicine [11]. With the use of these technologies, healthcare professionals will be able to monitor patients virtually, cut down on in-person visits, and give patients more individualized treatment.

Overall, the idea of a fast computer network infrastructure for healthcare systems based on a 6G future view is a significant development in the technology of healthcare, with the potential to enhance patient outcomes and completely transform the way healthcare is provided [12]. One of the most significant and quickly expanding sectors in the world is healthcare. Technology advancements have completely changed the healthcare industry, enabling patients to get more effective and efficient care. The creation of a quick computing network infrastructure for health systems based on a 6G future vision is the next significant step in this transformation [13]. Although it is still in the research stage, 6G wireless technology is anticipated to offer quicker and more dependable communication capabilities than the existing 5G [25–30] technology. It is estimated that 6G would be introduced around 2030 and feature data transmission rates of up to 1 terabyte per second (TBps), which would make it 50 times faster than 5G [31–34]. One sector that would gain substantially from 6G technology is indeed the healthcare sector. Healthcare professionals will be able to send data more quickly and accurately thanks to the new network, which will help them give patients better, more individualized treatment [14]. Remote monitoring is one application of 6G technology in healthcare. Healthcare professionals may remotely and in real-time check their patient's health state without having to make in-person visits. With 6G, remote monitoring can be carried out more quickly and accurately, which might help avoid significant health issues.

Telemedicine is another application for 6G technology in the medical field. Technology is used in telemedicine to offer patients virtual medical care.

Careful planning and consideration of a number of factors are necessary when creating a fast computer network architecture for healthcare systems. A few of the crucial components required to create such an infrastructure are as follows:

High-speed Internet connectivity: To enable prompt and dependable data transfer between healthcare professionals, patients, and other stakeholders, a rapid computer network architecture needs high-speed Internet access.

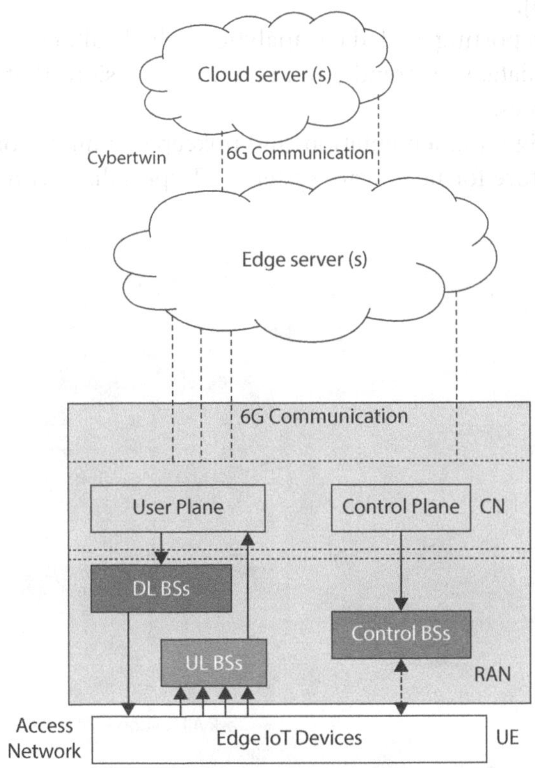

Figure 10.3 Network infrastructure. (Source: [16]).

Networking hardware supports data transfer across a network and comprises routers, switches, firewalls, and other networking devices [15].
Servers: Electronic health records (EHRs), medical imaging, and other clinical data all require servers in order to be stored and accessed.

Large volumes of clinical data must be stored and managed using storage technologies like storage area network (SAN) and network-attached storage (NAS).

To secure the network infrastructure from cyberattacks and guarantee the confidentiality, authenticity, and availability of patient data, the security architecture consists of firewalls, password security, and systems to detect intrusions.
Redundancy: Redundancy ensures that, in the case of hardware failure or other disturbances, the broadband network can continue to function. Power sources, backup servers, and data storage options are all included.
Interoperability standards: For the interchange of healthcare data between various systems and stakeholders, interoperability norms such as Health Level Seven (HL7) and Fast Healthcare Interoperability Resources (FHIR) are crucial [16].

Tools for reporting and data analytics help healthcare professionals study clinical data, spot trends, and take wise decisions that will enhance patient outcomes.

For the design, implementation, and upkeep of a quick computing network architecture for healthcare systems, IT specialists with expertise are a must [17].

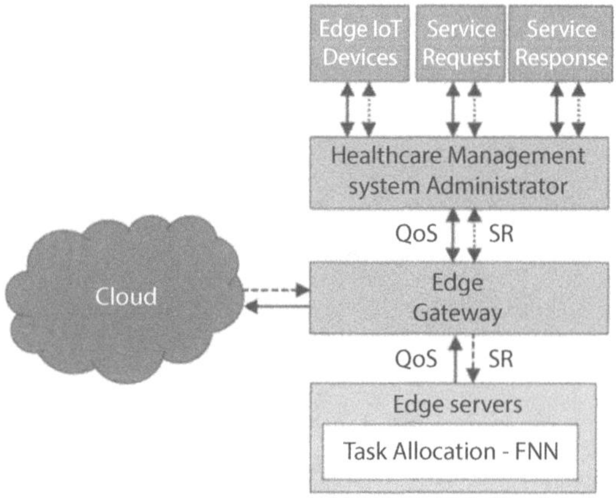

Figure 10.4 Cloud infrastructure. (Source: [17]).

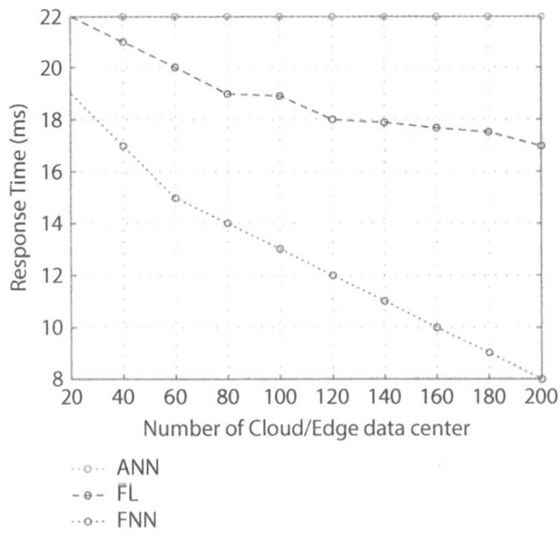

Figure 10.5 Plot. (Source: [18]).

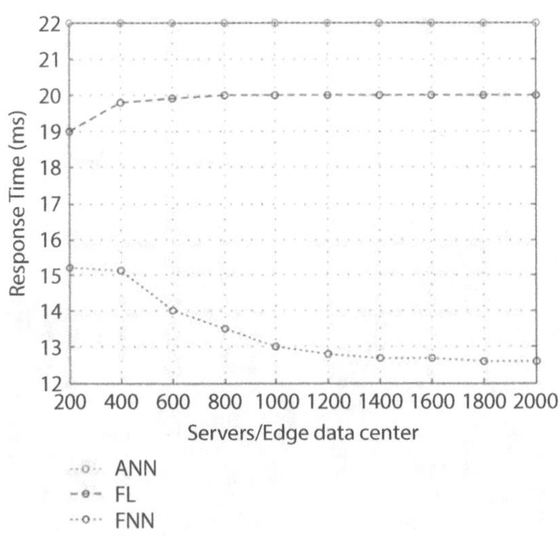

Figure 10.6 Plot. (Source: [18]).

The evolution graph has been properly executed between the response time and the number of cloud and data center that is required for this particular framework for the healthcare system. In order to implement this plot, different values have been taken which can appropriately be associated with the overall structure of the entire healthcare system through implementing the network process of 6G.

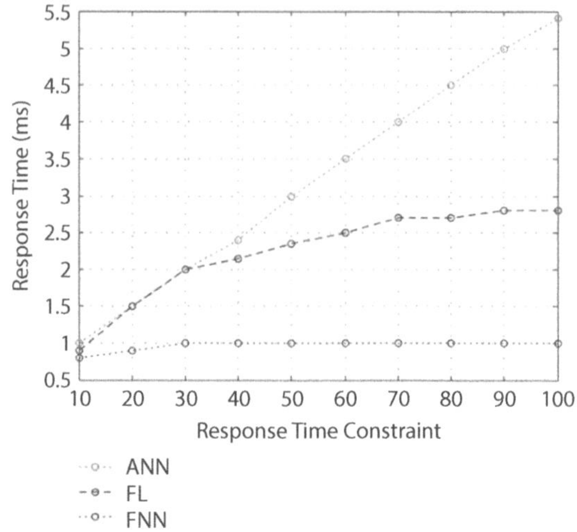

Figure 10.7 Plot. (Source: [18]).

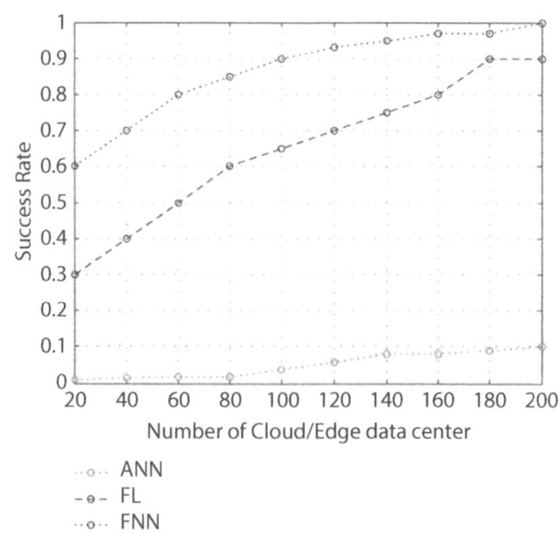

Figure 10.8 Plot. (Source: [18]).

In this plot, the axis is slightly different and the line that has been executed through implementing values are also slightly different from each other. Three different values have been properly executed: the first one is the response time with respect to the influence of the entire data center, the second one is the resource utilization with respect to the influence of the particular data center, and the third one is the success rate with respect to the influence of the data center [18]. All these three values have been properly executed with the help of different elements of the network infrastructure.

This graph has been executed between the response time along with the response time constraints. The first one deals with the response time with respect to the response time constraints, and the second one is the resource utilization with respect to the success rate.

The distributed resource allocation parameters of the FNN wireless health system are used in this study to distribute the best resources to the edge devices. FL changes are put into practice to accommodate the scattered settings of edge intelligence. The design of computing and storage reducing costs in the network edge and in hidden units has been a great success in terms of enhanced mean success rate, greater resource utilization, and better network throughput. Comparing conventional approaches to the FNN wireless healthcare model, dispersed deep learning models show improved scalability. Metaheuristic models may be used in the future to develop shear intelligence for identifying the best resource allocation for edge devices.

10.5 Conclusion

During pandemic and emergency situations, the 6G correspondence organizations representing things to come ought to be worked to help medical services with state-of-the-art correspondence innovation. In case of a pandemic, later on, 6G-upheld medical services correspondence can lessen the unfortunate results and deal with speedy responses. The healthcare system will undergo major changes as a result of technologies like IoMT, VLC, cordless sensor, PLS, and autonomous cars. Other technologies, such as waveforms, which are not currently covered by 6G aspirations but which may be useful in patient care may address issues concerning capacity, security, dependability, etc.

Together with this, medical technology is advancing quickly, from wireless IoMT to injectable IoBNT with neuralink to analyze brain activity and enhance the quality of life. These tools will help with early detection as well as remote delivery of routine healthcare during pandemic outbreaks. Yet, there is still work to be done in order to precisely integrate these tools into the public health system for a practical case. Moreover, communication technology research needs to be done on how to deal with psychological consequences that occur during lockdown. Ultimately, a complete clinical framework that can convey all expected administrations in emergency situations should be created.

References

1. Aggarwal, S., Kumar, N., Tanwar, S., Blockchain-envisioned UAV communication using 6G networks: Open issues, use cases and future directions. *IEEE IoT J.*, *8*, 7, 5416–5441, 2020. https://doi.org/10.1109/JIOT.2020.3020819.
2. Chavhan, S., Shift to 6G: Exploration on trends, vision, requirements, technologies, research, and standardization efforts. *Sustain. Energy Technol. Assess.*, *54*, 102666, 2022. https://doi.org/10.1452/564654.3020819.
3. Dao, N.N., Pham, Q.V., Tu, N.H., Thanh, T.T., Bao, V.N.Q., Lakew, D.S., Cho, S., Survey on aerial radio access networks: Toward a comprehensive 6G access infrastructure. *IEEE Commun. Surv. Tutor.*, *23*, 2, 1193–1225, 2021. https://doi.org/10.8789/148645131218.
4. Dua, S., Kumar, S.S., Albagory, Y., Ramalingam, R., Dumka, A., Singh, R., Rashid, M., Gehlot, A., Alshamrani, S.S., AlGhamdi, A.S., Developing a speech recognition system for recognizing tonal speech signals using a convolutional neural network. *Appl. Sci.*, *12*, 12, 6223, 2022. https://doi.org/10.25845/66559.
5. Friha, O. and Ferrag, M.A., Blockchain technology for 6G communication networks: A vision for the future, in: *Cybersecurity Issues in Emerging Technologies*, pp. 77–96, CRC Press, UK, 2021, https://doi.org/10.8569/54419.
6. Gehlot, A., Malik, P.K., Singh, R., Akram, S.V., Alsuwian, T., Dairy 4.0: Intelligent communication ecosystem for the cattle animal welfare with blockchain and IoT enabled technologies. *Appl. Sci.*, *12*, 14, 7316, 2022. https://doi.org/10.8965/2222fggas.
7. Imoize, A.L., Adedeji, O., Tandiya, N., Shetty, S., 6G enabled smart infrastructure for sustainable society: Opportunities, challenges, and research roadmap. *Sensors*, *21*, 5, 1709, 2021. https://doi.org/10.7896/7458549.
8. Janjua, M.B., Duranay, A.E., Arslan, H., Role of wireless communication in healthcare system to cater disaster situations under 6G vision. *Front. Commun. Netw.*, *1*, 610879, 2020. https://doi.org/10.9687/4448856465fsd.
9. Kaiser, M.S., Zenia, N., Tabassum, F., Mamun, S.A., Rahman, M.A., Islam, M.S., Mahmud, M., December. 6G access network for intelligent internet of healthcare things: Opportunity, challenges, and research directions, in: *Proceedings of International Conference on Trends in Computational and Cognitive Engineering: Proceedings of TCCE 2020*, pp. 317–328, Springer Singapore, Singapore, 2020, https://doi.org/10.9987/564487419.
10. Kulkani, N.P., Mantri, D.S., Prasad, N.R., Pawar, P.M., Prasad, R., 6G future vision: Requirements, design issues and applications, in: *6G Enabling Technologies*, pp. 23–43, River Publishers, India, 2023, https://doi.org/10.1111/415448851212665.
11. Kumari, A., Gupta, R., Tanwar, S., Amalgamation of blockchain and IoT for smart cities underlying 6G communication: A comprehensive review. *Comput. Commun.*, *172*, 102–118, 2021. https://doi.org/10.8789/5299418.

12. Mihai, S., Yaqoob, M., Hung, D.V., Davis, W., Towakel, P., Raza, M., Karamanoglu, M., Barn, B., Shetve, D., Prasad, R.V., Venkataraman, H., Digital twins: A survey on enabling technologies, challenges, trends and future prospects. *IEEE Commun. Surv. Tutor.*, 68, 1–16, 2022. https://doi.org/10.8754/41584511351.
13. Nayak, S. and Patgiri, R., 6G communication technology: A vision on intelligent healthcare, in: *Health Informatics: A Computational Perspective in Healthcare*, pp. 1–18, 2021, https://doi.org/10.8795/158945231681.
14. Nova, S.N., Rahman, M.S., Chakraborty, C., Patients' health surveillance model using IoT and 6G technology, in: *Green Technological Innovation for Sustainable Smart Societies: Post Pandemic Era*, pp. 191–209, 2021, https://doi.org/10.9687/2653329.
15. Ray, P.P., A perspective on 6G: Requirement, technology, enablers, challenges and future road map. *J. Syst. Archit.*, *118*, 102180, 2021. https://doi.org/10.9654/52659659.
16. Shahzadi, S., Iqbal, M., Chaudhry, N.R., 6g vision: Toward future collaborative cognitive communication (3c) systems. *IEEE Commun. Stand. Mag.*, *5*, 2, 60–67, 2021. https://doi.org/10.8547/1564684623.
17. Singh, R., Akram, S.V., Gehlot, A., Buddhi, D., Priyadarshi, N., Twala, B., Energy System 4.0: Digitalization of the energy sector with inclination towards sustainability. *Sensors*, *22*, 17, 6619, 2022. https://doi.org/10.8455/4861312312.
18. Yap, K.Y., Chin, H.H., Klemeš, J.J., Future outlook on 6G technology for renewable energy sources (RES). *Renewable Sustain. Energy Rev.*, *167*, 112722, 2022. https://doi.org/10.85478/56448451121.
19. Yadav, R. and Tripathi, A.A., Survey on hybrid, 3D, interference mitigation and secure data beamforming techniques for 5G system. *Wireless Pers. Commun.*, 114, 883–900, 2020. https://doi.org/10.1007/s11277-020-07397-w.
20. Yadav, R. and Tripathi, A., Enhanced optimization assisted interference mitigation with vertical beamforming in 3D MIMO-OFDMA for 5G wireless communication network. *Int. J. Pervasive Comput. Commun.*, *19*, 2, 191–210, 2023. https://doi.org/10.1108/IJPCC-01-2021-0024.
21. Yadav, R. and Tripathi., A., 3D MIMO beamforming using spatial distance SVM algorithm and interference mitigation for 5G wireless communication network. *J. Case Inf. Technol.*, *24*, 4, 1–26, 2022. http://doi.org/10.4018/JCIT.296717.
22. Yadav, R., Tripathi, A., Pathak, S., Gill, H.S., 5G and beyond networks for 3D MIMO using artificial intelligence in 5G network. *J. Phys. Conf. Ser.*, 2273, 1, 012007, IOP Publishing. 2022, May. http://doi.org/10.1088/1742-6596/2273/1/012007.
23. Yadav, R. and Tripathi, A., Design of a scheduling algorithm in 3D MIMO beamforming 5G systems for interference mitigation. *2021 7th International Conference on Advanced Computing and Communication Systems (ICACCS)*, Coimbatore, India, pp. 1690–1694, 2021.

24. Yadav, R., Raman, R., Rana, A., Gangodkar, D., Tiwari, M., Kiranmayee, P., A novel PSO-based channel allocation system for interference in 5G and higher-level wireless communication systems. *2022 11th International Conference on System Modeling & Advancement in Research Trends (SMART)*, Moradabad, India, pp. 644–648, 2022.
25. Yadav, R., Ritambhara, K.K., Vaigandla, Ghantasala, G.S.P., Singh, R., Gangodkar, D., The block chain technology to protect data access using intelligent contracts mechanism security framework for 5G networks. *2022 5th International Conference on Contemporary Computing and Informatics (IC3I)*, Uttar Pradesh, India, pp. 108–112, 2022.
26. Singh, R., Khurana, V., Sambasiva Reddy, M., Yadav, R., Jangir, R., Kapila, D., "Wireless communication design using neural networks and deep learning. *2022 International Conference on Innovative Computing, Intelligent Communication and Smart Electrical Systems (ICSES)*, Chennai, India, pp. 1–6, 2022.
27. Venkatanaresh, M. *et al.*, Effective proactive routing protocol using smart nodes system. *Measurement: Sensors*, 24, 100456, 2022. https://doi.org/10.1016/j.measen.2022.100456.
28. Shinde, V.B., Yadav, R., Singh, V., Prakash, A., Sarojwal, A., Akram, S.V., Linear Analysis of RC Tower with wind loading and telecommunication system. *2022 International Conference on Innovative Computing, Intelligent Communication and Smart Electrical Systems (ICSES)*, Chennai, India, pp. 1–6, 2022.
29. Kumari, P.R., Chaturvedi, A., Juyal, A., Pant, B., Mydhili, S.K., Yadav, R., Deep learning-based hybrid system for multiuser MIMO systems. *2022 5th International Conference on Contemporary Computing and Informatics (IC3I)*, Uttar Pradesh, India, pp. 1596–1601, 2022.
30. Singh, D., Keerthi Nayani, A.S., Sundar Rajan, M., Yadav, R., Alanya-Beltran, J., Chakravarthi, M.K., Implementation of virual instrumentation for signal acquisition and processing. *2022 International Conference on Innovative Computing, Intelligent Communication and Smart Electrical Systems (ICSES)*, Chennai, India, pp. 1–4, 2022.
31. Tie, P. *et al.*, Optimal design of supply chain inventory information forecasting and control system in cloud environment for biomedical instruments. *J. Eng.*, 11, 2022, 1067–1075, 2022. https://doi.org/10.1049/tje2.12177.
32. Wang, B. *et al.*, Vibration compensation for railway track displacement monitoring system using biomedical image processing concept. *J. Eng.*, *11*, 2022, 1076–1085, 2022. https://doi.org/10.1049/tje2.12178.
33. Sasikala, T.S. *et al.*, Improved RAL routing protocol to identify duplicate packets in QoS. *Measurement:Sensors*, 24, 100489, 2022. https://doi.org/10.1016/j.measen.2022.100489.
34. Wang, S. *et al.*, Wireless sensor network technology for vibration condition monitoring of mechanical equipment. *Electrica*, *23*, 2, 366–375, 2023.

11

Analysis of Multimodality Fusion of Medical Image Segmentation Employing Deep Learning

G. Santhakumar[1], Dattatray G. Takale[2], Swati Tyagi[3]*, Raju Anitha[4], Mohit Tiwari[5] and Joshuva Arockia Dhanraj[6]

[1]Electronics and Communication Engineering, Sri Krishna College of Technology, Coimbatore, Tamil Nadu, India
[2]Computer Engineering Vishwakarma Institute of Information Technology, SPPU, Pune, India
[3]University of Delaware, Newark, DE, USA
[4]Department of Computer Science & Engineering, Koneru Lakshmaiah Education Foundation, Vijayawada, India
[5]Department of Computer Science and Engineering, Bharati Vidyapeeth's College of Engineering, Delhi A-4, Rohtak Road, Paschim Vihar, Delhi, India
[6]Centre for Automation and Robotics (ANRO), Department of Mechatronics Engineering, Hindustan Institute of Technology and Science, Padur, Chennai, India

Abstract
Medical imaging methods using multiple modalities are used more frequently in both clinical settings and academic studies. The use of ensemble learning and associated multimodal image processing has grown quickly and has a special benefit for medical uses. This study suggested a deep learning (DL) convolutional neural network (CNN) method for fusing multimodal medical images that is effective. The multimodality medical images that were used as input for the experimental study included computed tomography (CT), magnetic resonance imaging (MRI), and positron emission tomography (PET). The proposed approach utilizes a Siamese convolutional network to generate a weight map that incorporates the movement of pixels from multiple medical images. To meet a level of accuracy similar to human visual recognition, the medical image fusion

**Corresponding author*: swatyagi@udel.edu
Joshuva Arockia Dhanraj: ORCID: https://orcid.org/0000-0001-5048-7775

Kapil Joshi and Somil Kumar Gupta (eds.) Human Cancer Diagnosis and Detection Using Exascale Computing, (171–184) © 2024 Scrivener Publishing LLC

operation is performed through a multiscale approach with the use of medical image pyramids. The decomposed coefficients are automatically adjusted using a comparison-based approach which is local in nature. The best fused multimodal medical images with the highest quality, quickest processing times, and best visualization in terms of both visual quality and objective evaluation criteria are produced experimentally using the suggested fusion methods.

Keywords: Multimodal fusion, deep learning, medical image segmentation

11.1 Introduction

As more sophisticated methods and tools have become available, the use of multiple modalities with a similar focus has become increasingly popular in the area of biomedical imaging. PET and CT acquisition, for instance, are now routinely performed in the clinical setting for a variety of uses [1, 26]. CT and MRI, which offer specifics on anatomical frameworks via elevated visibility and geometric determination to better characterize nodules, and functional imaging methods like PET, which lack anatomical description but offer numeric metabolic and operational information about diseases, can be used to better understand diseases [27]. The concurrent documenting of functional MRI (fMRI) and electroencephalography (EEG), which provides higher geometric determination and temporal determination on brain dynamics, is another frequently used multimodal imaging method in neuroscience research [2].

As a result, numerous analyses utilizing computer-aided detection systems and multimodal biomedical imaging have been created. The underlying assumption is that numerous imaging modalities contain a wealth of information that is distinct from and useful in conjunction with one another [29].

For instance, autonomous recognition of solitary pulmonary nodules was applied in one DL-based system [3] by first recognizing questionable areas from CT images, then integrating them with high-uptake regions found on PET images. Each modality exposes a distinct kind of biological data for tumor-induced tissue alterations and presents "somewhat distinct information processing tasks," as stated in a multimodal imaging study for brain tumor segmentation [4]. Similar ideas have been put forth in the context of ensemble learning [5], where the results of choices made by various techniques are combined by a "meta-learner" on the basis that the various priors employed by these techniques characterize various aspects or perspectives of the data [28].

Multimodal medical imaging generates an increasing quantity of data, and there are numerous methods for analyzing those data [16]. Based on scientific research in a segmentation assignment, we examine the variations among multimodal fusion methods for medical image processing in this study. A viewpoint on multimodal image analysis is given by James and Dasarathy in their review [6], who also note that any traditional image fusion technique entails "registration and fusion of features from the recorded images." Furthermore, networks depicting numerous streams of information "can be taken further and channels can be integrated at any point in the network," according to the assessment work of Litjens *et al.* [7].

Spatial domain and transform domain are two categories used to classify conventional medical picture fusion techniques. The focus of the early studies was on geometric domain-based medical image fusion approaches [30]. HIS and primary assessment are common techniques. Yet, spectral and spatial distortion of fused pictures is the result of the spatial domain technique [8]. The transform domain is now the primary area of study for improved fusion impacts. It conducts reconstruction methods after converting the original image into the frequency or other domains in order to integrate them. The four stages of the fusion procedure are signal, feature, symbol, and pixel level. Currently, the pixel level is extensively used, and the contour alteration, discrete wavelet, and pyramid transform are its characteristic examples [31]. Good structure and avoiding distortion are two benefits of the transform domain-based technique, but noise is also produced during the fusion processing [17]. Denoising is thus a problem for picture fusion [9]. It is clear from the papers established in the previous 2 years that there is almost no way for the suggested fusion algorithm to rely solely on the spatial domain. The PCA-DWT approach, for example, integrates transform and spatial domain techniques. A medical image fusion technique based on DL was developed in 2017 with the arrival of the DL boom [18].

In modern decades, medical image registration and segmentation have seen the widespread use of CNN, recurrent neural networks (RNN), U-Net networks, GAN, and other DL models, but only CNN and U-Net networks have been used for medical image fusing [32]. An image-processing neural network with three layers—a convolutional layer, a pooling layer, and a completely integrated layer—is known as CNN [19]. Caffe, TensorFlow, MatConvNet, and similar deep learning frameworks are used for medical picture fusion. The U-Net network is currently discovered to have been trained using the PyTorch DL technology.

11.1.1 Research Gap

The majority of the present study on DL-based multimodality medical image segmentation is restricted to two-dimensional (2D) images. The use of DL methods for multimodality picture segmentation on three-dimensional (3D) or higher-dimensional images is not well studied. A restricted amount of study has also been done on combining different DL approaches to enhance the efficacy of multimodality image segmentation. Moreover, more research needs to be done on how various data preprocessing methods affect how well multimodality picture segmentation works. Due to their dependence on a single type of data, current medical image segmentation methods are only partially effective in their segmentation and classification of medical images.

11.1.2 Research Aim

In an attempt to increase the precision of medical image segmentation and classification, the objective of this research is to examine the efficiency of multimodality fusion of medical image segmentation using DL methods.

The second goal of this study is to investigate solutions to problems that could arise when applying DL approaches to medical image segmentation, like the requirement for a substantial quantity of training data and the possibility of overfitting.

11.2 Literature Review

The most recent state-of-the-art success in image classification, segmentation, object detection, and tracking tasks has been demonstrated by DL-based methods. DL techniques have lately attracted a lot of attention in multimodal medical image segmentation because of their capacity for self-learning and generalization over vast amounts of data. In this article, we provide a summary of DL-based methods for the multimodal segmentation of medical images. First, we describe the fundamentals of multimodal medical picture segmentation and DL. We then show various DL network frameworks, examine their fusion techniques, and contrast the outcomes [10, 11]. Because it is straightforward and concentrates on the upcoming segmentation network design, the earlier fusion is frequently used [20]. The later fusion, yet, focuses more on the fusion approach to understand the intricate relationships between various modalities.

Researchers are now able to glean an increasing amount of information from medical pictures thanks to developments in automated diagnostic tools. Multimodality images have recently been employed in order to acquire medical images that are more informative. Compared with standard medical pictures, these images contain a great deal more information. The creation of multimodality images is a difficult job though. The suggested method first uses a non-subsampled contourlet transform (NSCT) domain to break the image up into subbands. The source images are then used to extract features using an extreme variant of Inception (Xception). The best characteristics are chosen using the multiobjective differential evolution. The merged coefficients are then obtained using the energy loss-based fusion functions and the coefficient of determination [21]. The inverse NSCT is then used to calculate the fused image. The suggested method surpasses the competing multimodality image fusion methods, according to comprehensive experimental findings.

Medical image fusion techniques are increasingly important for multiple clinical uses because they can integrate medical images from different patterns to increase the precision and dependability of a diagnosis. In an attempt to develop fused images with high visual clarity and distinct structural details, this study suggests a medical image fusion algorithm based on CNN. To create the weight map, the proposed technique combines the trained Siamese convolutional network with the pixel activity data from the original images. The original image is broken down in the background using a contrast pyramid [22]. A weighted fusion operator and different spatial frequency bands are used to merge the source images. The findings of comparative experiments demonstrate that the proposed fusion algorithm can efficiently maintain the source images' complex structural details while generating pleasing visual impacts for humans [33].

A state-of-the-art result for 3D biomedical segmentation has been attained through the gradual application of DL based on segmentation models to biomedical images [13]. Yet, the majority of current biomedical segmentation studies take into consideration the application cases by adjusting just one kind of medical images from the relevant examination technique [34]. Multiple image segmentation techniques are typically necessary for a final diagnosis when contemplating the clinical applications of radiology evaluation for diseases, particularly in the case of some serious illnesses like cancer [23]. As a result, we conduct studies to fully utilize the additional information of multimodal images by contemplating the instances of deploying multimodal images and investigating the efficient multimodality fusion relying on deep NN, alluding to the clinic observations of radiologists in image analysis [12].

As information sources are frequently flawed, it is important to consider their dependability when performing multisource information fusion jobs [14, 15]. The formalism of the Dempster–Shafer theory is used in this paper to integrate the outcomes of multi-MR image segmentation while taking into consideration the reliability of various modalities in relation to various categories [35]. The structure is made up of three components: an encoder–decoder feature extraction component, an apparent segmentation component that calculates a belief function for each modality at each voxel, and a multimodality evidence fusion component that gives each modality's verification a vector of discount rates and incorporates the ignored verification according to Dempster's rule [24]. To improve segmentation precision and reliability, the entire structure is evaluated by minimizing a fresh loss function relying on a discounted Dice index. The technique was assessed using a database of 1,251 individuals with brain tumors called BraTS 2021. Our approach employs a powerful novel concept for integrating multi-information inside the deep NN, and quantitative and qualitative outcomes demonstrate that it surpasses the current state of the art [37].

Today, getting pertinent medical information for clinical purposes depends heavily on medical images. Yet, it is necessary to evaluate and enhance medical image clarity. When reconstructing medical images, a number of variables have an impact on the image quality. Multimodality-based image fusion is useful for obtaining the most therapeutically pertinent information [25]. Each approach has its presumptions, advantages, and difficulties. In this article, some significant non-traditional work in multimodality-based image fusion is critically analyzed. Researchers frequently ask for assistance in understanding the above methods and selecting the best strategy; this is specific to their cause. As a result, this study provides a short introduction to both conventional and non-conventional multimodality-based image fusion techniques [36].

11.3 Research Methodology

Assume I1 and I2 display the original pictures. I1 and I2 are first divided into subbands using NSCT. Our main goal is to combine the corresponding subbands from the two original images. Utilizing the Inception (Xception) model's excessive iteration, the high subband is fused. The importance of the calculated fused high subbands is assessed using the coefficient of determination [38]. The local energy function is used to accomplish the fusion of low subbands. To calculate the multimodality fused image, inverse NSCT is used. The suggested model's step-by-step approach is shown in Figures 11.1 and 11.2.

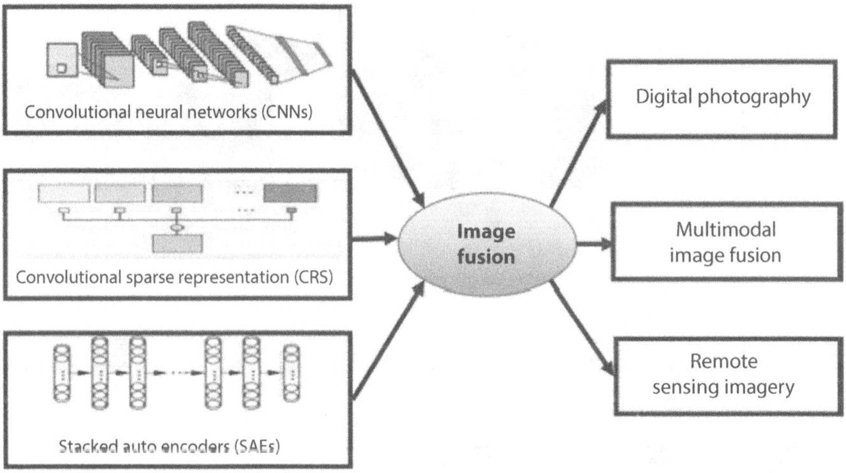

Figure 11.1 Design of DL-based image fusion.

Non-subsampled contourlet transform

The decomposition of the pictures into the wavelet domain is performed using the well-known NSCT. It is a transform that is shift-invariant and can offer extensive positional information [40]. This directionality effectively reduces the root mean square error when converting the transformed pictures to the original ones.

Feature extraction using the deep Xception method

The underfitting problem may affect CNN because not all possible features may be extracted. An extreme version of the Inception paradigm is employed to resolve this problem [39].

Feature selection using multiobjective differential evolution

The best features are chosen in this stage from the features acquired by the Xception method. The fitness function to choose the best features uses the fusion factor and entropy measures. Numerous numerically challenging issues can be resolved using a multiobjective differential evolution (Figure 11.2).

11.4 Results and Discussion

Efficiency contrast of multimodal fusion and single-modal systems

In Figure 11.3, the DICE coefficient of the two systems is summarized: On PET+CT+T1, category I, II, and III fusion networks have typical DICEs of

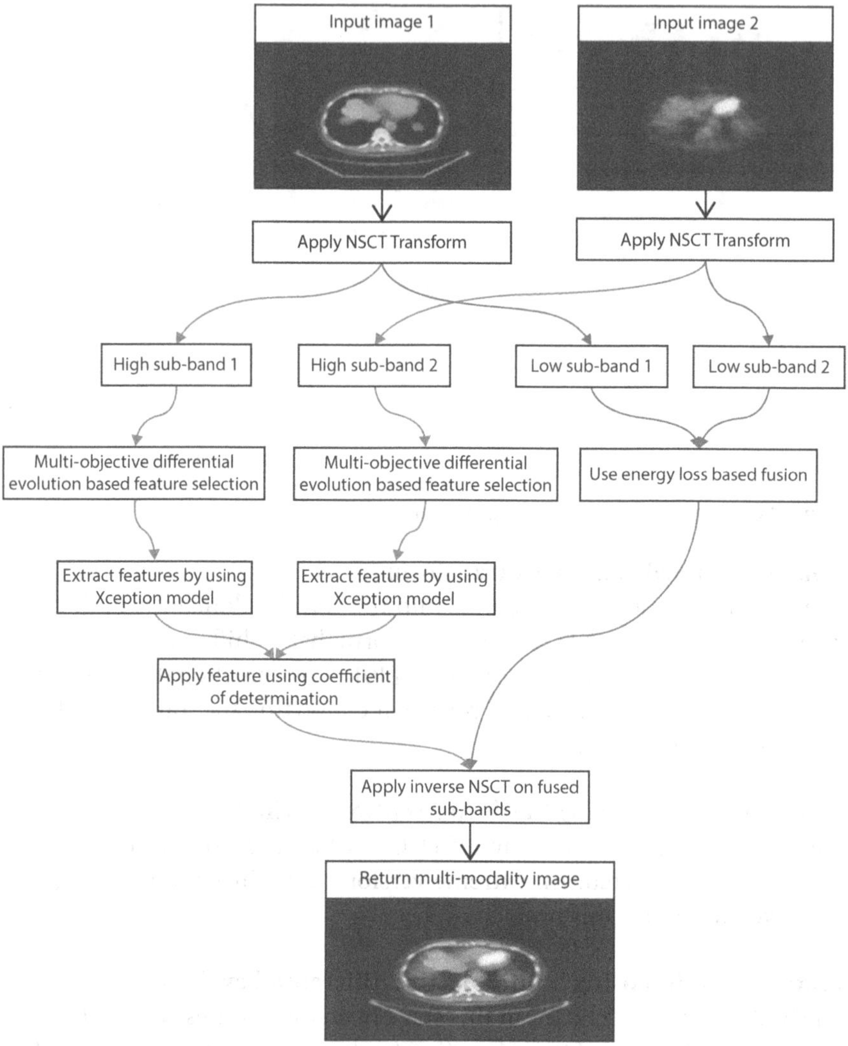

Figure 11.2 Diagrammatic flow of the suggested DL model for multimodality image fusion [11].

82%, 80%, and 77%, respectively. On PET+CT+T2, category I, II, and III fusion systems have average DICEs of 85%, 85%, and 84%, respectively. For PET, CT, T1, and T2 images, the average efficacy is 87%, 74%, 72%, and 91%. The statistics show that no network obtained an outcome greater than 80% and that all single-modality systems have smaller DICE than multimodal fusion systems. The systems that were evaluated and trained on T2-weighted MR performed the best.

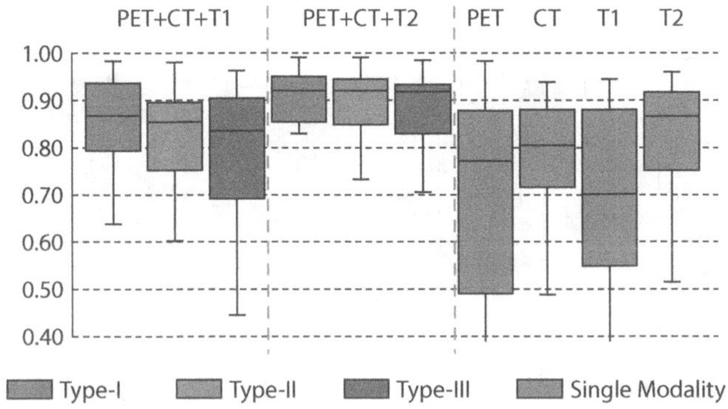

Figure 11.3 DICE coefficient of systems.

Efficiency evaluation using artificial, poor-quality images

By evaluating the systems on fabricated poor-resolution images with Gaussian noise, we were able to obtain label maps and associated estimation accuracies. For both original and low-resolution images with a noise magnitude *k* of 1, Figure 11.4 highlights the model findings. The statistics allow for the following three noteworthy conclusions of PET, CT T2.

Evaluation of efficiency using various modality combos

Based on assessments of the model performance variation among multimodal and single-modal systems and a careful analysis of the label maps from system outcomes, we have ascertained that more imaging modalities can contribute fresh knowledge to the segmentation task even with lower image resolution. Nevertheless, it is not clear how various modalities add to the multimodal systems. Put simply, if a particular combination of imaging

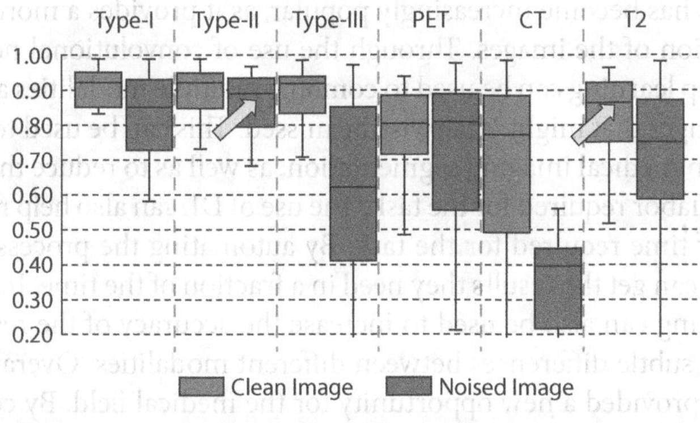

Figure 11.4 Efficiency on original and low-resolution images.

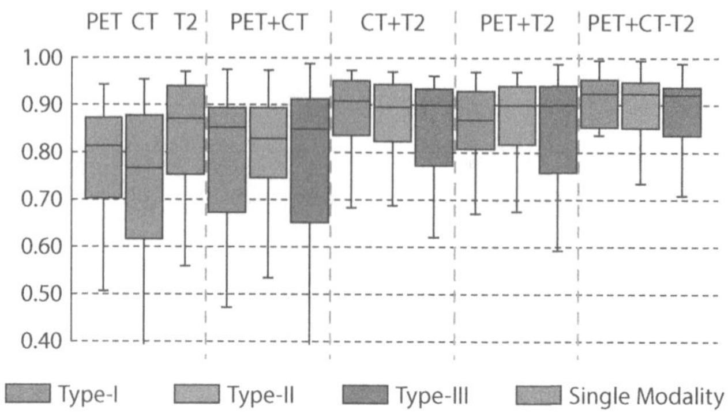

Figure 11.5 Statistics of these networks' efficiency.

modalities reliably produces little to no efficiency improvement when contrasted to its single-modality duplicate, we can infer that the additional modality is not aiding in the segmentation task. To achieve this, we used extra permutations of the imaging modalities described in the methods section to train and test the multimodal fusion networks. Figure 11.5 presents the statistics of these networks' achievements.

11.5 Conclusion

The use of deep learning in medical imaging segmentation has provided a new opportunity for the medical field to increase its accuracy and speed. By combining multiple modalities, such as MRI, CT, and PET scans, medical specialists can gain more information about a patient's condition and make more informed decisions. The use of deep learning to fuse multiple modalities has become increasingly popular, as it provides a more accurate segmentation of the images. Through the use of convolutional neural networks, deep learning can be used to combine multiple modalities and detect subtle changes that might otherwise be missed. This can be used to improve accuracy in medical imaging segmentation, as well as to reduce the amount of manual labor required for the task. The use of DL can also help reduce the amount of time required for the task. By automating the process, medical specialists can get the results they need in a fraction of the time. In addition, deep learning can also be used to increase the accuracy of the results, as it can detect subtle differences between different modalities. Overall, the use of DL has provided a new opportunity for the medical field. By combining multiple modalities, medical specialists can gain more information about a patient's condition and make more informed decisions. Additionally, deep learning can also minimize the quantity of time and effort needed for the task. In the future, deeper networks and more advanced techniques may be employed to further improve the accuracy and speed of segmentation.

References

1. Bagci, U., Udupa, J.K., Mendhiratta, N., Foster, B., Xu, Z., Yao, J., Mollura, D.J., Joint segmentation of anatomical and functional images: Applications in quantification of lesions from PET, PET-CT, MRI-PET, and MRI-PET-CT images. *Med. Image Anal.*, *17*, 8, 929–945, 2013.
2. Czisch, M., Wetter, T.C., Kaufmann, C., Pollmächer, T., Holsboer, F., Auer, D.P., Altered processing of acoustic stimuli during sleep: Reduced auditory activation and visual deactivation detected by a combined fMRI/EEG study. *Neuroimage*, *16*, 1, 251–258, 2002.
3. Teramoto, A., Fujita, H., Yamamuro, O., Tamaki, T., Automated detection of pulmonary nodules in PET/CT images: Ensemble false-positive reduction using a convolutional neural network technique. *Med. Phys.*, *43*, 6 Part 1, 2821–2827, 2016.
4. Menze, B.H., Jakab, A., Bauer, S., Kalpathy-Cramer, J., Farahani, K., Kirby, J., Van Leemput, K., The multimodal brain tumor image segmentation benchmark (BRATS). *IEEE Trans. Med. Imaging*, *34*, 10, 1993–2024, 2014.
5. Rokach, L., Ensemble-based classifiers. *Artif. Intell. Rev.*, *33*, 1–39, 2010. DOI 10.1007/s10462-009-9124-7.
6. James, A.P. and Dasarathy, B.V., Medical image fusion: A survey of the state of the art. *Inf. Fusion*, *19*, 4–19, 2014.
7. Litjens, G., Kooi, T., Bejnordi, B.E., Setio, A.A.A., Ciompi, F., Ghafoorian, M., Sánchez, C., I, A survey on deep learning in medical image analysis. *Med. Image Anal.*, *42*, 60–88, 2017.
8. James, A.P. and Dasarathy, B.V., Medical image fusion: A survey of the state of the art. *Inf. Fusion*, *19*, 4–19, 2014.
9. Iqbal, N., Saleem, S., Jehan, W., Ahmad, K., Reduction of speckle noise in medical images using stationary wavelet transform and fuzzy logic, in: *2017 International Symposium on Recent Advances in Electrical Engineering (RAEE)*, IEEE, pp. 1–6, 2017, October.
10. Zhou, T., Ruan, S., Canu, S., A review: Deep learning for medical image segmentation using multi-modality fusion. *Array*, *3*, 100004, 2019.
11. Kaur, M. and Singh, D., Multi-modality medical image fusion technique using multi-objective differential evolution based deep neural networks. *J. Ambient Intell. Hum. Comput.*, *12*, 2483–2493, 2021.
12. Wang, K., Zheng, M., Wei, H., Qi, G., Li, Y., Multi-modality medical image fusion using convolutional neural network and contrast pyramid. *Sensors*, *20*, 8, 2169, 2020.

13. Jia, X., Liu, Y., Yang, Z., Yang, D., Multi-modality self-attention aware deep network for 3D biomedical segmentation. *BMC Med. Inf. Decis. Making, 20*, 3, 1–7, 2020.
14. Huang, L., Denoeux, T., Vera, P., Ruan, S., Evidence fusion with contextual discounting for multi-modality medical image segmentation, in: *Medical Image Computing and Computer Assisted Intervention–MICCAI 2022: 25th International Conference, Singapore, September 18–22, 2022, Proceedings, Part V*, Springer Nature Switzerland, Cham, pp. 401–411, 2022, September.
15. Diwakar, M., Singh, P., Ravi, V., Maurya, A., A non-conventional review on multi-modality-based medical image fusion. *Diagnostics, 13*, 5, 820, 2023.
16. Panwar, V., Sharma, D. K., Kumar, K. P., Jain, A., Thakar, C. . Experimental investigations and optimization of surface roughness in turning of en 36 alloy steel using response surface methodology and genetic algorithm. *Mater. Today Proc.*, 46, 6474–6481, 2021.
17. Jain, A. and Pandey, A.K., Modeling and optimizing of different quality characteristics in electrical discharge drilling of titanium alloy (Grade-5) sheet. *Mater. Today Proc.*, 18, 182–191, 2019.
18. Jain, A., Yadav., A.K., Shrivastava, Y., Modelling and optimization of different quality characteristics in electric discharge drilling of titanium alloy sheet. *Mater. Today Proc.*, 21, 1680–1684, 2019.
19. Jain, A. and Pandey, A.K., Multiple quality optimizations in electrical discharge drilling of mild steel sheet. *Mater. Today Proc.*, 8, 7252–7261, 2019.
20. Jain, A., Kumar, C.S., Shrivastava, Y., Fabrication and machining of fiber matrix composite through electric discharge machining: A short review. *Mater. Today Proc.*, 51, 1233–1237, 2021.
21. Dhaundiyal, R., Tripathi, A., Joshi, K., Diwakar, M., Singh, P., Clustering based multi-modality medical image fusion. *J. Phys. Conf. Ser.*, IOP Publishing, 1478, 1, 012024, 2020, April.
22. Praveen, S., Tyagi, N., Singh, B., Karetla, G.R., Thalor, M.A., Joshi, K., Tsegaye, M., PSO-based evolutionary approach to optimize head and neck biomedical image to detect mesothelioma cancer. *BioMed. Res. Int., 2022*, 2022.
23. Joshi, K., Joshi, K.N., Diwakar, M., Image fusion using cross bilateral filter and wavelet transform domain. *Int. J. Eng. Adv. Technol. (IJEAT), 8*, 110–115, 2019.
24. Bagwari, S., Roy, A., Gehlot, A., Singh, R., Priyadarshi, N., Khan, B., LoRa based metrics evaluation for real-time landslide monitoring on IoT platform. *IEEE Access, 10*, 46392–46407, 2022.
25. Bagwari, S., Gehlot, A., Singh, R., Priyadarshi, N., Khan, B., Low-cost sensor-based and LoRaWAN opportunities for landslide monitoring systems on IoT platform: A review. *IEEE Access, 10*, 7107–7127, 2021.
26. Joshi, K., Joshi, K.N., Diwakar, M., Tripathi, N.A., Gupta, H., Multi-focus image fusion using non-local mean filtering and stationary wavelet transform. *Int. J. Innov. Technol. Explor. Eng. (IJITEE), 9*, 344–350, 2019.

27. Joshi, K., Diwakar, M., Joshi, N.K., Lamba, S., A concise review on latest methods of image fusion. *Recent Adv. Comput. Sci. Commun. (Formerly: Recent Patents Comput. Science)*, *14*, 7, 2046–2056, 2021.
28. Diwakar, M., Tripathi, A., Joshi, K., Sharma, A., Singh, P., Memoria, M., A comparative review: Medical image fusion using SWT and DWT. *Mater. Today Proc.*, *37*, 3411–3416, 2021.
29. Joshi, K., Kumar, M., Tripathi, A., Kumar, A., Sehgal, J., Barthwal, A., Latest trends in multi-modality medical image fusion: A generic review, in: *Rising Threats in Expert Applications and Solutions: Proceedings of FICR-TEAS 2022*, pp. 663–671, 2022.
30. Sangeetha Francelin Vinnarasi, F., Daniel, J., Anita Rose, J.T., Pugalenthi, R., Deep learning supported disease detection with multi-modality image fusion. *J. Xray Sci. Technol.*, *29*, 3, 411–434, 2021.
31. Jia, X., Liu, Y., Yang, Z., Yang, D., Multi-modality self-attention aware deep network for 3D biomedical segmentation. *BMC Med. Inf. Decis. Making*, *20*, 3, 1–7, 2020.
32. Huang, L., Denoeux, T., Vera, P., Ruan, S., Evidence fusion with contextual discounting for multi-modality medical image segmentation, in: *Medical Image Computing and Computer Assisted Intervention–MICCAI 2022: 25th International Conference, Singapore, September 18–22, 2022, Proceedings, Part V*, Springer Nature Switzerland, Cham, pp. 401–411, 2022, September.
33. Parvathy, V.S. and Pothiraj, S., Multi-modality medical image fusion using hybridization of binary crow search optimization. *Healthcare Manag. Sci.*, *23*, 661–669, 2020.
34. Diwakar, M., Singh, P., Ravi, V., Maurya, A., A non-conventional review on multi-modality-based medical image fusion. *Diagnostics*, *13*, 5, 820, 2023.
35. Subbiah Parvathy, V., Pothiraj, S., Sampson, J., A novel approach in multimodality medical image fusion using optimal shearlet and deep learning. *Int. J. Imaging Syst. Technol.*, *30*, 4, 847–859, 2020.
36. Zhu, Z., Chai, Y., Yin, H., Li, Y., Liu, Z., A novel dictionary learning approach for multi-modality medical image fusion. *Neurocomputing*, *214*, 471–482, 2016.
37. Lei, T., Wang, R., Wan, Y., Du, X., Meng, H., Nandi, A.K., *Medical image segmentation using deep learning: A survey*, arXiv preprint arXiv:2009.13120, 2020.
38. Gupta, M., Kumar, N., Gupta, N., Zaguia, A., Fusion of multi-modality biomedical images using deep neural networks. *Soft Comput.*, *26*, 16, 8025–8036, 2022.
39. Hesamian, M.H., Jia, W., He, X., Kennedy, P., Deep learning techniques for medical image segmentation: Achievements and challenges. *J. Digit. Imaging.*, *32*, 582–596, 2019.
40. Bhavana, V. and Krishnappa, H.K., A survey on multi-modality medical image fusion, in: *2016 International Conference on Wireless Communications, Signal Processing and Networking (WiSPNET)*, IEEE, pp. 1326–1329, 2016, March.

12

New Perspectives, Challenges, and Advances in Data Fusion in Neuroimaging

Pedada Sujata[1], Dattatray G. Takale[2], Swati Tyagi[3]*, Saniya Bhalerao[4], Mohit Tiwari[5] and Joshuva Arockia Dhanraj[6]

[1]Department of ECE, Lendi Institute of Engineering and Technology, Jonnada, Vizianagaram, India
[2]Computer Engineering Vishwakarma Institute of Information Technology, SPPU, Pune, India
[3]University of Delaware, Newark, DE, USA
[4]Department of Pharmaceutics, MET Institute of Pharmacy, Bhujbal Knowledge City, Adgoan, Nashik, India
[5]Department of Computer Science and Engineering, Bharati Vidyapeeth's College of Engineering, Paschim Vihar, Delhi, India
[6]Centre for Automation and Robotics (ANRO), Department of Mechatronics Engineering, Hindustan Institute of Technology and Science, Padur, Chennai, India

Abstract
In order to get around the inherent constraints of distinct imaging modalities, multimodal fusion in neuroimaging integrates data from various imaging modalities. Higher temporal and spatial precision, improved contrast, the correction of imaging distortions, and the bridging of physiological and cognitive data can all be achieved through neuroimaging fusion. This analysis aims to examine the fusion and optimization of the multimodal neuroimaging technique and to examine a multimodal neuroimaging-based technique for measuring brain fatigue. Four-dimensional consistency of local neural activities (FOCA) and local multimodal serial analysis (LMSA) are primarily presented to naturally merge electroencephalogram (EEG) and functional magnetic resonance imaging (fMRI). With the time precision relying on EEG and the space precision focused on fMRI, the time–space

**Corresponding author*: swatyagi@udel.edu
Joshuva Arockia Dhanraj: ORCID: 0000-0001-5048-7775

Kapil Joshi and Somil Kumar Gupta (eds.) Human Cancer Diagnosis and Detection Using Exascale Computing, (185–198) © 2024 Scrivener Publishing LLC

matching in the data fusion system has acceptable outcomes, with the time precision above 88% and the space precision above 89%.

***Keywords*:** Neuroimaging, multimodal data fusion, multimodal neuroimaging, electroencephalogram

12.1 Introduction

The integrated analysis of datasets containing various kinds of data is known as data fusion. The primary justification for this strategy is a thorough categorization of the sample, which is frequently impossible with just one type of data or one analytical technique. For instance, aggressive tumors are challenging to identify using a single measurement technique, like a data type, for several factors, like minimal precision and minimal benign accountability [6]. Thus, data fusion enables the acquisition of additional knowledge about a sample, improving predictions, such as a patient's diagnosis [24]. This study provides an outline of various data fusion strategies based on DL and traditional ML approaches for a variety of measurement techniques, such as mammography, fluorescence lifetime imaging microscopy, single photon emission computed tomography, and computed tomography.

Pixel-, feature-, and decision-level fusion are the three general subcategories of data fusion. Data from various sources are directly combined through pixel-level synthesis. Fusion at the feature level combines the features extracted from various data kinds using statistical and ML techniques [23].

Decision-level fusion is the term used to describe the fusion of factors linked to decision rules [3]. Biomedical data fusion usually entails several preprocessing stages, including dimensionality reduction, noise and background removal, temporal and spatial alignment, and management of missing data [6].

The Internet of Things and social networks are just a few of the modern low- and high-layer applications that have effectively implemented numerous heterogeneous networks [7]. Heterogeneous networks are being widely used, which has resulted in an extraordinary pace of data generation and collection. The characteristics of these data, which are frequently alluded to as big data, include high diversity, velocity, and veracity [8]. Additionally, these enormous datasets that include organized, semistructured, and unstructured data are multimodal. Additionally, each modality has information unique to that modality [9], regardless of source, type, or distribution. For instance, a sports news website utilizes texts to characterize a sport's substance and images to capture the action as it happens [25]. These texts and images are depictions of a single event in their original, unedited versions. When one modality is lacking, the plausible fusion of these multimodal data can aid in our understanding of the relevant occurrence [10]. Therefore, a key area of study in the field of big data is the integration of information in multimodal data, which provides opportunities to better understand shared- and cross-modal information [11]. This is because multimodal data are becoming more and more accessible and available.

A key technique in multimodal data mining is multimodal data fusion, which seeks to combine data from various sources, distributions, and types into a single global space where both intermodality and cross-modality can be uniformly depicted [12]. By utilizing modality-specific information, it can offer richer information than a singular modality [13]. The exploration of cross-modal and complementary information between modalities has previously been addressed by a few multimodal data fusion techniques [14]. For instance, Kettenring [15] suggested the multimodal canonical correlation evaluation for the cross-modal generalization data and the linear intermodality connection. In order to identify the factors from the multisource datasets, Valdes-Sosa *et al.* [16] suggested the partial least squares method of linear correlations over numerous factors. The multimodal component analysis of Groves *et al.* [17] is a probability approach that combines the independent factors of each various modality using the Bayesian framework. These multimodal data fusion methods are limited to large quantities of high-volume, high-velocity, and high-veracity multimodal data because they are based on superficial properties that cannot characterize the inherent interior patterns and exterior relations in multimodal data. Therefore, novel multimodal computing methods are needed in order to fully mine the structures in the multimodal data [18].

Like conventional big data, multimodal big data have high volumes, varieties, and speeds. The diversity of the multidimensional big data, however, stands out more than the other qualities. With each modality-independent distribution, multimodal big data are made up of multiple modalities that each hold a portion of the description of the same objects of interest [26]. Additionally, there are intricate connections between modalities. The efficiency of different multimodal applications can be further enhanced by the complete modeling of the fusion representations concealed in the cross-modality and intermodality [27].

Due to easier access to imaging devices, particularly hybrid systems like PET/MR [20], multimodal neuroimaging, or the continuous imaging measurement [19] or accumulation of distinct measurement, has emerged as a new study field. The joint analysis of the multimodal data was also made possible by new developments in neuroimaging computing techniques. The free and open-source software (FOSS) packages and interfaces for neuroimaging computing help to advance and expedite the conversion of multimodal neuroimaging studies from the laboratory to better clinical treatment [28].

12.1.1 Research Gap

The emphasis of the current data fusion study in neuroimaging has been on techniques for combining and analyzing data from various sources to learn new things about the brain and how it works [29]. Data fusion can be used to create new neuroimaging approaches and to boost existing neuroimaging methods, and it may even help us better understand neurodegenerative diseases. Unfortunately, there is a dearth of research on how data fusion can be used in these other areas of neuroimaging. This knowledge gap offers a chance to deepen our understanding of the potential of data fusion in neuroimaging and to create fresh, cutting-edge applications for this technology.

12.2 Literature Review

In order to get around the inherent constraints of individual imaging modalities, multimodal fusion in neuroimaging integrates data from various imaging modalities [1, 2]. Higher temporal and spatial precision, improved contrast, the correction of imaging distortions, and the bridging of physiological and cognitive data can all be achieved through neuroimaging fusion. Over 450 references from sources released between 1978 and 2020 were examined for this research. We offer a review that includes (1) a summary of the present multimodal fusion issues, (2) the present medical applications of fusion for neurological diseases, (3) the advantages and disadvantages of the imaging modalities that are currently available, (4) the basic fusion rules, (5) the techniques for evaluating the fusion quality, and (6) the applications of fusion for atlas-based segmentation and measurement [30]. All things considered, multimodal fusion offers important advantages in medical prognosis and brain study. Multimodal neuroimaging will advance if engineers, researchers, and clinicians are educated widely and conduct more studies.

Substantial quantities of data are produced every day as a result of the expansion of imaging modalities like photoacoustic tomography, CT, and tomography. Substantial biomedical datasets provide more details about pathologies, but they also pose new difficulties in thoroughly analyzing the data [30]. By combining numerous data outcomes to improve the coherence of the information, data fusion techniques advance our knowledge of the data. Data generation is only the first stage in the fusion procedure; other elements like noise, missing data, and high dimensionality are also important. An outline of the advancements in data preprocessing for data fusion is given in this article, along with new information about the subject [32].

Despite difficulties in gathering and combining non-redundant imaging data, multimodal neuroimaging has established itself as a cornerstone of basic and cognitive neuroscience in people. A complete physiological view of brain processes and measurements, frameworks, and normalization and the accessibility of biomarkers are just a few of the significant perspectives into brain processes and structures that multimodal data integration can provide in addition to complementarity in spatiotemporal resolution [4, 5]. In the context of each of these potential benefits, we address data acquisition and fusion in multimodal neuroimaging in this review [31]. When modeling and analyzing multimodal data using generative approaches, limitations—resulting from distinctions in the neuronal and structural underpinnings of each approach—must be taken into consideration. We draw the conclusion that multimodal data fusion can significantly enhance the value of neuroscience applications when these obstacles are properly addressed, making it an essential method for understanding the brain [33].

Human brain mapping is celebrating 21 years of research on cognitive function in the 21st century. This review examines imaging neuroscience and the main theories it has advanced; some theories herald intriguing new directions, while others have spectacularly failed. There is much to be proud of in terms of accomplishments because it is hard to picture contemporary neuroscience without brain imaging. Current research will be examined from the viewpoints of functional segregation and combination in the brain, giving particular interest to methods that approach questions about the dispersed and combined nature of neuronal processing [35].

Applying DL to the study of real-world images has seen tremendous success. In contrast, there are some difficulties in analyzing neuroimaging data, such as greater dimensionality, smaller sample sizes, a variety of heterogeneous modalities, and limited ground truth. The four distinct and significant categories of dynamic connectivity, multimodal fusion, interpretation/visualization, and classification/prediction are discussed in this article as they relate to DL techniques in the area of neuroimaging [34]. We address the advantages of combining data characteristics and model structures, highlight recent developments in each of these areas, and generate recommendations for the application of DL to neuroimaging data. We evaluate promising applications and significant obstacles for each group. Lastly, we cover all four areas in our discussion of the future paths of neuroimaging DL for medical applications, a subject of a great deal.

12.3 Research Methodology

12.3.1 Human Brain Temporal and Spatial Data Mining Using FOCA and Data Fusion

The combined spatial information currently utilizes MRI data, which gives incredibly precise spatial data information for EEG source positioning, offering evidence with a superior spatial resolution. The spatial positional discrepancy between EEG and fMRI methods is the primary impediment to spatial information [21]. The disparity in their temporal resolutions is the main temporal level constraint of the combination of EEG and fMRI. Researchers are inclined to rely on the integration of multimodal temporal–spatial data, with model-driven and non-model-driven data fusion strategies [36] being the two commonly used methods from the viewpoint of sharing and fusing temporal–spatial data. Figure 12.1 displays the data-gathering process for the neuroimaging methods EEG and fMRI.

In addition, the number of voxels, repetition time, and time points are all set to 25, 2, and 250, respectively, in the simulation evaluation of FOCA.

12.3.2 Construction of the Multimodal Neuroimaging Data Fusion

Only one spatial information register cannot guarantee that the elements are similar events for EEG and fMRI neuroimaging technologies. The registration may not succeed despite the time dimension disparity between EEG and fMRI [22]. Additionally, while focusing on the combined information of the two modalities during the data information fusion procedure between EEG and fMRI, it is also important to reduce the uncertainty of shared data information. The data fusion among the two shows the exact time course in the exact location from the standpoint of data sharing [37]. As a result, registrations for time and room are required. Based on this,

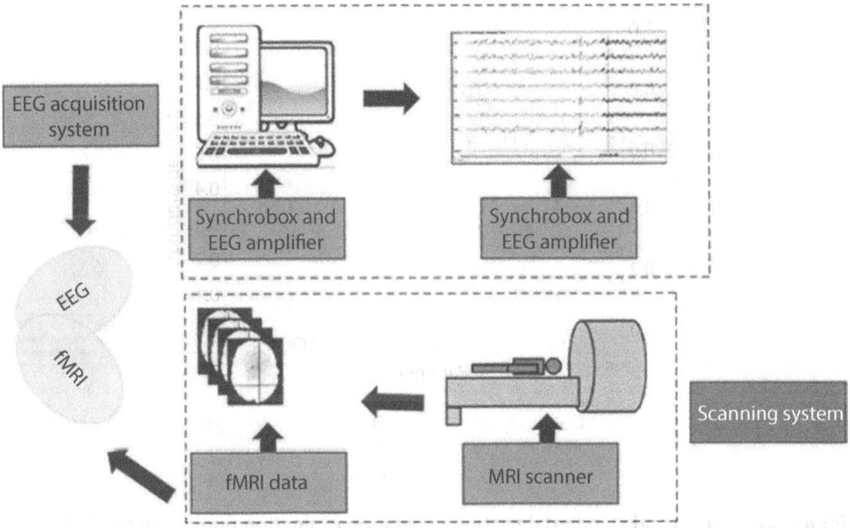

Figure 12.1 Data collection of neuroimaging techniques.

a data fusion method that can differentiate between time and location is constructed using the multimodal data fusion methodology. Different temporal and space data fusion techniques are used in this system to register between modalities [39]. The system also has several levels of credibility, starting with time–space misregistration and ending with time–space registration.

12.4 Results and Discussion

When the time, space, and time–space are coherent, inconsistent, and consistent, correspondingly, in Figure 12.2, the letters A to D and A′ to D′ stand for the standard deviation and mean value correlating to the FOCA index.

Figure 12.2 illustrates how, regardless of time and space, the value equivalent to the FOCA index varies among the values of the time (Ct) and the space correlation coefficient (Cs). The values of Ct, Cs, and FOCA are therefore the nearest under the assumption of time–space coherence. In the situation of time–space coherence, the simulation findings are extremely steady. Through data analysis, it was discovered that the local voxel behaviors' temporal and spatial consistencies are well handled by the FOCA index. Thus, it is hypothesized that this index will reveal and

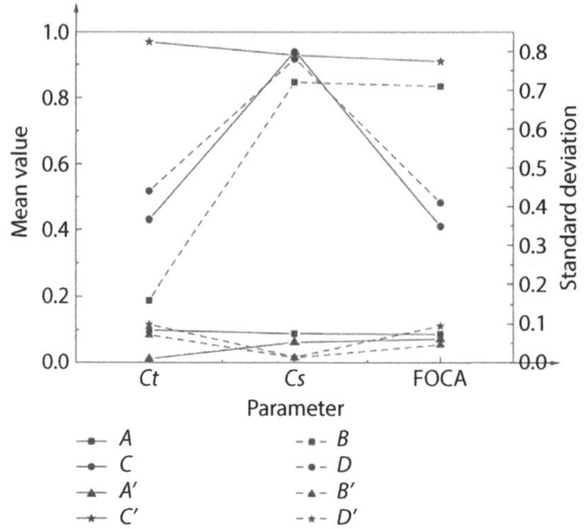

Figure 12.2 Mean and standard deviation simulation evaluation findings of the FOCA index.

describe the temporal–spatial coherence traits of local areas if it is applied to the fMRI neuroimaging technique.

12.4.1 EEG–fMRI Shared Multimodal Simulation Evaluation

The correlation between the regression coefficients of the LMSA and the GLM approach and the variations in the signal-to-noise ratios is displayed in Figure 12.3, which is positive. The suggested LMSA approach completely analyzes the time-related data information and takes into consideration the unpredictability of relying on the data fusion evaluation of EEG and fMRI. The findings of the simulation analysis discussed above demonstrate the importance of this technique's inclusion in addressing the issue of low signal-to-noise ratio.

12.4.2 Implementation of Multimodal Neuroimaging Data Fusion

Figure 12.4 displays the variations in the related coefficients of the techniques, including emiCCA, lCCA, and kCCA, given various function factors. The time-consuming variations generated by these three techniques, given various data dimensions and data points, are depicted in Figure 12.5.

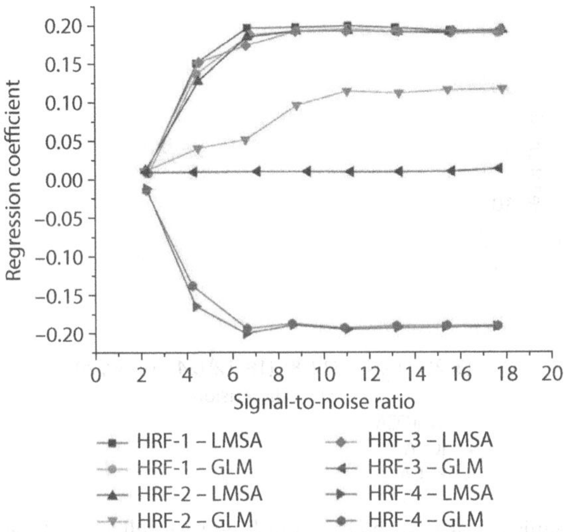

Figure 12.3 Findings of LMSA and GLM simulation analyses at various signal-to-noise ratios.

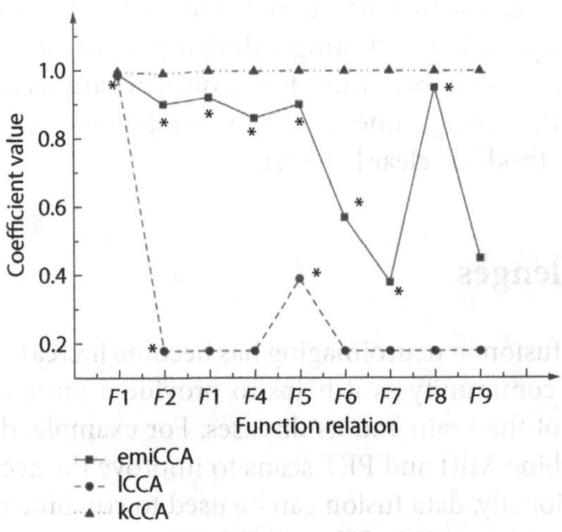

Figure 12.4 Variations in emiCCA, lCCA, and kCCA coefficients correlating to various function factors.

The coefficient related to emiCCA is the most relevant, as shown in Figures 12.4 and 12.5, in addition to any linear or non-linear connections. In contrast, the coefficient pertaining to the independent random factor is not relevant. While kCCA essentially gives an appropriate word number of

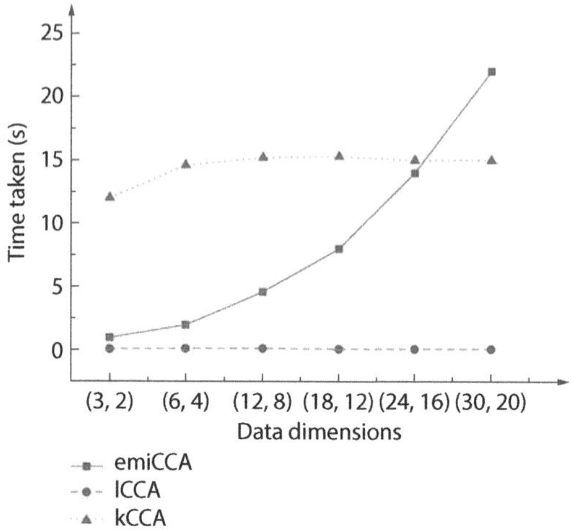

Figure 12.5 The emiCCA, lCCA, and kCCA techniques result in two time-consuming shifts: (a) various data dimensions and (b) distinct data points.

1 for any function, lCCA can acquire relevant correlation coefficients for quadratic functions. The time usage related to emiCCA is dispersed among the other techniques, demonstrating a similar pattern based on time utilization variations among these three techniques in various data extensions. The findings of the average time spent and correlation coefficient show that the emiCCA method has clear benefits.

12.5 Challenges

The use of data fusion in neuroimaging has become increasingly important to the medical community as it helps to provide a more comprehensive understanding of the brain and its diseases. For example, data fusion can be used to combine MRI and PET scans to improve the accuracy of brain imaging. Additionally, data fusion can be used to combine multiple imaging modalities such as MRI, CT, and SPECT to create a more complete picture of the brain. As the capabilities of data fusion in neuroimaging continue to grow, so too do the challenges associated with its use [38]. One of the primary challenges is the need for reliable data sources. As data fusion combines multiple sources of data, it is critical that the data are accurate and up to date. Additionally, data fusion requires the development of robust algorithms to ensure that only relevant and reliable data are combined. In order to overcome these challenges, new perspectives and advances in data fusion are needed. For example, machine learning techniques such as deep learning can be used to better identify and analyze the data used in data fusion. Additionally, new algorithms and software tools can be developed to improve the accuracy and reliability of data fusion. Finally, advances in data security and privacy can help to ensure that the data used in data fusion are properly protected. As data fusion involves combining multiple sources of data, it is important to ensure that the data are secure from unauthorized access. Additionally, data privacy regulations should be in place to ensure that the data are only used for its intended purpose [40]. Overall, data fusion in neuroimaging holds great potential for improving the accuracy and reliability of medical diagnosis and treatment. However, in order for this potential to be realized, new perspectives, challenges, and advances must be made to ensure that data fusion is used correctly and securely. By doing so, data fusion can help to improve the accuracy and reliability of medical diagnosis and treatment and provide a more complete picture of the brain and its diseases.

12.6 Conclusion

Data fusion in neuroimaging has opened new possibilities for exploring the brain. It has allowed researchers to correlate physiological signals with brain activity and its associated behaviors. Furthermore, it has allowed for the development of more sophisticated techniques for analyzing the brain's complex network of neurons and synapses. Data fusion in neuroimaging is revolutionizing how we understand and treat neurological conditions. By combining brain imaging data with other types of physiological data, researchers are able to gain a more comprehensive picture of the brain's structure. This improved understanding of the brain has implications for diagnosing and treating neurological diseases, like epilepsy, autism, and Alzheimer's. Additionally, data fusion in neuroimaging is enabling researchers to gain insight into the effects of aging on the brain. The future of data fusion in neuroimaging looks bright. New advances in technology are allowing researchers to explore the brain at unprecedented levels of detail and accuracy. This has enabled a much greater understanding of the brain's complex network of neurons and synapses. Furthermore, new techniques are being developed to improve the accuracy and reliability of data fusion methods. Data fusion in neuroimaging is an exciting and rapidly evolving field of research. It provides researchers with unprecedented information about the brain and its associated behaviors. As new techniques and technologies are developed, they will continue to provide new perspectives and opportunities for understanding the brain and its disorders. It will also lead to improved treatments for neurological conditions and new insights into the effects of aging on the brain.

References

1. Zhang, Y.D., Dong, Z., Wang, S.H., Yu, X., Yao, X., Zhou, Q., Gorriz, J.M., Advances in multimodal data fusion in neuroimaging: Overview, challenges, and novel orientation. *Inf. Fusion*, *64*, 149–187, 2020.
2. Wang, S., Celebi, M.E., Zhang, Y.D., Yu, X., Lu, S., Yao, X., Tyukin, I., Advances in data preprocessing for biomedical data fusion: An overview of the methods, challenges, and prospects. *Inf. Fusion*, *76*, 376–421, 2021.
3. Uludağ, K. and Roebroeck, A., General overview on the merits of multimodal neuroimaging data fusion. *Neuroimage*, *102*, 3–10, 2014.
4. Friston, K.J., Modalities, modes, and models in functional neuroimaging. *Science*, *326*, 5951, 399–403, 2009.
5. Yan, W., Qu, G., Hu, W., Abrol, A., Cai, B., Qiao, C., Calhoun, V.D., Deep learning in neuroimaging: Promises and challenges. *IEEE Signal Process Mag.*, *39*, 2, 87–98, 2022.
6. Wang, S., Celebi, M.E., Zhang, Y.D., Yu, X., Lu, S., Yao, X., Tyukin, I., Advances in data preprocessing for biomedical data fusion: An overview of the methods, challenges, and prospects. *Inf. Fusion*, *76*, 376–421, 2021.
7. Zhang, C., Patras, P., Haddadi, H., Deep learning in mobile and wireless networking: A survey. *IEEE Commun. Surv. Tutor.*, *21*, 3, 2224–2287, 2019.
8. Gao, J., Li, P., Chen, Z., A canonical polyadic deep convolutional computation model for big data feature learning in internet of things. *Future Gener. Comput. Syst.*, *99*, 508–516, 2019.
9. Li, Y., Yang, M., Zhang, Z., A survey of multi-view representation learning. *IEEE Trans. Knowl. Data Eng.*, *31*, 10, 1863–1883, 2018.
10. Lahat, D., Adali, T., Jutten, C., Multimodal data fusion: An overview of methods, challenges, and prospects. *Proc. IEEE*, *103*, 9, 1449–1477, 2015.
11. Khaleghi, B., Khamis, A., Karray, F.O., Razavi, S.N., Multisensor data fusion: A review of the state-of-the-art. *Inf. Fusion*, *14*, 1, 28–44, 2013.
12. Poria, S., Cambria, E., Bajpai, R., Hussain, A., A review of affective computing: From unimodal analysis to multimodal fusion. *Inf. Fusion*, *37*, 98–125, 2017.
13. Wagner, J., Andre, E., Lingenfelser, F., Kim, J., Exploring fusion methods for multimodal emotion recognition with missing data. *IEEE Trans. Affect. Comput.*, *2*, 4, 206–218, 2011.
14. Sui, J., Adali, T., Yu, Q., Chen, J., Calhoun, V.D., A review of multivariate methods for multimodal fusion of brain imaging data. *J. Neurosci. Methods*, *204*, 1, 68–81, 2012.

15. Kettenring, J.R., Canonical analysis of several sets of variables. *Biometrika, 58*, 3, 433–451, 1971.
16. Valdés-Sosa, M.M.E. and Cohen, M.F.G.R., Concurrent EEG/fMRI analysis by multiway Partial Least Squares. *Neuroimage, 22*, 3, 1023–1034, 2004.
17. Groves, A.R., Beckmann, C.F., Smith, S.M., Woolrich, M.W., Linked independent component analysis for multimodal data fusion. *Neuroimage, 54*, 3, 2198–2217, 2011.
18. Zhang, Q., Yang, L.T., Chen, Z., Deep computation model for unsupervised feature learning on big data. *IEEE Trans. Serv. Comput., 9*, 1, 161–171, 2015.
19. Knopman, A.A., Wong, C.H., Stevenson, R.J., Homewood, J., Mohamed, A., Somerville, E., Bleasel, A.F., The relationship between neuropsychological functioning and FDG-PET hypometabolism in intractable mesial temporal lobe epilepsy. *Epilepsy Behav., 44*, 136–142, 2015.
20. Bisdas, S., Nägele, T., Schlemmer, H.P., Boss, A., Claussen, C.D., Pichler, B., Ernemann, U., Switching on the lights for real-time multimodality tumor neuroimaging: The integrated positron-emission tomography/MR imaging system. *Am. J. Neuroradiol., 31*, 4, 610–614, 2010.
21. Rashdan, M., Dual-time resolution time-based transceiver for low-power serial interfaces. *Analog Integr. Circuits Signal Process, 92*, 81–89, 2017.
22. Zieleniewska, M., Duszyk, A., Różański,.P., Pietrzak, M., Bogotko, M., Durka, P., Parametric description of EEG profiles for assessment of sleep architecture in disorders of consciousness. *Int. J. Neural Syst., 29*, 03, 1850049, 2019.
23. Panwar, V., Sharma, D.K., Kumar, K.V.P., Jain, A., Thakar, C., Experimental investigations and optimization of surface roughness in turning Of EN 36 alloy steel using response surface methodology and genetic algorithm. *Mater. Today:. Proc.*, 46, 6474–6481, 2021.
24. Jain, A. and Pandey, A.K., Modeling and optimizing of different quality characteristics in electrical discharge drilling of titanium alloy (Grade-5) sheet. *Mater. Today:. Proc.*, 18, 182–191, 2019.
25. Jain, A., Yadav, A.K., Shrivastava, Y., Modelling and optimization of different quality characteristics in electric discharge drilling of titanium alloy sheet. *Mater. Today Proc.*, 21, 1680–1684, 2019.
26. Jain, A. and Pandey, A.K., Multiple quality optimizations in electrical discharge drilling of mild steel sheet. *Mater. Today Proc.*, 8, 7252–7261, 2019.
27. Jain, A., Kumar, C.S., Shrivastava, Y., Fabrication and machining of fiber matrix composite through electric discharge machining: A short review. *Mater. Today Proc.*, 51, 1233–1237, 2021.
28. Dhaundiyal, R., Tripathi, A., Joshi, K., Diwakar, M., Singh, P., Clustering based multi-modality medical image fusion. *J. Phys. Conf. Ser.*, 1478, 1, 012024, 2020, April. IOP Publishing.
29. Praveen, S., Tyagi, N., Singh, B., Karetla, G.R., Thalor, M.A., Joshi, K., Tsegaye, M., PSO-based evolutionary approach to optimize head and neck biomedical image to detect mesothelioma cancer. *BioMed. Res. Int.*, 2022, 2022.

30. Joshi, K., Joshi, K.N., Diwakar, M., Image fusion using cross bilateral filter and wavelet transform domain. *Int. J. Eng. Adv. Technol. (IJEAT)*, 8, 110–115, 2019.
31. Bagwari, S., Roy, A., Gehlot, A., Singh, R., Priyadarshi, N., Khan, B., LoRa Based Metrics Evaluation for Real-Time Landslide Monitoring on IoT Platform. *IEEE Access*, 10, 46392–46407, 2022.
32. Bagwari, S., Gehlot, A., Singh, R., Priyadarshi, N., Khan, B., Low-cost sensor-based and LoRaWAN opportunities for landslide monitoring systems on IoT platform: A review. *IEEE Access*, 10, 7107–7127, 2021.
33. Joshi, K., Joshi, K.N., Diwakar, M., Tripathi, N.A., Gupta, H., Multi-focus image fusion using non-local mean filtering and stationary wavelet transform. *Int. J, Innov. Technol. Explor. Eng. (IJITEE)*, 9, 344–350, 2019.
34. Joshi, K., Diwakar, M., Joshi, N.K., Lamba, S., A concise review on latest methods of image fusion. *Recent Adv. Comput. Sci. Commun. (Formerly: Recent Patents Comput. Science)*, 14, 7, 2046–2056, 2021.
35. Diwakar, M., Tripathi, A., Joshi, K., Sharma, A., Singh, P., Memoria, M., A comparative review: Medical image fusion using SWT and DWT. *Mater. Today:. Proc.*, 37, 3411–3416, 2021.
36. Joshi, K., Kumar, M., Tripathi, A., Kumar, A., Sehgal, J., Barthwal, A., Latest trends in multi-modality medical image fusion: A generic review, in: *Rising Threats in Expert Applications and Solutions: Proceedings of FICR-TEAS 2022*, pp. 663–671, 2022.
37. Parvathy, V.S. and Pothiraj, S., Multi-modality medical image fusion using hybridization of binary crow search optimization. *Healthcare Manag. Sci.*, 23, 661–669, 2020.
38. Subbiah Parvathy, V., Pothiraj, S., Sampson, J., A novel approach in multimodality medical image fusion using optimal shearlet and deep learning. *Int. J. Imaging Syst. Technol.*, 30, 4, 847–859, 2020.
39. Zhu, Z., Chai, Y., Yin, H., Li, Y., Liu, Z., A novel dictionary learning approach for multi-modality medical image fusion. *Neurocomputing*, 214, 471–482, 2016.
40. Parvathy, V.S. and Pothiraj, S., Multi-modality medical image fusion using hybridization of binary crow search optimization. *Healthcare Manag. Sci.*, 23, 661–669, 2020.

13

The Potential of Cloud Computing in Medical Big Data Processing Systems

A. Mallareddy[1], M. Jaiganesh[2], Sophia Navis Mary[3], Manikandan K.[4], Umakant Bhaskar Gohatre[5] and Joshuva Arockia Dhanraj[6,7]*

[1]*Department of Information Technology, CVR College of Engineering, Vastunagar, Mangalpalli, Ibrahimpatnam, Telangana, India*
[2]*Department of Information Technology, Karpagam College of Engineering, Myleripalayam, Coimbatore, Tamil Nadu, India*
[3]*Department of MCA, Ethiraj College for Women, Chennai, Tamil Nadu, India*
[4]*School of Computer Science and Engineering, Vellore Institute of Technology (VIT), Vellore, Tamil Nadu, India*
[5]*Department of Electronics and Telecommunications Engineering, Smt. Indira Gandhi College of Engineering, Navi Mumbai, Maharashtra, India*
[6]*Centre for Automation and Robotics (ANRO), Department of Mechatronics Engineering, Hindustan Institute of Technology and Science, Padur, Chennai, India*
[7]*University Center for Research & Development (UCRD) Chandigarh University, Mohali, Punjab, India*

Abstract

In the realm of healthcare, information technology has indeed been extensively employed and evolved, and it has formed a significant role in the advancement of healthcare treatment. Cloud computing innovation has advanced fast consecutive times, injecting fresh life into the growth of clinical and medical data. Cloud computing makes the utilization of the Internet as a transporter to deliver dynamic, scalable, and adaptable operations. The construction of a local clinical cooperation cloud computing system allows the medical data system to efficiently combine the health details of patients from various clinical facilities and offer prompt and sharing collaborating functions. Among the most difficult issues is processing big data, which necessitates a specialized technique. This work presents a novel fuzzy rule-oriented classifier to meet this difficulty and offer medical services. The suggested approach is dependent on the development of early clusters, retrieving

**Corresponding author*: joshuva1991@gmail.com; ORCID: 0000-0001-5048-7775

Kapil Joshi and Somil Kumar Gupta (eds.) Human Cancer Diagnosis and Detection Using Exascale Computing, (199–214) © 2024 Scrivener Publishing LLC

and processing cloud settings containing big data. In the suggested method, a fuzzy rule-oriented classifier is thus constructed for an effective decision for data categorization. Membership operations have been meant for fuzzification and defuzzification procedures to execute inference from acquired data. The suggested technique is assessed using several measures, including average reaction duration, accuracy, calculation expense, classification duration, and incorrect positive proportion. The collected findings verify the efficiency of the suggested method in terms of several performance assessment criteria in a cloud computing context.

***Keywords*:** Processing, big data, cloud computing, medical, and healthcare

13.1 Introduction

Healthcare attempts to preserve and enhance individual health through illness diagnosis, therapy, and control [1]. Healthcare suppliers all around the globe have been transitioning to software programs as a service, which is offered by the majority of cloud suppliers [2]. Since medical data are private, many parties must safely transmit patient and medical data to offer superior-quality treatment [3]. A cloud platform is an effective approach to preserving and processing medical data because it is accessible in big data volumes and numerous types [4]. The majority of software programs are now implemented in data facilities [5]. Cloud computing is indeed a dominating paradigm for doing complicated computations because it can effectively conduct larger-scale data calculations by offering scalable assets [6]. According to major assessment companies such as Gartner, Inc. and business data companies such as IDC, big data and cloud computing constitute developing innovations in the present business intelligence sector [7].

Cloud computing is indeed the best framework for larger-scale storage and complicated processing like big data analytics (BDA) [8]. Its benefits comprise scalability, adaptability, safety, simultaneous computing, and asset virtualization [9]. Cloud computing has the potential to minimize the expenses of automated processes, information technology, and infrastructure management while boosting operating effectiveness and user accessibility [10].

As previously noted, medicine is among the industries that generate massive amounts of data. Identification of patient groups and connections is required in the evaluation of huge collections of medical records [11]. This includes creating multiple designs based on statistical concepts or machine learning approaches [12]. Among the key issues that companies face is the requirement to safeguard the privacy of medical data [13]. Because healthcare produces complicated datasets, big data solutions must manage such data. Big data use facilitates the examination of computing biomedicine, genetic, and related medical data [14]. Big data innovations have been said to possess a lot of possibilities in the realm of healthcare. In healthcare, the combination of BDA and multiple systems would yield outstanding outcomes [15].

In this area, we will look at the security concepts that are required for data management. For medical data, they require a protected cloud-oriented platform [16]. Systems that are both energy-efficient and cost-effective are required for larger-scale data administration. Cloud computing offers numerous benefits, including expense savings, scalability, natural adaptability, power efficiency, and flexibility [17]. Figure 13.1 depicts the way the data are encrypted using identity-oriented encryption whenever the transmitter encrypts and transmits it to the cloud server.

Depending on the data acquired at a centralized repository like cloud servers, an effective data retrieving system could additionally construct instances of unidentified patients experiencing a specific collection of ailments (as described by the physician) or give other medical-based trends [18]. Among the most difficult issues in the setting of computation of the cloud is categorizing the acquired data based on its setting. Numerous research ideas have utilized different data mining methods for retrieving and processing big data [19]. For handling the diverse kind of data in this context, these recommendations include categorization, grouping, and connection criteria [20]. In response to these recommendations, this article proposes a novel BDA approach to deliver medical services [21]. This research has modified the widely known expectation-maximization (EM) method [22] to hold the data on the cloud to offer medical facilities, taking into account various clouds depending on various data groups. A fuzzy rule-oriented classifier is subsequently set forth to store fuzzy data and retrieve data from the cloud quickly and efficiently [23]. The first research, which was described in [24], is expanded in this publication, which also provides a thorough explanation of each stage of the research process.

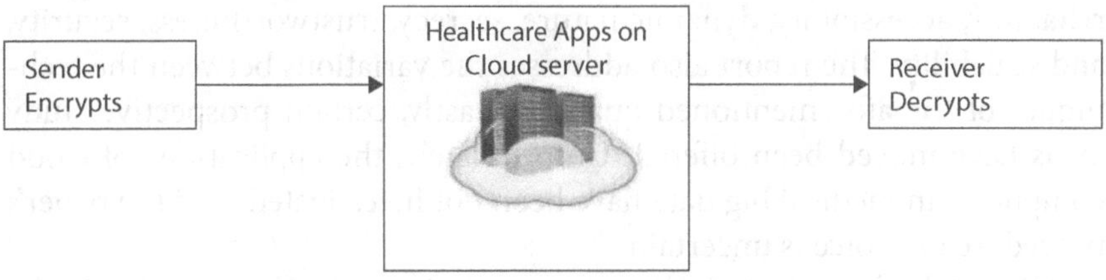

Figure 13.1 Secured cloud computing model for big data.

In this study, as opposed to [24], a more thorough literature analysis is conducted. The contrasts between the suggested system and the present plans about several evaluation metrics have indeed been underlined. The suggested system has also undergone a thorough evaluation using a variety of evaluation measures in various simulated scenarios, and it has been contrasted to reference designs in both centralized and distributed cloud contexts.

13.2 Literature Review

This part discusses certain selected works on cloud computing and various relevant publications to emphasize the purpose of authoring this paper [25]. In addition, several review papers related to the subject area were analyzed to illustrate the reason for producing this work as well as a few of their shortcomings. Numerous scholars have proposed cloud computing as an innovative and significant commercial model for biological data exchange.

Anuja and Jeyamala [26] examined the privacy concerns and answers for cloud-based medical image storage and exchange. They have also explored possible solutions to these problems. They classified security measures and proposed several novel ones to tackle the storage difficulties of medical photos in the cloud. On a routine basis, the researchers have categorized the security options to achieve authenticity, secrecy, access management, and strong availability in distinct lists. According to the findings of their research, the main disadvantage of the cloud is security.

Among the most important difficulties in cloud computing is evaluating the confidence level to allow users to choose trustworthy services [27]. As a result, Chiregi and Navimipour [28] offered a comprehensive examination of the most recent methods in this subject. Additionally, they examined cloud confidence evaluation strategies and classified them into two broad categories: centralized and distributed methods. They have also identified various confidence characteristics such as authenticity, confidentiality, reliability, accessibility, dynamic nature, secrecy, trustworthiness, security, and scalability. The report also addresses the variations between the techniques of the aforementioned qualities. Lastly, certain prospective study areas have indeed been offered. Unfortunately, the applications of cloud computing in medical big data have been not investigated, and the paper's procedure of choice is uncertain.

Ali *et al.* [29] conducted a literature analysis on cloud computing in the medical field. They reviewed 316 publications and narrowed them down to 88 to offer a paradigm containing three aspects: cloud-based medical potential, challenges, and uses. Suggestions for prospective study and practice have also been presented in the fields of value-added medical facilities for medical decision-making, safety, and confidentiality; medical surveillance characteristics; and cloud-based service delivery methods. Yet, the use of cloud computing in medical big data is not investigated. Furthermore, there is no evidence of cloud computing's performance in medicine.

Lastly, formal validation is a critical topic in the design of complicated data networks. As a result, using formal validation methodologies in cloud services is required to improve the system's accuracy. Souri *et al.* [30] developed an SLR approach for evaluating the present technological study in cloud formal validation. Additionally, the study divides formal validation methodologies into three categories: specification and procedure algebra, model verifying, and theorem stating. The validation techniques are contrasted using technical characteristics like specification techniques, modeling, validation instruments, and validation methods. The primary characteristics of the chosen studies, in addition to a few suggestions for prospective study, have indeed been explored.

13.3 Materials and Method

Figure 13.2 displays the network structure employed in the suggested system. The data collection layer, the transmitting layer, and the computing layer are the three layers that make up this structure [31].

The data collection layer is in charge of compiling patient information from various regions. The body sensing system, automobile ad hoc network, and system of gadgets existing in residences or different hospitals could all produce these data [32]. Body detectors or devices installed in automobiles have been used to produce the data via the vehicular system [33]. The majority of these vehicles are paramedics and healthcare vans, but if the patients' cars have the right monitors, data could also be transmitted from them [34]. Gadgets in these systems either transmit data independently or can select a network head who is in charge of managing data transfer for each of these connections [35]. Gadgets, body sensor systems, and automobiles can create an intra- or intercoalition and select a cluster head (CH) [36] for the transfer of mobile data, as illustrated in Figure 13.2.

The subclouds are indeed a set of distinct variables that comprise the majority of illnesses, and as illustrated in Figure 13.3, these subclouds were subsequently separated into several groups [37]. The suggested scheme's

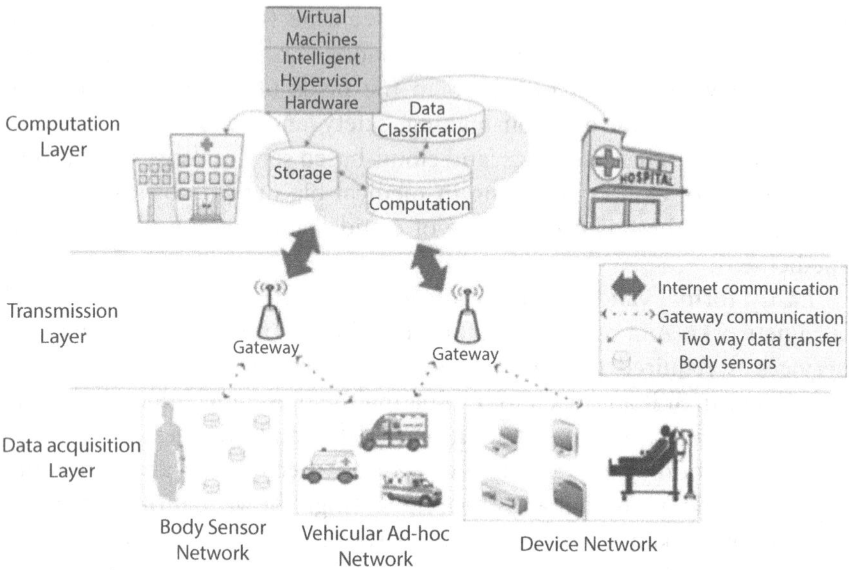

Figure 13.2 The suggested framework of the network model.

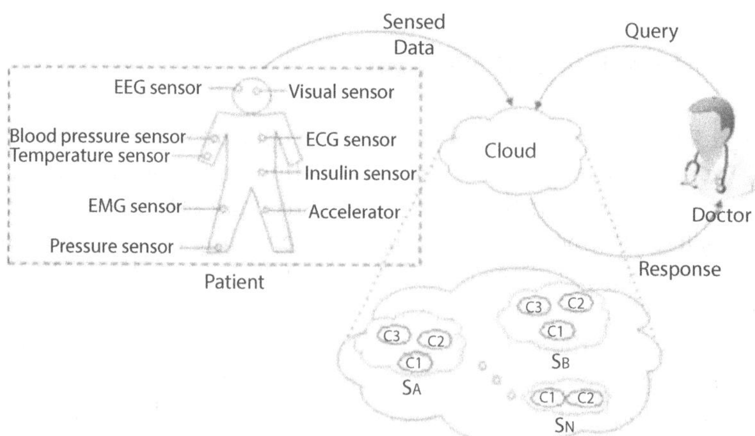

Figure 13.3 The suggested scheme's data flow.

data flow is depicted in Figure 13.3. As previously mentioned, the patient's data are collected utilizing a variety of sensors and saved in the cloud. The medical professional then looks for inquiries in the cloud. Depending on the revised EM technique, clustering is carried out by determining the participation of every number with the designated groups and upgrading the clusters as necessary. For instance, the age cloud subcloud SA can be divided into three clusters reflecting distinct age classes, like children, grownups, and senior citizens. To categorize fuzzy data and recover fuzzy questions as described by the professional, a fuzzy rule-oriented classifier has also been developed [38].

The training collection's groups are made via initial cluster creation. These groups house the fresh data [39]. The professional's symptoms that have been unable to be precisely measured are labeled as fuzzy symptoms, and their grouping is explained. The identical method is used in these groups to quantify the sufferers' fuzzy data [40]. Ultimately, a system is created that can get a catalog of potential sufferers for a given ailment based on the indications that an expert has defined (Figure 13.4).

Algorithm 1: Initial Cluster Formation.

Input: Initial Cluster Set(A), Number of new data values(N)
Output: Classified data; Revised Cluster Set

procedure Classify$A$
  A = [A_1 A_2 A_3 ... A_k]
  for (i = 1; i ≤ N; i++) **do** ▷ E-STEP
    for (j = 1; j ≤ k; j++) **do**
      Calculate μ_j for each cluster using (1)
    end for
    Classify the cluster set for each i according to algorithm 2
  end for
  Calculate the membership matrix M according to (2)
  for (i = 1; i ≤ N + k; i++) **do** ▷ M-STEP
    Revise the centroid of each cluster set using (3)
    Store the new centroid in C_i
  end for
  New centroids for each cluster are stored as C = [C_1 C_2 C_3 ...C_k]
  max = 0
  for (i = 1; i ≤ k; i++) **do** ▷ Update Centroids
    t = $|C_i - A_i|$
    if ($t > max$) **then**
      max ← t
    end if
  end for
  if (max > ϕ) **the**
    CLASSIFY(C)
  else
    return(C)
  end if
end procedure

Figure 13.4 Algorithm of cluster formation [40].

13.4 Result and Discussion

This part investigates the performance assessment of the suggested system in terms of numerous criteria, which have been described further below.

Figure 13.5 depicts the effect of work arrival rate fluctuation on average reply duration using varied levels of σ, μ, and load modification (η) on the cloud.

The collected findings indicate that as the task arrival ratio increases, so does their response duration with varying levels of σ and μ. When the task arrival premium changes, so does the burden on the cloud, which is controlled in terms of setting awareness of retrieving and processing data. At varying choices η, the mean response duration increases, while the variance σ increases (Figure 13.5(a)–(c)). σ and μ are calculated depending on the mean and variance from the average value of response duration for various task arrival rates. η is calculated by dividing the number of demands handled by the overall tasks arriving in a set amount of duration. According to these numbers, with a considerable departure from the average value, the estimates of average response duration rise. This is because the classifier created in the suggested approach may not perform effectively for big collections of datasets in terms of variation from the mean value. Because the data acquired for the medical service are diverse, the average reaction duration in the cloud context increases with the task arrival rate.

Table 13.1 shows the detailed computations and outcomes of these processes. Figure 13.6 depicts the effect of task arrival rate on accuracy percentage using various values of η, σ, and μ on the cloud.

The outcomes reveal that as the task arrival rate and stress on the cloud grow, so does the accuracy of retrieving and processing the data. This is because a rise in the task arrival rate increases the likelihood of fragile cluster development, which might lead to incorrect choices at different

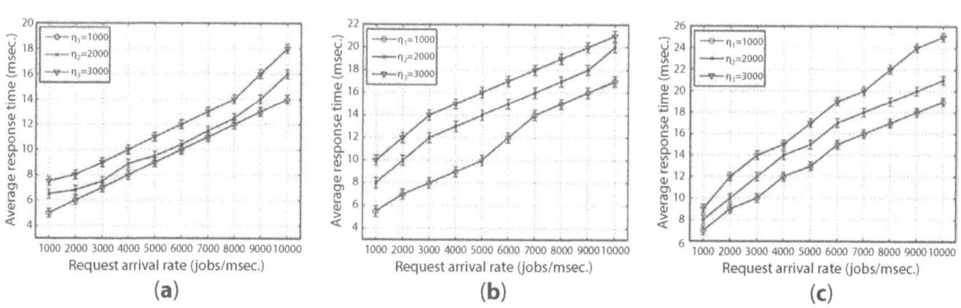

Figure 13.5 Change in average response duration as a function of (a) σ = 0.2, μ = 1,000; (b) σ = 0.4, μ = 1,000; and (c) σ = 0.6, μ = 1,000.

Table 13.1 The detailed computations and outcomes of these processes.

Early	5	15	55					
Training collection				67	22	11	3	
Repetition				E-stage				M-stage
1	M = 1 0 0	0 1 0	0 0 1	0.17 0.35 0.49	0.40 0.50 0.11	0.49 0.45 0.05	0.50 0.42 0.08	$C_1 = 12$ $C_2 = 26$ $C_3 = 54$
2	M = 1 0 0	0 1 0	0 0 1	0.19 0.33 0.48	0.46 0.49 0.05	0.50 0.44 0.06	0.49 0.42 0.10	$C_1 = 16$ $C_2 = 26$ $C_3 = 55$
3	M = 1 0 0	0 1 0	0 0 1	0.20 0.31 0.48	0.49 0.49 0.02	0.49 0.45 0.06	0.47 0.42 0.11	$C_1 = 18$ $C_2 = 26$ $C_3 = 56$
4	M = 1 0 0	0 1 0	0 0 1	0.22 0.30 0.49	0.50 0.49 0.01	0.49 0.45 0.06	0.47 0.43 0.11	$C_1 = 20$ $C_2 = 25$ $C_3 = 57$
5	M = 1 0 0	0 1 0	0 0 1	0.23 0.29 0.49	0.50 0.49 0.01	0.48 0.46 0.06	0.46 0.43 0.11	$C_1 = 21$ $C_2 = 25$ $C_3 = 58$

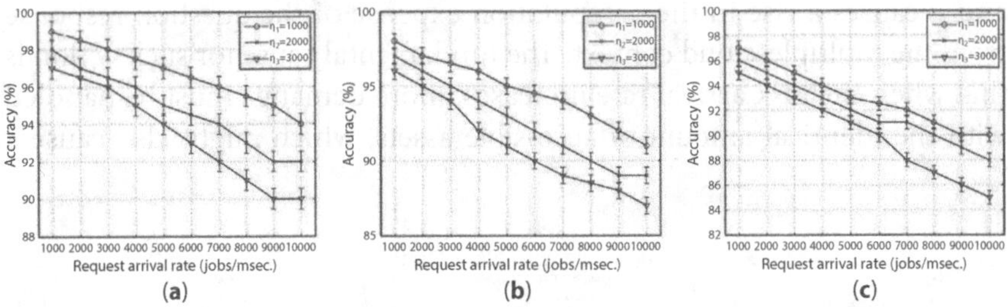

Figure 13.6 Accuracy percentage variation with (a) $\sigma = 0.2, \mu = 1{,}000$; (b) $\sigma = 0.4, \mu = 1{,}000$; and (c) $\sigma = 0.6, \mu = 1{,}000$.

phases of the suggested system. As a result, the accuracy of data retrieving decreases as the task arrival rate increases. According to the data, there is a variation from the average value μ following a rise in the task arrival rate, which leads to a rise in the σ divergence. Because of the substantial variance from the average value, fragile clusters might form. As a result, it might be hard to establish precise conclusions regarding the precise forecast of rule-oriented classifier functioning.

As shown in Figure 13.6(a)–(c), increasing the values reduces the accuracy of correctly predicting a patient's condition from a wide range of information sources in the cloud system. To calculate the accuracy, distinct instances from the rule-oriented repository have been collected concerning diverse sets of data resources from distinct persons, and a cloud repository is built. With this cloud repository, physicians seated in remote locations examine patients' medical data, giving them the freedom to obtain data regarding different patients anytime from anywhere. Furthermore, the suggested approach uses effective E- and M-steps to classify data into multiple categories, which have been then examined to make the best choices in duration intervals.

The effect of task arrival speed on the computational expense of setting awareness of data retrieving from the cloud is depicted in Figure 13.7. The computational expense is calculated based on several assets used to execute the distinct demands issued by users.

The collected outcomes reveal that as the work arrival rate and pressure rise, so does the computational expense. The computation expense is the overall expense associated with the use, accessibility, and usage of network assets in the cloud computing context. The larger the question processing computation expense, the larger the stress σ and task arrival rate. The larger the load and task arrival rate, the larger the calculation expense connected with question processing. As illustrated in Figure 13.7, changing the η, σ, and μ causes a rise in the computation expense of the question response from the multiple-cloud context. The fundamental cause for such action is that when the task arrival rate increases, more demands must be handled with the identical amount of accessible assets, which might also cause a

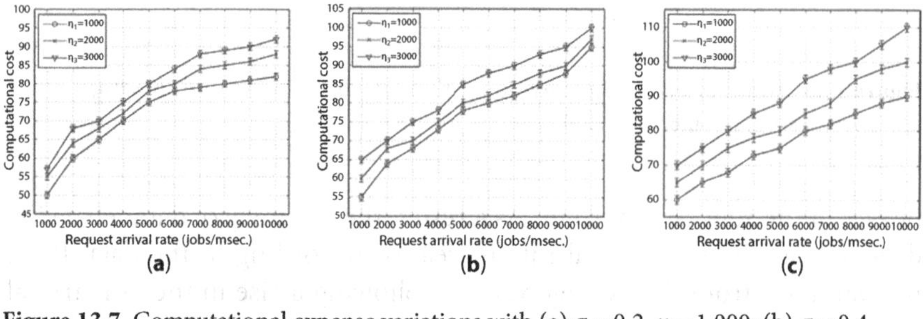

Figure 13.7 Computational expense variations with (a) σ = 0.2, μ = 1,000; (b) σ = 0.4, μ = 1,000; and (c) σ = 0.6, μ = 1,000.

performance barrier in a certain portion of the system. This raises the computational price of the suggested strategy regarding the task arrival rate.

Figures 13.8 and 13.9 calculate the false-positive proportion at $\sigma = 0.4$ and $\mu = 1{,}000$ in centralized and scattered sites with varied data volumes. It should be mentioned that these incorrect positive reports are assessed by an expert.

According to the figures, as the volume of the data increases, so does the false-positive proportion in all of the methods employing distinct classifiers. Nonetheless, when contrasted with the various approaches, the suggested fuzzy rule-oriented classifier has the lowest false-positive proportion. This

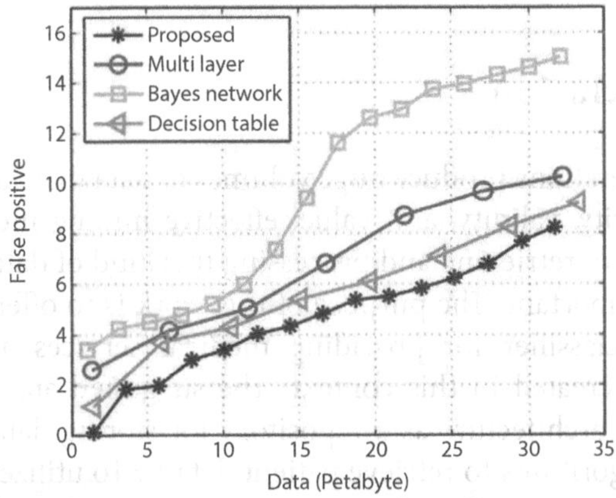

Figure 13.8 The false-positive rate in a centralized place.

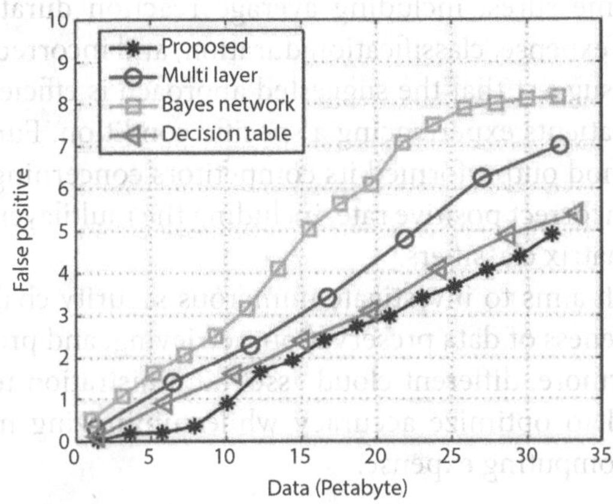

Figure 13.9 The false-positive rate in a distributed place.

is primarily because the suggested technique employs a rule-oriented classifier, which allows the decision support network to easily classify data. Furthermore, the level of false-positive proportion has been larger in centralized locations than in spread locations (as shown in Figures 13.8 and 13.9). This is mostly because data at a spread site are present at numerous sites, with a larger possibility of finding it than at a centralized site.

As a result, the suggested fuzzy rule-oriented classifier reduces the false-positive proportion in cloud-oriented architecture. This research contrasted the suggested fuzzy rule-oriented classifier to the current multilayer, Bayes system, and decision matrix classifiers. The outcomes show that the suggested fuzzy rule-oriented classifier beats the other classifiers in terms of false-positive proportion.

13.5 Conclusion

As medical operations produce huge volumes of data that vary in quantity, diversity, velocity, validity, and value, effective mining methods for setting awareness of retrieving and processing this kind of data have become increasingly important. The purpose of this work is to offer a novel fuzzy rule-oriented classifier for providing medical services and classifying the huge data created in this context. The suggested approach employs cloud-oriented architecture as a repository for storing data and employs quantitative algorithms to retrieve patient details. To utilize analytics, EM and fuzzy rule-oriented classifiers are used to create algorithms for group creation and retrieving the data. The suggested method is contrasted to existing systems, and its performance has been evaluated using a variety of evaluation measures, including average reaction duration, accuracy, computational expense, classification duration, and incorrect positive rate. The outcomes suggest that the suggested approach is efficient in identifying potential patients experiencing a specific condition. Furthermore, the suggested method outperformed its competitors concerning classification duration and incorrect positive rate, including the multilayer, Bayes model, and decision matrix classifiers.

This research aims to investigate numerous security challenges related to setting awareness of data preservation, retrieving, and processing in the future. Furthermore, different cloud asset administration techniques will be investigated to optimize accuracy while minimizing mean response duration and computing expense.

References

1. Santos, M.A., Munoz, R., Olivares, R., Rebouças Filho, P.P., Del Ser, J., de Albuquerque, V.H.C., Online heart monitoring systems on the internet of health things environments: A survey, a reference model and an outlook. *Inf. Fusion, 53*, 222–239, 2020.
2. Diwakar, M., Tripathi, A., Joshi, K., Memoria, M., Singh, P., Latest trends on heart disease prediction using machine learning and image fusion. *Mater. Today:. Proc., 37*, 3213–3218, 2021.
3. Singh, D., Singh, R., Gehlot, A., Akram, S.V., Priyadarshi, N., Twala, B., An imperative role of digitalization in monitoring cattle health for sustainability. *Electronics, 11*, 17, 2702, 2022.
4. Dhaundiyal, R., Tripathi, A., Joshi, K., Diwakar, M., Singh, P., Clustering-based multi-modality medical image fusion. *J. Phys. Conf. Ser.*, 1478, 1, 012024, 2020. IOP Publishing.
5. Baral, M.M. and Verma, A., Cloud computing adoption for healthcare: An empirical study using SEM approach. *FIIB Business Rev., 10*, 3, 255–275, 2021.
6. Liu, Y., Liang, S., He, C., Zhou, Z., Fang, W., Li, Y., Wang, Y., A Cloud-computing and big data-based wide area monitoring of power grids strategy, in: *IOP Conference Series: Materials Science and Engineering*, vol. 677, IOP Publishing, p. 042055, 2019, December.
7. Sharma, M., Rastogi, R., Arya, N., Akram, S.V., Singh, R., Gehlot, A., Joshi, K., LoED: LoRa and edge computing based system architecture for sustainable forest monitoring. *IJETT, 70*, 5, 88–93, 2022.
8. Ahamad, S., Roshan, A., Lourens, M., Shekher, V., Joshi, K., Alanya-Beltran, J., The critical role played by big data management in effectively addressing security and overall privacy concerns through correlation analysis, in: *2022 2nd International Conference on Advance Computing and Innovative Technologies in Engineering (ICACITE)*, IEEE, pp. 130–134, 2022, April.
9. Hashem, I.A.T., Yaqoob, I., Anuar, N.B., Mokhtar, S., Gani, A., Khan, S.U., The rise of "big data" on cloud computing: Review and open research issues. *Inf. Syst., 47*, 98–115, 2015.
10. Sharma, M., Rastogi, R., Arya, N., Akram, S.V., Singh, R., Gehlot, A., Joshi, K., LoED: LoRa and edge computing based system architecture for sustainable forest monitoring. *IJETT, 70*, 5, 88–93, 2022.
11. Singh, D., Singh, R., Gehlot, A., Akram, S.V., Priyadarshi, N., Twala, B., An imperative role of digitalization in monitoring cattle health for sustainability. *Electronics, 11*, 17, 2702, 2022.
12. Kirola, M., Memoria, M., Dumka, A., Joshi, K., A comprehensive review study on optimized data mining, machine learning, and deep learning techniques for breast cancer prediction in a big data context. *BPJ, 15*, 1, 13–25, 2022.
13. Batko, K. and Ślęzak, A., The use of big data analytics in healthcare. *J. Big Data, 9*, 1, 3, 2022.

14. Singh, R., Gehlot, A., Mittal, M., Samkaria, R., Singh, D., Chandra, P., Design and development of a cloud-assisted robot, in: *Smart and Innovative Trends in Next Generation Computing Technologies: Third International Conference, NGCT 2017, Dehradun, India, October 30-31, 2017, Revised Selected Papers, Part II 3*, Springer, Singapore, pp. 419–429, 2018.
15. Shahbaz, M., Gao, C., Zhai, L., Shahzad, F., Hu, Y., Investigating the adoption of big data analytics in healthcare: The moderating role of resistance to change. *J. Big Data*, *6*, 1, 1–20, 2019.
16. Singh, R., Gehlot, A., Rashid, M., Saxena, R., Akram, S.V., Alshamrani, S.S., AlGhamdi, A.S., Cloud server and internet of things assisted system for stress monitoring. *Electronics*, *10*, 24, 3133, 2021.
17. Sharma, S.D., Sharma, S., Singh, R., Gehlot, A., Priyadarshi, N., Twala, B., Stress detection system for working pregnant women using an improved deep recurrent neural network. *Electronics*, *11*, 18, 2862, 2022.
18. Joshi, K., Joshi, K.N., Diwakar, M., Tripathi, N.A., Gupta, H., Multi-focus image fusion using non-local mean filtering and stationary wavelet transform. *IJITEE*, *9*, 344–350, 2019.
19. Joshi, K., Diwakar, M., Joshi, N.K., Lamba, S., A concise review of the latest methods of image fusion. *Recent Adv. Comput. Sci. Commun. (Formerly: Recent Patents Comput. Science)*, *14*, 7, 2046–2056, 2021.
20. Dumka, A., Verma, P., Singh, R., Kumar Bisht, A., Anand, D., MoaiteqAljahdali, H., Aparicio Obregón, S., A novel deep learning based healthcare model for COVID-19 pandemic stress analysis. *CMC*, *72*, 3, 6029–6044, 2022.
21. Praveen, S., Tyagi, N., Singh, B., Karetla, G.R., Thaler, M.A., Joshi, K., Tsegaye, M., PSO-based evolutionary approach to optimize head and neck biomedical image to detect mesothelioma cancer. *BioMed. Res. Int.*, *2022*, 1–12, 2022.
22. Fong, S., Wong, R., Vasilakos, A.V., Accelerated PSO swarm search feature selection for data stream mining big data. *IEEE Trans. Serv. Comput.*, *9*, 1, 33–45, 2015.
23. Diwakar, M., Tripathi, A., Joshi, K., Sharma, A., Singh, P., Memoria, M., A comparative review: Medical image fusion using SWT and DWT. *Mater. Today:. Proc.*, *37*, 3411–3416, 2021.
24. Jindal, A., Dua, A., Kumar, N., Vasilakos, A.V., Rodrigues, J.J., An efficient fuzzy rule-based big data analytics scheme for providing healthcare-as-a-service, in: *2017 IEEE International Conference on Communications (ICC)*, IEEE, pp. 1–6, 2017, May.
25. Joshi, K., Kumar, M., Tripathi, A., Kumar, A., Sehgal, J., Barthwal, A., Latest trends in multi-modality medical image fusion: A generic review, in: *Rising Threats in Expert Applications and Solutions: Proceedings of FICR-TEAS 2022*, pp. 663–671, 2022.

26. Anuja, M. and Jeyamala, C., A survey on security issues and solutions for storage and exchange of medical images in the cloud. *IJETEE, 11*, 6, 27–32, 2015.
27. Chiregi, M. and Navimipour, N.J., Trusted services identification in the cloud environment using the topological metrics. *Karbala Int. J. Mod. Sci., 2*, 3, 203–210, 2016.
28. Chiregi, M. and Navimipour, N.J., A comprehensive study of the trust evaluation mechanisms in cloud computing. *J. Serv. Sci. Res., 9*, 1–30, 2017.
29. Ali, O., Shrestha, A., Soar, J., Wamba, S.F., Cloud computing-enabled healthcare opportunities, issues, and applications: A systematic review. *Int. J. Inf. Manag., 43*, 146–158, 2018.
30. Souri, A., Navimipour, N.J., Rahmani, A.M., Formal verification approaches and standards in the cloud computing: A comprehensive and systematic review. *Comput. Stand. Interfaces, 58*, 1–22, 2018.
31. Madan, P., Singh, V., Chaudhari, V., Albagory, Y., Dumka, A., Singh, R., AlGhamdi, A.S., An optimization-based diabetes prediction model using CNN and bi-directional LSTM in a real-time environment. *Appl. Sci., 12*, 8, 3989, 2022.
32. Dua, S., Kumar, S.S., Albagory, Y., Ramalingam, R., Dumka, A., Singh, R., AlGhamdi, A.S., Developing a speech recognition system for recognizing tonal speech signals using a convolutional neural network. *Appl. Sci., 12*, 12, 6223, 2022.
33. Rajput, S.K., Patni, J.C., Alshamrani, S.S., Chaudhari, V., Dumka, A., Singh, R., Alghamdi, A.S., Automatic vehicle identification and classification model using the YOLOv3 algorithm for a toll management system. *Sustainability, 14*, 15, 9163, 2022.
34. Rana, A., Rawat, A.S., Afifi, A., Singh, R., Rashid, M., Gehlot, A., Alshamrani, S.S., A long-range internet of things-based advanced vehicle pollution monitoring system with node authentication and blockchain. *Appl. Sci., 12*, 15, 7547, 2022.
35. Cheng, X., Zhang, R., Yang, L., Wireless toward the era of intelligent vehicles. *IEEE IoT J., 6*, 1, 188–202, 2018.
36. Mukhtaruzzaman, M. and Atiquzzaman, M., Clustering in vehicular ad hoc network: Algorithms and challenges. *Comput. Electr. Eng., 88*, 106851, 2020.
37. Kumar, N., Kaur, K., Jindal, A., Rodrigues, J.J., Providing healthcare services on-the-fly using multi-player cooperation game theory in the Internet of Vehicles (IoV) environment. *Digit. Commun. Netw., 1*, 3, 191–203, 2015.
38. Omidvar, M., Zarei, E., Ramavandi, B., Yazdi, M., Fuzzy bow-tie analysis: Concepts, review, and application, in: *Linguistic Methods Under Fuzzy Information in System Safety and Reliability Analysis*, 2022.

39. Kabir, S., Walker, M., Papadopoulos, Y., Rüde, E., Securius, P., Fuzzy temporal fault tree analysis of dynamic systems. *Int. J. Approximate Reasoning, 77*, 20–37, 2016.
40. Kabir, S. and Papadopoulos, Y., A review of applications of fuzzy sets to safety and reliability engineering. *Int. J. Approximate Reasoning, 100*, 29–55, 2018.

14

Deep Learning (DL) on Exascale Computing to Speed Up Cancer Investigation

D. Rubidha Devi[1], S. Ashwini[2*], Samreen Rizvi[3], P. Venkata Hari Prasad[4], Mohit Tiwari[5] and Joshuva Arockia Dhanraj[6]

[1]*Department of CSE, Sastra Deemed University, Kumbakonam, India*
[2]*Department of Computing Technologies, School of Computing, SRM Institute of Science and Technology Kattankulathur Campus, Chennai, India*
[3]*TCS, Noida, UP, India*
[4]*Department of Computer Science and Engineering, Koneru Lakshmaiah Education, Foundation Vaddeswaram, Guntur, India*
[5]*Department of Computer Science and Engineering, Bharati Vidyapeeth's College of Engineering, Delhi, Paschim Vihar, Delhi, India*
[6]*Centre for Automation and Robotics (ANRO), Department of Mechatronics Engineering, Hindustan Institute of Technology and Science, Padur, Chennai, India*

Abstract

Cancer deep learning climate, benchmarks, and work processes will consolidate the force of exascale registering with brain network-based AI to address a scope of inexactly associated issues in cancer research. This application region presents novel difficulties to the exascale processing climate. Here, this exploration distinguishes one test in CANDLE work processes: saving brain network model portrayals to steady capacity. Deep learning, through brain organizations, has exhibited an exceptional capacity to mechanize numerous standard undertakings when given adequate information for preparing. What the brain network can learn from the training data is greatly influenced by its design, which includes the number of layers, the types of layers, and the connections between layers. The pattern for brain network models, particularly those prepared on Picture Net, has been becoming always significant and more intricate. The outcome has been always expanding

**Corresponding author*: ashwinisekar.achu@gmail.com; ORCID: 0000-0001-5111-337X
Joshuva Arockia Dhanraj: ORCID: 0000-0001-5048-7775

Kapil Joshi and Somil Kumar Gupta (eds.) Human Cancer Diagnosis and Detection Using Exascale Computing, (215–226) © 2024 Scrivener Publishing LLC

precision on benchmark datasets with the expense of expanded computational requests.

Keywords: Deep learning (DL), cancer, drug, patients, exascale

14.1 Introduction

Deep learning has shown great promise in accelerating cancer investigations. One area where deep learning has been particularly successful is in medical imaging. For example, deep learning models can be trained to quickly and accurately identify abnormal cells in medical images such as X-rays, CT scans, and MRI scans. These models can assist radiologists in identifying potential cancerous cells, reducing the amount of time needed to examine medical images manually [1]. Deep learning algorithms can be trained to detect patterns and mutations in large amounts of genomic data, allowing for more efficient and accurate diagnosis of cancer and personalized treatment plans. Overall, the use of deep learning in cancer investigation has the potential to significantly speed up the diagnosis and treatment of cancer, ultimately leading to better patient outcomes.

Prescient computational models for patients with cancer can later on help counteraction and therapy choices by illuminating decisions to accomplish the most ideal clinical result. The public precision medication drive in 2015 marked a significant development in precision medicine and inspired important campaigns aimed at and promoting precision oncology, including the precise forecasting of treatment results. Limitations in data and computation are anticipated to push this goal. While this was going on, the horizon of thinking in the current sciences was shifting as the constraints and changes involved in exascale handling were approaching, caused by the accelerated rise in data volumes and anticipated new information sources catalyzed by new advancements and drives like the PMI [2]. This interagency collaboration framework made it possible for the NCI along with the DOE to work closely together. These three pilot studies' clear-cut objectives were to advance unresolved areas of figuring advances in three distinct fields of malignant development research: (1) cell level: improve the ability of patient-driven preclinical models to identify novel treatments; (2) nuclear level: continue to handle the basic investigation of intractable goals; and (3) people level: acquire crucial insights into the factors that influence the development of human disease. In a similar vein, the pilot studies would develop novel weakness prediction systems to gauge confidence in the repeated knowledge model assumptions [3]. A team-based strategy is used in each and every one of the pilot projects conducted as part of JDACS4C's collaborative efforts, demonstrating the effectiveness of such well-coordinated activities. Pilot 1 (cell level), driven by profound learning, combines data in novel ways to support computationally long-sighted models for growth response to novel encouraging trained pros. Exploratory data, expansion, and computerized logic are combined in pilot 2 (subnuclear level), opening up new avenues for the study of decided-to-leave-related tumors. Pilot 3 (people level) engages in exact disease monitoring to alter malignant growth care by utilizing man-made knowledge and patient data at phenomenal scales.

14.2 Literature Review

Cancer is an incredibly complicated infection, which upsets essential natural cycles at a key level, prompting rebel cells to undermine the soundness of the person. Fortunately, significant technological advancements in chosen-to-leave-nuclear gene sequencing, subnuclear or cell imaging, and high-volume screening methods have made it possible to test the disorder's complex structure at a previously unheard-of level. This provides a window into the strategy for treating the illness at previously unheard-of time and spatial scales. Huge databases that can be examined using computerized artificial intelligence (ML) methods have been made possible by the use of these advancements [4]. Multiple persistent problems can be changed by computer-based intelligence (ML). In order to promote cancer research using machine learning, the U.S. Department of Energy established the Exascale Computing Project (ECP), concentrating on the growing effectiveness of ML systems and the expanding capacities of large-scale computing facilities (Flame). CANDLE is creating software architecture to enable flexible deep learning using DOE supercomputing capabilities. While it is explicitly stated that the FLAME project will support significant learning in each of the three cancer trials in the short term, its longer-term goal is to support a broad range of fundamental learning applications throughout DOE's science spaces [5]. Deep learning systems are under dynamic improvement by different examination networks in two businesses. Every one of these systems varies concerning the AI assignments they focus on, their convenience, information prehandling, and target issues. Most structures were architected for a solitary hub execution and a couple of dispersed memory multi-hub executions have as of late arisen, yet these executions are focused on more modest center counts and product bunch conditions. In addition, these executions depend on keeping away from correspondence by putting away information on nearby circles. Executions focusing on elite execution figuring frameworks will require novel strategies to completely take advantage of the framework interconnect data transfer capacity and geographies, as well as the deep memory orders.

The least complex, however generally expensive, techniques for hyperparameter improvement incorporate comprehensive space search (the savage power strategy), straightforward inclination plunge, various slope plummet, and irregular hunt. However, these pursuit algorithms can be tuned to execute rapidly (arbitrary hunt) or to track down the ideal arrangement (comprehensive inquiry), and the negligible improvement concerning used assets is not productive for issues with O(109) or more prominent sensible discrete boundary blends. There are two fundamental weaknesses involving a group of discrete hyperparameters selected by the client using logic for decreasing incidents: 1) It necessitates that the customer cast doubt on topological efficacies and efficiencies, and 2) it is limited to a somewhat narrow range of models [6] (i.e., it is convincing a confounded calculation into obliged limits). In any case, this is nonetheless significantly less unpredictable than the O(1021) volatility that is feasible in the recurrent pattern of CANDLE work processes, even after taking into account the appropriate reductions possible employing point drop. We could obtain two or three crucial levels of search space. The given network hyperparameters are improved by hypertune using Bayesian optimization. This application of Bayesian improvement is successful because it avoids having to calculate numerous complicated auxiliaries [7]. Discovering an orientation from an unexpected model can be compared to the calculation; many hyperparameters are chosen, followed by a different one, and if the second group is preferred over the first, a computation concentrates in that direction. This system excels due to its extensibility and ability to discover reasonable plans with basically less time to interact than formative calculations. However, it can also "skip around," not selecting a particular set of values or eliminating itself past an intriguing least. Formative calculations are an alternative theory. The NeuroEvolution of Spreading Topographies (Smooth) computation is one of the innate algorithms for hyperparameter search that is most noticeable and powerful. The Smooth system starts by creating a genome and then creates a general community using that genome shortly after [8]. The algorithm often selects out of the general population the most inappropriate people (those with the highest error rate or setback). The desired result is then produced by combining individuals from the

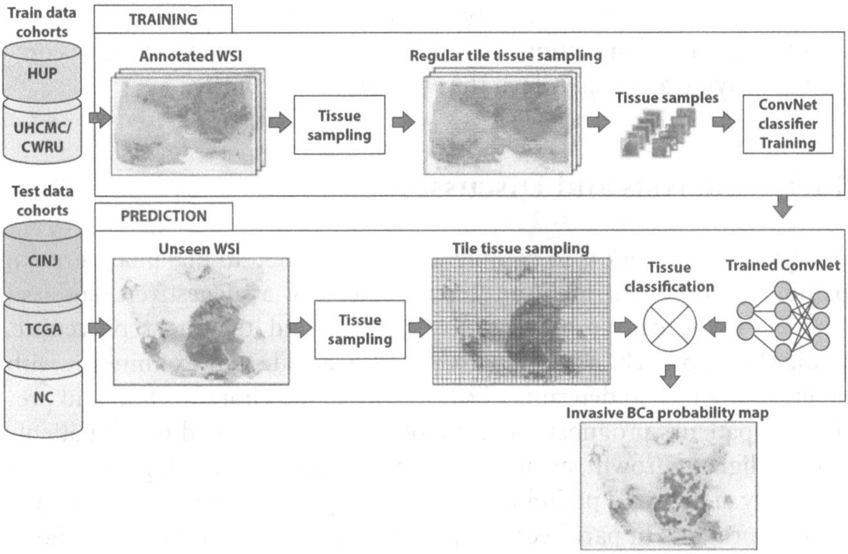

Figure 14.1 DL techniques for cancer investigation. (Source: [6]).

remaining subgroup. It accomplishes this on two levels: inside each central point (neuron) and in conjunction with the association's geology. One is frequently prepared to discover a passionately convincing game plan using this ancestral style calculation. There are, nonetheless, a few disadvantages to the Slick algorithm. The essential component that would most restrict us in our application is Perfect's adjustment of intrahub loads and boundaries [9]. While this can be useful by decreasing misfortune at the "beginning stage" of preparing, it likewise fills in as a geography-explicit component that fairly blocks the examination of unadulterated topological qualities and shortcomings. The other restricting component is the above expected to produce the organization without any preparation. Figure 14.1 shows DL techniques for cancer investigation.

14.3 Research Methodology

A secondary descriptive analysis method is used to gather relevant and actual information related to the topic. Deep learning models can also be used to predict the likelihood of cancer recurrence and to assist with treatment planning. Another promising application of deep learning in cancer investigation is the analysis of genomic data. The Public Foundations of

Success, a major driving force, organizes specialized missions and acts as a significant partner in cutting-edge entertainment via expert exascale computing, playing a crucial role in the abandoned-plan cycle.

14.4 Analysis and Discussion

The goal of this work is to comment on data related to malignant growth pathology. A patient might undergo a biopsy, or a suggestive tissue test, as part of the cancer prevention assurance and treatment procedure. Using this approach, a pathologist prepares a slide and examines it with an enlarging tool to determine how to handle the viral infection and predict the patient's prognosis. These biopsies are performed on all patients with malignant growth, creating a sizable number of pathology images. A summary of digitized pathology slides or a high-level topic of pathology is making progress in part because quantitative analyses of digitized whole-slide images produce insights that are typically repeatable and detailed.

$$a_j^l = K\,(\sum_k w_{jk}^l a_k^{l-1} + b_j^l$$

The widespread acceptance of computerized entire slide imaging is the enthusiasm being sparked by the FDA's endorsement of its primary diagnostic usage. It is generally predicted that the majority of new pathology images will be digital within the next 5 to 10 years. Growth-infiltrating lymphocytes, which are safe cell types that move into cancer to try to combat the illness, are a key component in these images [10]. Numerous cases prevent the assessment of TILs from having prognostic value, since understanding patient's safe reaction to growth is turning out to be progressively significant with the development of disease immunotherapy. TILs can be measured through picture examination and profound learning calculations. Each subsequent picture is commonly gigapixel in scale and envelops 100,000 to a million cell cores.

```
foreach i in [0:N-1] {
  sds_kv_put("key"+i, "value1") =>
  sds_kv_get("key"+i, 100);
}
```

Bench 1

```
foreach i in [0:N-1] {
  file f<"key"+i> = write("value");
  string s = read(f);
}
```

In the area of profound learning, the emphasis has been placed on achieving better accuracy or a reduction in mean-squared errors for specific endeavors while ignoring various factors that are essential to the process of action, such as assumption time. Formative smoothing out has been used to both arrange the association's geology and advance the heaps in the association [11]. Later research contends that short connections can perform almost as well as deeper ones, even with less computing complexity, and that deeper connections are less efficient. Additionally, a comparable result without the use of multiobjective advancement demonstrates that an evolutionary improvement strategy can accurately build simple connections as shown in Figure 14.2.

For a specific set of data, a profound learning method can be used three times, and HPC can be applied to any of the three stages. The three phases are organizing, preparing, and sending. The topography of the association and its hyperparameters are rearranged for the dataset during the initial step. The most notable approach for this step is for a professional who is using the profoundly improving method for Manually fine-tuning the association's configuration, consistently starting from another common collaboration plan and performing intuition-coordinated (to an extent not precisely abandoned) acclimations of different limits until the association's accuracy is increased. It is fully anticipated that this manual procedure would take months [12]. It has been demonstrated that using HPC alongside crucial simulated intelligence methodology can both increase

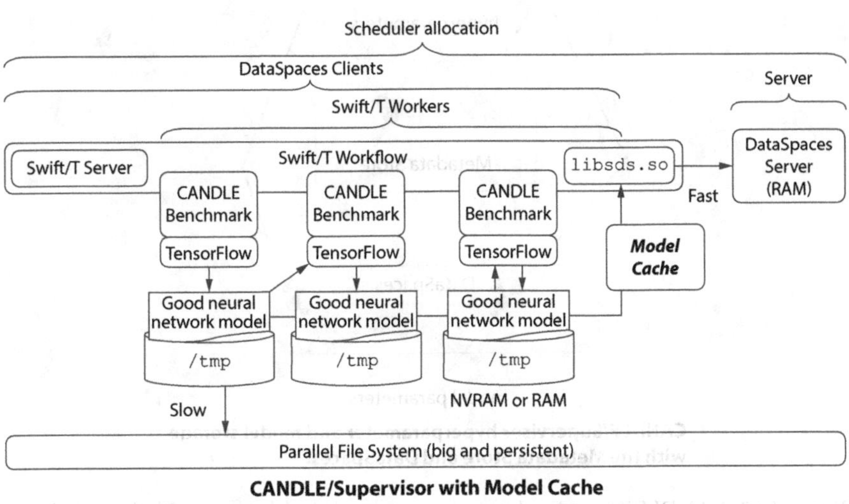

Figure 14.2 CANDLE/supervisor with the model cache. (Source: [11]).

the introduction of the association and reduce the possibility of orchestration down to hours, frequently beyond what a space expert could accomplish. Figure 14.3 shows the evidence of supervisor hyperparameter and model storage with the metadata store and data space. There are several methods for setting up hyperparameters for machine learning on HPC, which include using inherited calculations, Bayesian upgrades, and support vector machines to support the premise for great hyperparameter sets. To decide on the best arrangement for the deep learning network, which frequently necessitates examining hundreds of thousands to a billion of conceivable association plans, HPC is ideally suited to handle this period of profound advancement [13]. The organization of the club is synchronized in a variety of methods in the following stage.

With all centers working with different teams of data and weight exchange revitalizes, the planning data is passed through the network in bunches in one procedure. This approach is termed data parallelism, and yet, it has been shown to work against scaling mathematically while remaining aware of mathematical execution [14]. In a different method known as model parallelism, the layers of the association can be circled over multiple GPUs and various center points to build up the association as a whole. In any case, the scalability of this method is severely constrained

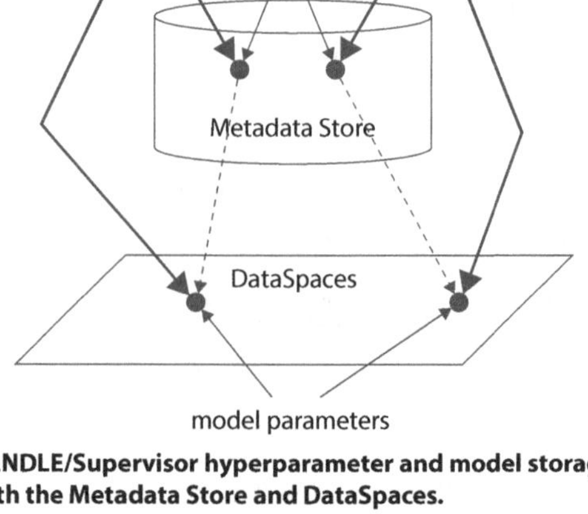

Figure 14.3 CANDLE/supervisor hyperparameter and model storage with the metadata store and data spaces. (Source: [13]).

because it has not yet been demonstrated that powerful associations that span entire supercomputers outperform these connections that can reside in a single center. The association is sent into action to look at verified data in the third and final step, which is known as inferencing or estimating. The presumption of HPC can be important, especially when simulation parallelism is typical for very large datasets. In any event, this is frequently not a realistic application of deep learning on HPC because the majority of space professionals do not move toward power-class HPC [15]. However, there are some narrowly defined situations where HPC would be useful for making assumptions. For greater impact, employing HPC to develop a model that can quickly and precisely represent data on non-HPC buildings is a potential roadblock for both HPC and design specialists.

14.5 Conclusion

Compartments can extraordinarily improve the capacity of clients to get to complex programming applications and work processes. In this paper, specialists used a compartment to deal with the sending of a confusing disease-based application suite called Light for sensible clients. An MPI-based workflow framework, rich Python and R libraries with tensor flow, improvements, etc., and Python-based application benchmarks are just a few of the cooperating elements that this system uses. The work interaction was at first planned to run on petascale DOE supercomputers; nonetheless, we used holders to redeploy the structure on a more unassuming bundle regularly used by prosperity specialists. The JDACS4C involvement offers important insights into the future of PC-based information for disease study and the crucial role that absurdly large-scale enrolment will play in illuminating and embellishing that future. Due to multidisciplinary participation and access to cutting-edge figuring tools, ideas have quickly been transformed into starter practices. Computer-based intelligence is being utilized to direct exploratory plans to utilize important research center assets, to foster new abilities for subatomic reproduction, and to smooth out and further develop efficiencies in the procurement of clinical information. The JDACS4C cooperation laid out an establishment for group science and is empowering development at the crossing point of cutting-edge figuring innovations and cancer research. These pilot projects are only the beginning of ridiculously large-scale enrolments in disease study and man-made knowledge. This study has significant ramifications for disease research. In particular, disease investigators continue to research and support novel markers to improve patient outcomes to a prudent degree.

Research demonstrates, for instance, that higher TIL densities are associated with favorable clinical outcomes and, for various disease types, extended sans malignant growth periods. This study uses a high-precision, high-speed methodology to update representations for numerous images. Along these lines, these photographs and their clarifications can then be used to accelerate disease research.

References

1. Al-Saadi, A., Ahn, D.H., Babuji, Y., Chard, K., Corbett, J., Hategan, M., Herbein, S., Jha, S., Laney, D., Merzky, A., Munson, T., Exaworks: Workflows for exascale, in: *2021 IEEE Workshop on Workflows in Support of Large-Scale Science (WORKS)*, IEEE, pp. 50–57, 2021 November, https://doi.org/10.1109/WORKS54523.2021.00012.
2. Bhatia, H., Aydin, F., Carpenter, T.S., Lightstone, F.C., Bremer, P.T., Ingólfsson, H.I., Nissley, D.V., Streitz, F.H., The confluence of machine learning and multiscale simulations. *Curr. Opin. Struct. Biol.*, *80*, 102569, 2023. https://doi.org/10.8875/dasdw78555.
3. Bhattacharya, T., Brettin, T., Doroshow, J.H., Evrard, Y.A., Greenspan, E.J., Gryshuk, A.L., Hoang, T.T., Lauzon, C.B.V., Nissley, D., Penberthy, L., Stahlberg, E., AI meets exascale computing: Advancing cancer research with large-scale high-performance computing. *Front. Oncol.*, *9*, 984, 2019. https://doi.org/10.1142/nklmm4512.
4. Chang, C., Deringer, V.L., Katti, K.S., Van Speybroeck, V., Wolverton, C.M., Simulations in the era of exascale computing. *Nat. Rev. Mater.*, 1–5, 2023. https://doi.org/10.8545/78545212.
5. Devarajan, H., Zheng, H., Kougkas, A., Sun, X.H., Vishwanath, V., Dlio: A data-centric benchmark for scientific deep learning applications, in: *2021 IEEE/ACM 21st International Symposium on Cluster, Cloud and Internet Computing (CCGrid)*, IEEE, pp. 81–91, 2021 May, https://doi.org/10.8545/yeuytjn7854.
6. Dua, S., Kumar, S.S., Albagory, Y., Ramalingam, R., Dumka, A., Singh, R., Rashid, M., Gehlot, A., Alshamrani, S.S., AlGhamdi, A.S., Developing a speech recognition system for recognizing tonal speech signals using a convolutional neural network. *Appl. Sci.*, 12, 12, 6223, 2022. https://doi.org/10.7854/4784112.
7. Iqbal, M.J., Javed, Z., Sadia, H., Qureshi, I.A., Irshad, A., Ahmed, R., Malik, K., Raza, S., Abbas, A., Pezzani, R., Sharifi-Rad, J., Clinical applications of artificial intelligence and machine learning in cancer diagnosis: Looking into the future. *Cancer Cell Int.*, *21*, 1, 1–11, 2021. https://doi.org/10.8547/8451598513.

8. dev Sharma, S. and Saxena, A., The smart analysis of environmental pollution widespread in the forest areas using analytical discussion based deep learning, in: *2023 IEEE International Conference on Integrated Circuits and Communication Systems (ICICACS)*, IEEE, pp. 1–6, 2023 February, https://doi.org/10.85475/4789412.
9. Nicolae, B., Li, J., Wozniak, J.M., Bosilca, G., Dorier, M., Cappello, F., Deepfreeze: Towards scalable asynchronous checkpointing of deep learning models, in: *2020 20th IEEE/ACM International Symposium on Cluster, Cloud and Internet Computing (CCGRID)*, IEEE, pp. 172–181, 2020 May, https://doi.org/10.7845/uhgf6671234012.
10. Patton, R.M., Johnston, J.T., Young, S.R., Schuman, C.D., Potok, T.E., Rose, D.C., Lim, S.H., Chae, J., Hou, L., Abousamra, S., Samaras, D., Exascale deep learning to accelerate cancer research, in: *2019 IEEE International Conference on Big Data (Big Data)*, IEEE, pp. 1488–1496, 2019 December, https://doi.org/10.6324/66989562.
11. Rokade, A., Singh, M., Malik, P.K., Singh, R., Alsuwian, T., Intelligent data analytics framework for precision farming using IoT and regressor machine learning algorithms. *Appl. Sci.*, 12, 19, 9992, 2022. https://doi.org/10.1106/daw756456452.
12. Sastry, R. V. L. S. N., Kapila, D., Jaiswal, S., Sargunam, S., Akram, S.V., Kumar, K.S., Critically analysing the concept of deep learning and how it impacts organizational performance, in: *2022 2nd International Conference on Advance Computing and Innovative Technologies in Engineering (ICACITE)*, IEEE, pp. 321–324, 2022, April, https://doi.org/10.8547/56123134684.
13. Sharpless, N.E. and Kerlavage, A.R., The potential of AI in cancer care and research. *Biochim. Biophys. Acta (BBA) Rev. Cancer*, *1876*, 1, 188573, 2020. https://doi.org/10.8547/4685462.
14. Singh, R., Gehlot, A., Rashid, M., Saxena, R., Akram, S.V., Alshamrani, S.S., AlGhamdi., A.S., Cloud server and internet of things assisted system for stress monitoring. *Electronics*, 10, 24, 3133, 2021. (2). 2021. https://doi.org/10.8965/545484812.
15. Yoon, H.J., Gounley, J., Gao, S., Alawad, M., Ramanathan, A., Tourassi, G., Model-based hyperparameter optimization of convolutional neural networks for information extraction from cancer pathology reports on HPC, in: *2019 IEEE EMBS International Conference on Biomedical & Health Informatics (BHI)*, IEEE, pp. 1–4, 2019. https://doi.org/10.9654/58461513.

15

Current Breakthroughs and Future Perspectives in Surgery Based on AI-Based Computing Vision

Suneet Gupta[1], Madhu Kumar Vanteru[2], Sanjeevkumar Angadi[3], Manikandan K.[4], Mohit Tiwari[5] and Joshuva Arockia Dhanraj[6,7*]

[1]Department of CSE, Alliance College of Engineering and Design, Alliance University, Bangalore, India
[2]Department of ECE, Balaji Institute of Technology and Science, Warangal, India
[3]Computer Science and Engineering, Nutan College of Engineering and Research, Talegaon Dabhade, Pune, India
[4]School of Computer Science and Engineering, Vellore Institute of Technology (VIT), Vellore, Tamil Nadu, India
[5]Department of Computer Science and Engineering, Bharati Vidyapeeth's College of Engineering, Delhi, Paschim Vihar, Delhi, India
[6]Centre for Automation and Robotics (ANRO), Department of Mechatronics Engineering, Hindustan Institute of Technology and Science, Padur, Chennai, India
[7]University Center for Research & Development (UCRD) Chandigarh University, Mohali, Punjab, India

Abstract

Artificial intelligence (AI) and computer vision have become increasingly important in various fields of medicine, including surgery. AI-based computing vision systems have shown great potential in assisting surgeons during surgery, improving surgical outcomes, and reducing the risks of complications. In this abstract, we will discuss some of the current breakthroughs and future perspectives in surgery based on AI-based computing vision. One of the most significant breakthroughs in this field has been the development of image-guided surgery. Using preoperative imaging, AI-based computing vision systems can create a three-layered guide of the patient's life structures, allowing surgeons to accurately plan and execute surgical procedures. These systems can also help surgeons identify and avoid

**Corresponding author*: Joshuva1991@gmail.com; ORCID: 0000-0001-5048-7775

Kapil Joshi and Somil Kumar Gupta (eds.) Human Cancer Diagnosis and Detection Using Exascale Computing, (227–238) © 2024 Scrivener Publishing LLC

critical structures, such as nerves and blood vessels, during the surgery. Another breakthrough has been the development of surgical robots, which use AI-based computing vision to assist surgeons during procedures. These robots can provide high-resolution, 3D imaging and can be used to control surgical instruments with greater precision and accuracy than human hands.

Keywords: Artificial Intelligence (AI), surgery, computing, vision

15.1 Introduction

Artificial intelligence (AI)-based computing vision systems can also be used to perform minimally invasive surgeries, reducing the need for large incisions and improving patient recovery times. In the future, AI-based computing vision systems are expected to play an even greater role in surgery. These systems may be able to predict surgical outcomes based on patient data and help surgeons make more informed decisions during procedures. They may also be able to learn from past surgeries and develop new techniques and strategies for improving surgical outcomes. Surgery is an inherently complex and challenging field that requires precision, skill, and expertise. The development of AI and computer vision technologies has shown great potential in assisting surgeons during procedures, improving surgical outcomes, and reducing the risks of complications [1]. AI-based computing vision systems can create a three-layered guide to a patient's life systems and provide high-resolution, 3D imaging, allowing surgeons to plan and execute surgical procedures with greater precision and accuracy. These systems can also assist in identifying and avoiding critical structures, such as nerves and blood vessels, during the surgery.

In this article, research developed some of the current breakthroughs and future perspectives in surgery based on AI-based computing vision. Researchers will examine the use of image-guided surgery and surgical robots and their impact on surgical outcomes. Additionally, we will explore the potential for AI-based computing vision systems to predict surgical outcomes based on patient data and learn from past surgeries to develop new techniques and strategies. Overall, the integration of AI-based computing vision in surgery can change the field and work on quiet results. AI-based computing vision systems are expected to become even more advanced and integrated into surgical practice [2]. These systems may be able to assist in more complex surgical procedures, provide real-time feedback to surgeons, and even perform surgeries autonomously. As innovation keeps advancing, it can upset the field of medical procedure and work on persistent results.

15.2 Literature Review

Mechanical developments have been connected to clinical advantages in the field of medical procedures. The route and arranging of intricate medical procedures have been made conceivable using both preoperative and intraoperative imaging strategies, like ultrasonography, registered tomography, and attractive reverberation imaging. Furthermore, the advancement of careful gadgets and instruments connected with endoscopic medical procedures has contributed fundamentally to the presentation and entrance of MIS. Postoperative consideration has likewise been worked on through modern sensors and screens. Following the presentation of these actions, artificial intelligence will assume a fundamental part in intraoperative careful navigation and robotization.

At the point when the fate of a medical procedure is compared to mechanical development in cars, we accept that independent medical procedures will be sitting tight for us past picture route a medical procedure. There is no question that man-made intelligence-based picture acknowledgment will turn into a fundamental central innovation to acknowledge independent medical procedures. In the vehicle field, independence level 1 is characterized as "vehicle is controlled by the driver, but some driving assist features may be included in the vehicle design." Also, man-made intelligence-based picture routes and robot-helped medical procedures actually fall under independence level 1. For medical procedures to accomplish a higher degree of independence, man-made intelligence ought to essentially examine and yield careful advances, life structures, instruments, and so on, with constant and vigorous precision in each circumstance [3]. A lot more elevated level of independence should be expected to supplant the administrator's capability, and normally, the latest test in the field of simulated intelligence in medical procedure will point somewhat to supplant the capability of right hand and degree. The effect of man-made intelligence put together careful framework disappointments with respect to patients should be limited. Artificial intelligence-based careful frameworks ought to be confirmed and guaranteed with full thought of the relative multitude of potential dangers. As of now, it is important to consider fitting techniques for every artificial intelligence-based careful framework, other than clinical preliminaries, to assess its security and adequacy.

There have been several studies and reviews examining the current breakthroughs and future perspectives in surgery based on AI-based computing vision. Here are some of the key findings:

Image-guided surgery: A systematic review published in the *Journal of Neurosurgery* found that image-guided surgery using AI-based computing vision systems can improve surgical outcomes and reduce the risk of complications. The study concluded that this technology should be considered a standard of care in neurosurgery [4].
Surgical robots: A review published in the journal *Surgical Oncology* found that surgical robots using AI-based computing vision systems can improve surgical precision, reduce the risk of complications, and improve patient outcomes. The study concluded that robotic surgery has the potential to revolutionize the field of surgery.
Predictive analytics: A review published in the *Journal of Healthcare Engineering* found that AI-based computing vision systems can be used to analyze patient data and predict surgical outcomes with a high degree of accuracy [5]. The study concluded that this technology has the potential to improve surgical decision-making and patient outcomes.
Learning from past surgeries: A study published in the *Journal of Laparoendoscopic & Advanced Surgical Techniques* found that AI-based computing vision systems can analyze large datasets of laparoscopic surgeries to identify patterns and trends. The study concluded that this technology has the potential to improve surgical techniques and reduce the risk of complications.
Augmented reality: A review published in the *Journal of Medical Systems* found that augmented reality technology using AI-based computing vision systems can provide real-time guidance to surgeons during procedures, improving surgical precision and reducing the risk of complications [6]. The study concluded that this technology has the potential to revolutionize surgical practice.

The mindful utilization of new advancements and steady structure of trust among people and artificial intelligence, for example, the impact of overdependence on the AI-based careful framework and adverse consequences on careful instruction, ought to be thought of. The treatment of short- or long-haul antagonistic occasions brought about by simulated intelligence based on a medical procedure ought to likewise be guaranteed [7]. To resolve these issues, it is upheld that wide arrangements overseeing the obtaining, stockpiling, sharing, and utilization of information should be created and settled upon by specialists, engineers, administrators, ethicists, patients, and so forth.

Albeit physical designs are simple for specialists to remember, they can likewise be perceived by simulated intelligence with high precision as well as the other way around for troublesome targets. The more troublesome

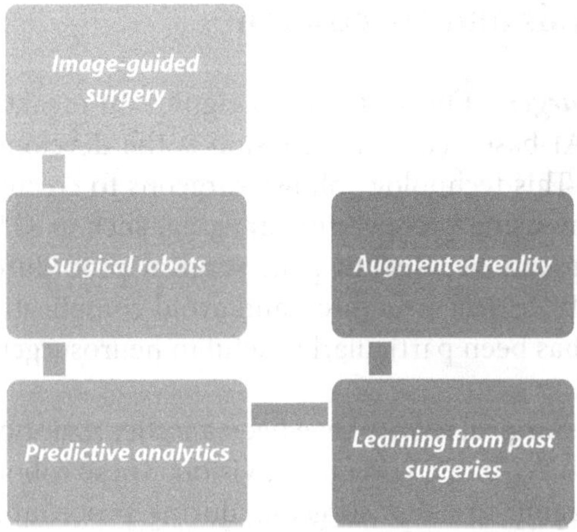

Figure 15.1 Key findings of AI-based computing vision. (Source: [8]).

the physical designs for specialists to perceive, for example, small nerves and vessels covered by fat tissue, the more important it is for man-made intelligence-based picture routes. The interpretation of focal points is one of the impending difficulties that are hard for even specialists to perceive and causing computer-based intelligence to learn them. Coordinating with different advances, for example, indocyanine green (ICG) and close infrared light, could be important to further develop the acknowledgment of exactness for troublesome targets [8]. Figure 15.1 shows the major key findings of AI based computing vision. Overall, the literature suggests that AI-based computing vision systems have the potential to work on careful results and lessen the gamble of confusion. As innovation keeps on developing, it can possibly upset the field of medical procedure and work on understanding the results.

15.3 Research Methodology

Secondary descriptive analysis has been done for this research to gather factual information regarding the research topic. Overall, AI-based computing vision systems have already shown great promise in surgery, and their future applications are expected to have a significant impact on patient outcomes and the practice of surgery. As innovation keeps on propelling, we can hope to see considerably more forward leaps in this field, prompting more secure and more viable surgical procedures.

15.4 Analysis and Discussion

Image-guided surgery: One of the most significant breakthroughs in surgery based on AI-based computing vision is the development of image-guided surgery. This technology allows surgeons to create a 3D map of a patient's anatomy using preoperative imaging, such as CT scans or MRI scans. This map can be used to plan surgical procedures with greater accuracy, identify critical structures, and avoid complications [9]. Image-guided surgery has been particularly useful in neurosurgery and orthopedic surgery.

Surgical robots: Surgical robots have been another major breakthrough in surgery based on AI-based computing vision. These robots use high-resolution, 3D imaging to assist surgeons during procedures, allowing for greater precision and accuracy. They can also perform minimally invasive surgeries, reducing the need for large incisions and improving patient recovery times. Robotic surgery has been particularly useful in urology, gynecology, and cardiothoracic surgery.

Predictive analytics: AI-based computing vision systems can analyze patient data to predict surgical outcomes and identify potential complications before they occur. This technology can be used to develop personalized treatment plans for patients and improve surgical decision-making [10].

Learning from past surgeries: AI-based computing vision systems can learn from past surgeries to develop new techniques and strategies for improving surgical outcomes. This technology can break down huge datasets of surgeries to distinguish examples and patterns, which can be utilized to illuminate future surgeries.

Augmented reality: Augmented reality technology is being developed to provide surgeons with real-time, interactive guidance during procedures. This technology can overlay digital information onto the surgeon's field of view, providing information on anatomy and surgical instruments.

Conclusion requires the capacity to handle various sorts of data about patients and distinguish anomalies with high exactness and reproducibility. In traditional determination, doctors process different bits of patient data utilizing their insight and additionally experience and identify anomalies in patients utilizing their faculties or through analytic hardware. This strategy at times neglects to distinguish anomalies in patients or results in some unacceptable choices being made. Also, the symptomatic capacity is reliant upon the experience of the doctor [11]. Consequently, man-made intelligence is supposed to have symptomatic execution with reproducibility

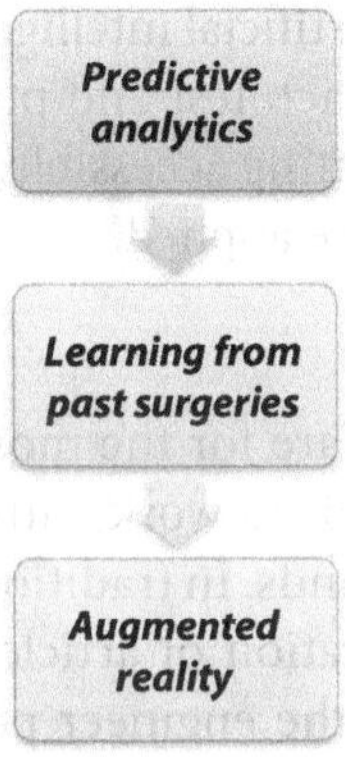

Figure 15.2 AI-based technologies. (Source: [12]).

and precision equivalent to or better than that of talented doctors and to make up for contrasts in doctor insight. Current man-made intelligence for determination is effectively being created to perform analytic imaging with registered tomography and tissue areas.

Specifically, convolutional brain networks perform well in the ILSVRC consistently; accordingly, convolutional brain networks are the most utilized for analytic imaging and proceed as well as or better than gifted doctors. Additionally, frameworks have been created to anticipate radiation or anti-cancer medication awareness utilizing convolutional brain organizations. Notwithstanding analytic imaging, computer-based intelligence is likewise being created to analyze infections, for example, malignant growth by means of AI of blood parts [12]. Nevertheless, constraints in estimation awareness and specialized ancient rarities, for example, clamor, are obstructions to determination utilizing blood parts. The advancement of further developed estimation innovation, as well as further developed AI models, would be expected for a determination that applies AI to blood parts. Figure 15.2 shows how the AI-based technologies amended for surgeries.

As previously mentioned, the ongoing use of computer-based intelligence for conclusion fundamentally works on the exactness of each test. Conversely, for the ID of sickness from different side effects in a patient and the consequences of tests, an extensive variety of information, not explicit information, and high-level data handling are important. To satisfy this need, Watson is one example of an artificial intelligence companion that can parse natural language and use expert systems to make complex judgments as it learns about a subject [13].

Accordingly, for findings, artificial intelligence is fundamentally evolved to work on the exactness of each test and pursue proper choices utilizing the huge amount of related writing accessible, and various calculations reasonable for each interaction are applied.

Treatment

For treatment, careful robots are for the most part being created. Careful robots are reasonable for itemized work with exact developments that are beyond the scope of human hands. In traditional careful robot calculations, characterization and identification of articles expected during a medical procedure are performed by the engineer physically making elements of the district of interest; in any case, with the coming of profound learning, convolution brain networks are being applied for the grouping and location of items. Moreover, constant expectations are likewise being made with repetitive brain organizations. Customary careful robots are worked by a doctor; notwithstanding, careful robots that work consequently without activity by a doctor are likewise being created [14]. Subsequently, the advancement of man-made intelligence has additionally prompted the improvement of robots that help doctors during medical procedures. Furthermore, in drug treatment, simulated intelligence-based applications are being presented in determination and follow-up as opposed to in the treatment cycle. Different man-made intelligence applications have been presented in the medication improvement cycle to foster helpful medications. In the medication improvement process, designers need to handle a gigantic measure of data to find only a couple of promising mixtures from

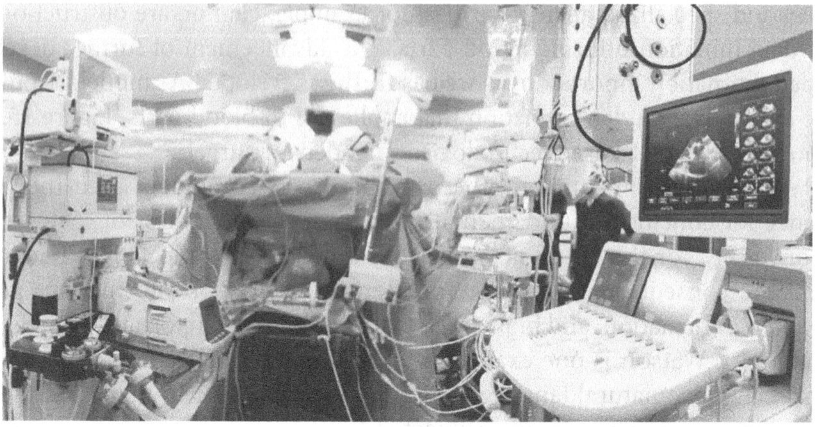

Figure 15.3 AI-based surgery treatment. (Source: [15]).

millions to a huge number of up-and-comer compounds [15]. Different kinds of computer-based intelligence assume dynamic parts in handling these data, as portrayed exhaustively later in this audit. Figure 15.3 shows how the surgeries and the treatment happening through AI.

Follow-up

In medication, regardless of what sort of sickness or what kind of therapy is given, follow-up is pretty much generally important. Furthermore, the future of the planet has expanded by 20 years over the most recent 50 years, and as the populace ages, the gamble of having persistent illnesses increments. Against this foundation, wearable gadgets outfitted with computer-based intelligence that can continually screen ailments and promptly identify any anomaly in wearers are effectively being created. Specifically, wearable gadgets are supposed to be utilized in cardiology, where the state of the patient might change quickly and there is an immediate connection with mortality status [16]. The greater part of the applications for follow-up endorsed by the FDA in 2017–2020, including the ECG application on the Apple™ Watch, is wearable cardiology gadgets. Some of the calculations in wearable gadgets are applied to counterfeit brain organizations or versatile calculations.

Artificial intelligence has advanced with the times and has been used in applications in drug improvement and medical care. These applications are consistently creating results, and the utilization of artificial intelligence is becoming laid out. The execution of artificial intelligence in the public eye should defeat issues, for example, how to foster driving organizations and train information researchers. Notwithstanding, organization improvement might in any case confront a few hindrances, for example, executing simulated intelligence, work, and cost. Later on, to work on human well-being, we should not just foster computer-based intelligence but also contemplate the concurrence of people with simulated intelligence.

15.5 Conclusion

The integration of AI-based computing vision in surgery has shown great potential in improving surgical outcomes and reducing the risks of complications. Current breakthroughs, such as image-guided surgery, surgical robots, predictive analytics, learning from past surgeries, and augmented reality, have demonstrated the potential for AI-based computing vision to revolutionize the field of surgery. These technologies have already shown promising results in improving surgical precision, reducing the risk of complications, and improving patient outcomes. Looking into the future,

AI-based computing vision systems are expected to become even more advanced and integrated into surgical practice. The potential for these systems to assist in more complex surgical procedures, provide real-time feedback to surgeons, and even perform surgeries autonomously is invigorating. As innovation keeps on developing, it can possibly change the field of medical procedure and work on quiet results. It is critical to guarantee that the integration of AI-based computing vision systems in surgery is done in a safe, responsible, and ethical manner, with careful consideration given to issues such as patient privacy, data security, and the need for human oversight. A few issues should be tended to before man-made intelligence can be consistently coordinated into the fate of a medical procedure regarding specialized plausibility, exactness, well-being, cost, and moral and legitimate contemplations.

References

1. Arinez, J.F., Chang, Q., Gao, R.X., Xu, C., Zhang, J., Artificial intelligence in advanced manufacturing: Current status and future outlook. *J. Manuf. Sci. Eng.*, *142*, 11, 658–696, 2020. https://doi.org/10.1115/1.4047855.
2. Asai, A., Konno, M., Taniguchi, M., Vecchione, A., Ishii, H., Computational healthcare: Present and future perspectives. *Exp. Ther. Med.*, *22*, 6, 1–13, 2021. https://doi.org/10.1452/48563.
3. Dimitriadou, E. and Lanitis, A., A critical evaluation, challenges, and future perspectives of using artificial intelligence and emerging technologies in smart classrooms. *Smart Learn. Environ.*, *10*, 1, 1–26, 2023. https://doi.org/10.7858/85636212.
4. Duggal, A.S., Singh, R., Gehlot, A., Rashid, M., Alshamrani, S.S., AlGhamdi., A.S., Digital taste in mulsemedia augmented reality: Perspective on developments and challenges. *Electronics*, 11, 9, 1315, 2022. https://doi.org/10.1147/589654.
5. Fatima, A., Shafi, I., Afzal, H., Díez, I.D.L.T., Lourdes, D.R.S.M., Breñosa, J., Espinosa, J.C.M., Ashraf, I., Advancements in dentistry with artificial intelligence: Current clinical applications and future perspectives. *Healthcare*, 10, 11, 2188, 2022. MDPIhttps://doi.org/10.5487/85693147.
6. Hunde, B.R. and Woldeyohannes, A.D., Future prospects of computer-aided design (CAD)–A review from the perspective of artificial intelligence (AI), extended reality, and 3D printing. *Results Eng.*, 14, 1, 100478, 2022. https://doi.org/10.1458/856994.
7. Joshi, K., Kumar, M., Tripathi, A., Kumar, A., Sehgal, J., Barthwal, A., Latest trends in multi-modality medical image fusion: A generic review, in: *Rising Threats in Expert Applications and Solutions*, pp. 663–671, 2022, https://doi.org/10.1489/523697412.

8. Kitaguchi, D., Takeshita, N., Hasegawa, H., Ito, M., Artificial intelligence-based computer vision in surgery: Recent advances and future perspectives. *J. Gastrointest. Surg.*, *6*, 1, 29–36, 2022. https://doi.org/10.15236/8523694.
9. Praveen, S., Tyagi, N., Singh, B., Karetla, G.R., Thalor, M.A., Joshi, K., Tsegaye, M., PSO-based evolutionary approach to optimize head and neck biomedical image to detect mesothelioma cancer. *BioMed. Res. Int.*, 9, 2, 236–288, 2022. https://doi.org/10.5369/16564654.
10. Quero, G., Mascagni, P., Kolbinger, F.R., Fiorillo, C., De Sio, D., Longo, F., Schena, C.A., Laterza, V., Rosa, F., Menghi, R., Papa, V., Artificial intelligence in colorectal cancer surgery: Present and future perspectives. *Cancers*, *14*, 15, 3803, 2022. https://doi.org/10.1541/484121357384.
11. Rovira-Sugranes, A., Razi, A., Afghah, F., Chakareski, J., A review of AI-enabled routing protocols for UAV networks: Trends, challenges, and future outlook. *Ad Hoc Networks*, *130*, 102790, 2022. https://doi.org/10.5412/546555.
12. Sharma, A.K., Ghodke, P.K., Goyal, N., Nethaji, S., Chen, W.H., Machine learning technology in biohydrogen production from agriculture waste: Recent advances and future perspectives. *Bioresour. Technol.*, 111, 85, 128076, 2022. https://doi.org/10.1311/32135.
13. Sharma, M., Rastogi, R., Arya, N., Akram, S.V., Singh, R., Gehlot, A., Buddhi, D., Joshi., K., LoED: LoRa and edge computing based system architecture for sustainable forest monitoring. *IJETT*, 70, 5, 88–93, 2022. https://doi.org/10.1458/5585455.
14. Sharma, V.K., Singh, R., Gehlot, A., Buddhi, D., Braccio, S., Priyadarshi, N., Khan, B., Imperative role of photovoltaic and concentrating solar power technologies towards renewable energy generation. *Int. J. Photoenergy*, 6, 1254–1259, 2022. https://doi.org/10.2548/546355.
15. Singh, R., Akram, S.V., Gehlot, A., Buddhi, D., Priyadarshi, N., Twala, B., Energy System 4.0: Digitalization of the energy sector with inclination towards sustainability. *Sensors*, 17, 45, 2, 6619, 2022. https://doi.org/10.5255/415455.
16. Zhang, C. and Lu, Y., Study on artificial intelligence: The state of the art and future prospects. *J. Ind. Inf. Integr.*, *23*, 100224, 2021. https://doi.org/10.2541/144255.

16

MRI-Based Brain Tumor Detection Using Machine Learning

Vivek Kumar[1]*, Pinki Chugh[1], Bhuprabha Bharti[2], Anchit Bijalwan[3], Amrendra Tripathi[4], Ram Narayan[1] and Kapil Joshi[1]

[1]*Department of CSE, Uttaranchal Institute of Technology, Uttaranchal University, Dehradun, India*

[2]*Hindustan College of Science and Technology, Mathura, India*

[3]*Department of Cyber Security, School of Computing and Innovative Technologies, British University Vietnam, Hanoi, Vietnam*

[4]*School of Computing, UPES, Dehradun, India*

Abstract

One of the most frequently diagnosed tumors in people of all ages is a brain tumor. All facets of human life have been impacted by technological advancements. For instance, technology's usage in medicine has significantly benefited human society. Brain tumors are currently the most dangerous disease in the world. Tumors can harm healthy brain tissue or raise intracranial pressure, both of which have an effect on the brain. Therefore, a tumor cell's rapid development could result in death. Consequently, making an early diagnosis of a brain tumor is more important because it can spare the patient from negative consequences. Processing medical photographs is essential for assisting people in recognizing various disorders. An important aspect of brain tumor classification is dependent on the doctor's skill and knowledge. The field of image classification technology has advanced significantly in recent years, and the most widely used and superior method that has been deemed best in this field is the SVM classifier. For this reason, SVM classifier is utilized in this study to classify a brain tumor. This article focuses on using technology to help treat brain tumors, one of the most frequent and dangerous diseases ever. Images from the MRI sequence were used as the input image in a segmentation and detection approach for brain cancers in order to pinpoint the tumor area. The major objective is to identify whether the brain has a brain tumor or is healthy.

**Corresponding author*: vivek11krr@gmail.com

Kapil Joshi and Somil Kumar Gupta (eds.) Human Cancer Diagnosis and Detection Using Exascale Computing, (239–252) © 2024 Scrivener Publishing LLC

Keywords: Magnetic resonance imaging, brain tumor detection, image segmentation, feature extraction, SVM classifier

16.1 Introduction

One important organ in charge of the central nervous system is the brain. By joining the bone marrow, the human brain completes the function of the central nervous system. Controlling how the human body behaves falls under the purview of the brain. It gathers data from various senses, makes decisions, and then communicates those decisions to the body. The brain, with the assistance of neurons, is the focal point of the human body's administrative system and is in charge of all bodily functions. One of the most well-liked subjects in the academic world right now is research on brain tumors [1]. The segmentation of tumor regions and the classification of the tumor are, in general, the components of malignant tumor classification. The central nervous system contains this important organ. As a result, brain tumors can result in life-threatening illnesses, making early identification crucial. The characteristics that should be used to categorize brain tumors are crucial in establishing which class the tumor belongs to [2]. Cancerous cells can develop out of control in any organ or body component to form a tumor. According to the characteristics and competing treatments, the tumor is divided into various types. A brain tumor is regarded as the riskiest and most meticulous tumor kind, necessitating a thorough examination by a physician who can accurately classify the tumor [3]. The most popular non-invasive scanning method now employed by radiologists is magnetic resonance imaging, as it allows for the detection of small structural changes that are difficult to see with computed tomography-based imaging. Both professional radiologists and doctors find the manual processing of MRI scans to be time-consuming, particularly in complex instances. Radiologists are frequently required to compare tumor tissues with surrounding areas in difficult instances, improving images to increase perceptual quality prior to tumor type categorization. Large amounts of data cannot be processed in this manner, and manual processes cannot be repeated. The most important diagnostic step for the patient's health is the early diagnosis of brain tumors with high prediction accuracy. For the quick and accurate detection of malignancies, novel concepts and methods are urgently desired. Every computer-aided radiology system that uses artificial intelligence and its primary enablers, machine learning and deep learning algorithms, must convert data into valuable information through feature extraction [4]. The brain, a delicate organ, controls how individuals behave and move their bodies. It governs all of our perceptions, memories, and feelings. Every organ and bodily part has a direct nerve link to the brain, which enables the brain to communicate with the nerves to regulate the parts. An abnormal cell formation in the human brain is known as a brain tumor. In various parts of the world, there are numerous different types of brain tumors. Brain tumors can be classified as malignant (cancerous) or benign (non-cancerous), depending on the type. Brain tumors can develop from brain tumors or cancers that have already spread to other parts of the body. Strong headaches, blurred vision, loss of balance, mental disorientation, and seizures are the main signs and symptoms of brain tumors [5]. Chemotherapy, radiation therapy, and surgery are all forms of treatment for brain tumors in humans. The human brain is extremely difficult to analyze and has billions of active cells. Figure 16.1 depicts the human brain in both its normal and tumor-free states.

Brain analysis typically favors MRI scanning. The capacity to clearly see the soft tissue is one of the benefits of scanning. Because unionizing radiation is used to visualize the brain areas, there are no negative effects. The brain's aberrant cell development is frequently located via an MRI scan [6]. A computer aid is already an important part of daily clinical practice when processing diagnostic data. Consider how a substantial volume of pictures is processed and analyzed, for example, to provide high-quality information for disease diagnosis and treatment.

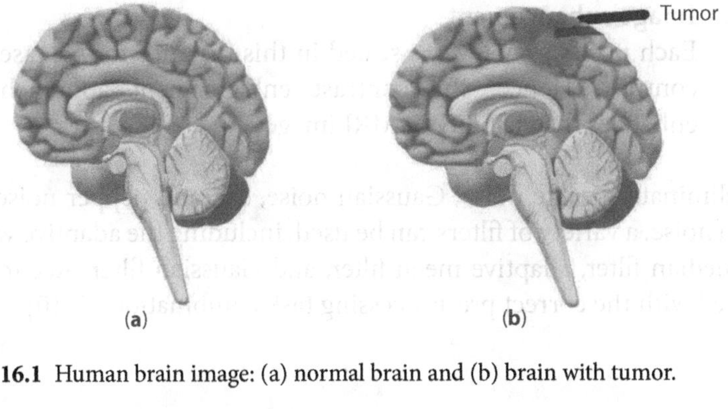

Figure 16.1 Human brain image: (a) normal brain and (b) brain with tumor.

16.2 Pre-Processing

Pre-processing, or increasing the quality of an image to be utilized further by removing unwanted picture information, is the first step in the detection technique because raw photographs already contain noise. This unwanted image information is referred to as the image noises. If this issue is not appropriately addressed, the categorization may contain a number of errors. The brain images from magnetic resonance imaging are acquired and sent as input to the pre-processing stage. Pre-processing is necessary because it allows for improvements in photo statistics that improve the picture's shape and capabilities, both of which are probably essential for similar processing. The noise must be delayed for similar processing because extreme accuracy is required. Moreover, pre-processing strategy parameters are regularly changed to improve the quality of the input photographs [7].

The following is a definition of the pre-processing functions:

a. **Conversion from RGB to grayscale**
   This conversion suggests that the image might be composed of different tones of gray. Although some MRI scans are primarily RGB data, the grayscale image contains the grayscale values. Consequently, grayscale representations of these photographs must be created.
b. **Employing median filtering to reduce noise**
   The filtering procedure is referred to as getting rid of the noise that is present in the image. During the process of converting a picture from RGB to grayscale, some noise may contaminate the image. Filtering is used to reduce the noise as a result. Moreover, it is used to remove noise from transformed photographs, such as salt and pepper [8].
c. **Image enhancement**
   Each pixel's gray level is scaled in this instance to increase contrast. Hence, the contrast enhancement approach enhances the visibility of MRI images.

To eliminate speckle noise, Gaussian noise, salt and pepper noise, and Poisson noise, a variety of filters can be used, including the adaptive wiener filter, median filter, adaptive mean filter, and Gaussian filter. Accuracy is increased with the correct pre-processing task combination [9, 10].

16.3 Segmentation

The preprocessed image is divided into segments each representing a separate region. Using input photographs, segmentation extracts the necessary region. As a result, accurately segmenting lesion sites is a more important endeavor. Semi- and completely automated approaches are used since the manual segmentation procedure is flawed. Image segmentation is the process of dividing a picture into mutually exclusive, comprehensive sections that are homogeneous and according to some predetermined standard. In the context of a brain tumor, segmentation entails separating aberrant from normal brain tissue [11]. Image segmentation is a well-known research issue and a current hot topic in the study of images. The term "image segmentation" describes the process of breaking apart a picture into various fragments based on attributes including color, grayscale, spatial texture, and geometric shapes. These traits must show continuity or similarity within the same region while highlighting clear differences between locations. The image segmentation approach is gradually refined to produce ever-more accurate segmentation results with a substantial rise in the suggested network structure [12]. As seen in Figure 16.2, one of the segmentation methods frequently employed in image processing applications is K-means clustering.

The primary goal of this segmentation algorithm's clustering operation is to distinguish between a set of items that belong to one group and objects that belong to other groups based on shared traits [13]. The better

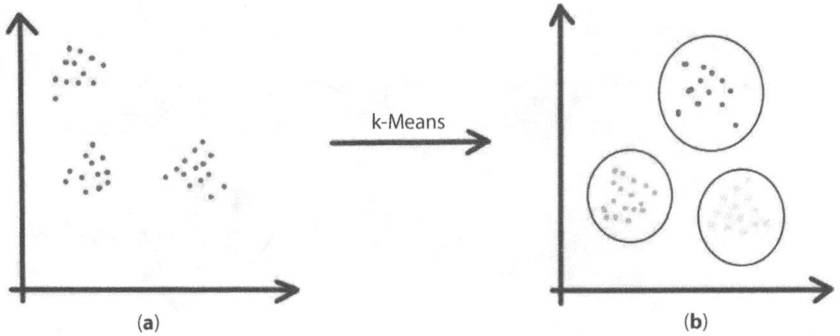

Figure 16.2 K-means clustering.

the clustering findings may be obtained, the more homogeneity (or resemblance) there is inside a group and the more difference there is between groups.

Defining centroids for every cluster was the biggest target. The centroids are to be kept adeptly as different positions yield different results. The desirable option is to keep them at maximum difference as possible. This results in the following phase joining all the points from a given dataset to the closest centroid. The first stage is completed as there is no open point. Here, the barycenter of the clusters produced by the earlier phase was utilized to create k new centroids [14, 15]. Fresh binding is required to be established among the identical data set points and the closest new centroid as soon as these k new centroids are determined. A loop is thus created, causing the k new centroids to continuously change locations until they reach the level where no more modifications are possible.

16.4 Feature Extraction

Shape features are applied to the segmented objects or regions in the scene after the picture segmentation stage is complete. In order to process the images further, feature extraction is utilized to extract hidden and visible attributes from images. Dimensionality reduction and information extraction from rich data containing medical images, such as radiography, magnetic resonance imaging, and computerized tomography, are two of these.

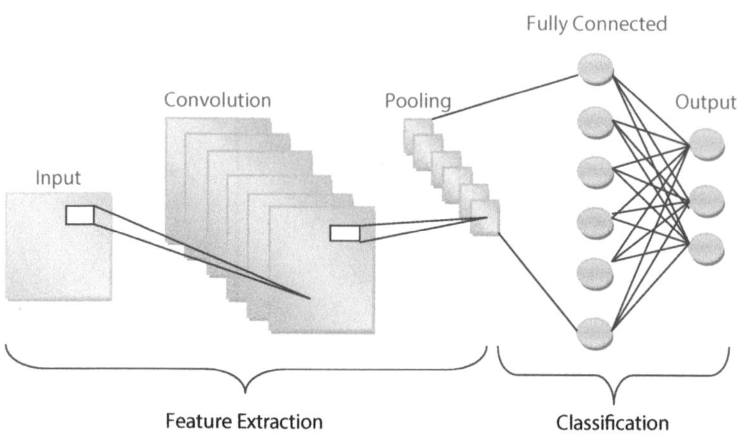

Figure 16.3 CNN architecture.

Although these modalities comprise a variety of information kinds, the pertinent and necessary information is extracted using the feature extraction technique [16, 17]. Deep learning is a branch of machine learning. Deep learning has the benefit of teaching the system to extract features on its own as it is trained [18, 19]. The structure of a convolutional neural network (CNN) is shown in Figure 16.3. Using kernels or convolutional filters, the CNN topologies of the deep learning network can independently extract visual characteristics. One of the key advantages of convolutional neural networks is their capacity to automatically extract features, which does away with the need for a separate feature extractor.

Typically, a CNN has three layers:

a. **Convolutional layer**

   A convolutional layer is a type of layer in a CNN that applies a set of learnable filters or kernels to the input data. As the filters slide over the input data, it performs a dot product between the filter weights and the input values at each position, producing a 2D activation map of the filtered outputs. The convolution operation results in an output feature map that represents a learned representation of the input data's spatial features. The learnable filters are typically small in spatial size but are applied to the entire input depth, allowing them to learn local features that can be combined to form more complex patterns.

   Convolutional layers are often followed by non-linear activation functions like rectified linear unit (ReLU) and pooling layers that help reduce the output dimensionality and control overfitting. The convolutional layers are trained using backpropagation and stochastic gradient descent to minimize the difference between the predicted output and the true output.

   Convolutional layers are widely used in image and video processing tasks like object detection, segmentation, and recognition.

b. **Pooling layer**

   A pooling layer is a type of layer in a CNN that operates on the output of a convolutional layer. The pooling layer reduces the dimensionality of the output feature map by downsampling its spatial size while retaining the most important information. The pooling layer works by partitioning the output feature map into non-overlapping subregions, called pooling regions or windows, and applying an aggregation function to each window. The most common aggregation functions used in pooling layers are max pooling and average pooling.

In max pooling, the maximum value of each pooling region is selected, while in average pooling, the average value of each pooling region is computed. The pooling operation helps in reducing the sensitivity of the model to small variations in the input and improves its ability to generalize to new data. Moreover, it also helps in reducing the computational cost and the number of parameters in the network. Pooling layers are typically applied after each convolutional layer in a CNN. The pooling layer's output is then passed to the next convolutional layer or a fully connected layer. The pooling layer does not have any trainable parameters and is therefore only responsible for downsampling the output feature map.

c. **Fully connected layer**

A fully connected (FC) layer is a type of layer commonly used in neural networks for tasks such as image classification and regression. In an FC layer, all the neurons are connected to all the neurons of the previous layer. This results in the production of a new output created by passing through an activation function, combining with a weight and bias from the previous layer. The weights and biases in the FC layer are learned during training using backpropagation in order to optimize the network for a given task.

In typical neural network architecture, FC layers are usually used at the end of the network to map the extracted features to the output of the network. For example, in an image classification task, the FC layer might take the flattened output from the convolutional layers and map it to a set of output neurons corresponding to different classes.

16.5 SVM Classifier

Support vector machine (SVM) is a supervised learning algorithm used for classification and regression tasks. SVMs are used for binary classification tasks, where the goal is to classify data into one of two classes as shown in Figure 16.4.

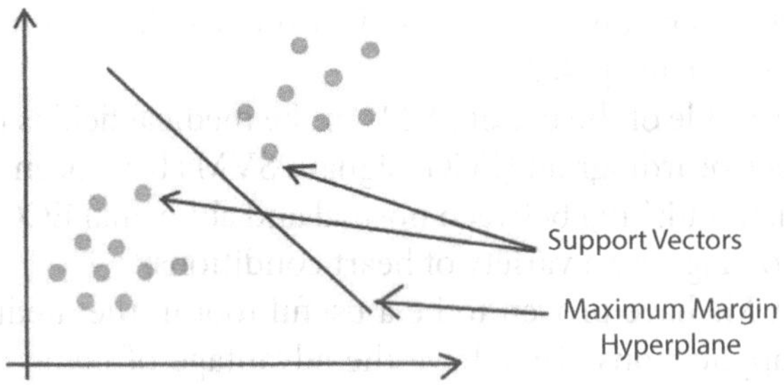

Figure 16.4 Support vector machine.

The basic idea behind SVMs is to find a hyperplane in a high-dimensional space that separates the data into two classes with the maximum possible margin. The margin is the distance between the hyperplane and the closest data points from each class. By maximizing the margin, SVMs aim to create a decision boundary that is robust to noise and generalizes well to new data [20, 21].

In cases where a linear decision boundary is not sufficient to separate the data, SVMs can use a technique called kernel trick to transform the input data into a higher-dimensional space where a linear boundary is more likely to exist. This allows SVMs to classify data that is not linearly separable.

During training, the SVM algorithm learns the optimal values of the parameters that define the hyperplane by minimizing a loss function that penalizes misclassifications. The choice of loss function and hyperparameters, such as the regularization parameter and the kernel function, can have a significant impact on the performance of the classifier.

SVMs have been shown to perform well on a wide range of classification tasks, including text classification, image classification, and bioinformatics. They are also popular because of their ability to handle high-dimensional data and their strong theoretical foundation [22, 23].

SVMs have been used in a variety of applications in the medical field, including diagnosis, classification, and prediction tasks.

One example of the use of SVMs in medical diagnosis is the detection of breast cancer from mammography images. SVMs have been shown to be effective in distinguishing between benign and malignant breast masses, achieving high levels of sensitivity and specificity.

SVMs have also been used for prediction tasks in the medical field, such as predicting the progression of Alzheimer's disease from MRI scans. In this case, SVMs were trained on MRI scans from patients with different stages of Alzheimer's disease and used to predict the progression of the disease in new patients [24, 25].

Another example of the use of SVMs in the medical field is in the classification of electrocardiogram (ECG) signals. SVMs have been shown to be effective in distinguishing between normal and abnormal ECG signals and can be used to diagnose a variety of heart conditions.

Overall, SVMs have proven to be a useful tool in the medical field for a variety of applications. They have the advantage of being able to handle high-dimensional data and to model complex relationships between variables. However, as with any machine learning algorithm, care must be taken to ensure that the results are accurate and reliable and that the algorithm is properly validated on new data.

For this purpose, we approximate each component by the evaluation of a facility and plot each datum item as a point in n-dimensional space. In keeping with that idea, we carry out grouping after finding a hyperplane that effectively divides the two classes [26].

16.6 Methodology

Pre-processing, picture segmentation, feature extraction, and a classifier are used in the method for the identification and classification of brain cancers. The method for brain tumor detection is shown in Figure 16.5.

Image dataset: Digital photographs selected for testing, training, and assessing the effectiveness of machine learning algorithms are included in an image dataset.
Image pre-processing: This system uses a scanned, noisy MRI picture as its input. Hence, the first thing we want to do is clean up the input image's noise.
Segmentation: The straightforward region-based picture segmentation method is called region growing. Given that it involves choosing initial

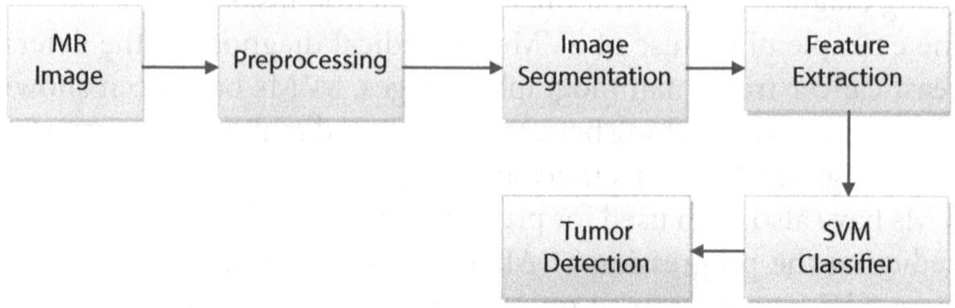

Figure 16.5 Method for brain tumor detection.

seed points for image segmentation, it is also categorized as a pixel-based image segmentation technique.
Feature extraction: The image edges are detected using feature extraction. It is the process of gathering more in-depth details about an image, like shape, texture, color, and contrast.
SVM classifier: It is a supervised learning technique mostly utilized for classifying data into several categories. A set of label data is used to train SVM.
Tumor identification: We are now extracting features from a collection of previously acquired brain MRIs. An information base is developed for comparison.

16.7 Conclusion

This research gives a detailed analysis of previous studies regarding the usage of deep learning to assess brain tumors using MRI images to classify them into tumorous and non-tumorous cases. MRI is the best detecting technique for tumors. The physical properties of brain tumors are not enough for disease detection. Brain tumor detection, segmentation, and classification are the three stages to generate computer-based techniques for finding tumors from images. The best method for image collection analysis is CNN; in comparison to manual techniques, it provides better accuracy, less noise, and quick processing time.

References

1. Khan, A.H., Abbas, S., Khan, M.A., Farooq, U., Khan, W.A., Siddiqui, S.Y., Ahmad, A., Intelligent model for brain tumor identification using deep learning. *Appl. Comput. Intell. Soft Comput.*, 2022, 8104054, 2022.
2. Ozyurt, F., Sert, E., Avci, E., Dogantekin, E., Brain tumor detection based on Convolutional Neural Network with neutrosophic expert maximum fuzzy sure entropy. *Measurement*, 147, 106830, 2019. Elsevier.
3. Rammurthy, D. and Mahesh, P.K., Whale Harris hawks optimization based deep learning classifier for brain tumor detection using MRI images. *J. King Saud Univ. - Comput. Inf. Sci.*, 34, 6, 3259–3272, 2022.
4. Qureshi, S.A., Ahmed Raza, S.E., Hussain, L., Malibari, A.A., Nour, M.K., ul Rehman, A., Al-Wesabi, F.N., Hilal, A.M., Intelligent ultra-light deep learning model for multi-class brain tumor detection. *Appl. Sci.*, 12, 8, 3715, 2022.

5. Shah, H.A., Saeed, F., Yun, S., Park, J.-H., Paul, A., Kang, J.-M., A robust approach for brain tumor detection in magnetic resonance images using finetuned efficient net. *IEEE Access*, 10, 65426–65438, 2022.
6. Hannan, S.A., Hivre, M., Lata, M., Krishna, B.H., Sathyasiva, Arshad, M.W., Brain damage detection using machine learning approach. *IJHS*, 6, S8, 4910–4924, 2022.
7. Kshirsagar, P.R., Rakhonde, A.N., Chippalkatti, P., *MRI image based brain tumor detection using machine learning*, vol. 81, pp. 3672–3680, The Mattingley Publishing Co., Inc, 2020.
8. Abd Khalid, N.E., Ismail, M.F., AB Manaf, M.A., Fadzil, A.F.A., Ibrahim, S., MRI brain tumor segmentation: A forthright image processing approach. *BEEI*, 9, 3, 1024–1031, 2020.
9. Munir, K., Elahi, H., Ayub, A., Frezza, F., Rizzi, A., Cancer diagnosis using deep learning: A bibliographic review. *Cancers*, 11, 9, 1235, 2019. MDPI-.
10. Geetha, A. and Gomathi, N., A robust grey wolf-based deep learning for brain tumour detection in MR images. *Biomed. Eng. / Biomedizinische Technik*, 65, 2, 191–207, 2020.
11. Lathera, M. and Singh, P., Investigating brain tumor segmentation and detection techniques. *International Conference on Computational Intelligence and Data Science*, vol. 167, pp. 121–130, 2019.
12. Liu, X., Song, L., Liu, S., Zhang, Y., A review of deep-learning-based medical image segmentation methods. *Sustainability*, 13, 3, 1224, 2021.
13. Baji, F.S., Abdullah, S.B., Abdulsattar, F.S., K-Mean clustering and local binary pattern techniquesfor automatic brain tumor detection. *Bull. Electr. Eng. Inform.*, 12, 3, 1586–1594, 2023.
14. Avcı, H. and Karakaya, J., A novel medical image enhancement algorithm for breast cancer detection on mammography images using machine learning. *Diagnostics*, 13, 3, 348, 2023.
15. Wahyuni, S.N., Khanom, N.N., Astuti, Y., K-Means algorithm analysis for election cluster prediction. *JOIV*, 7, 1, 1–6, 2023.
16. Iqbal, S., Siddiqui, G.F., Rehman, A., Hussain, L., Saba, T., Prostate cancer detection using deep learning and traditional techniques. *IEEE Access*, 9, 27085–27100, 2021.
17. Modiya, P. and Vahora, S., Brain tumor detection using transfer learning with dimensionality reduction method. *Int. J. Intell. Syst. Appl. Eng.*, 10, 2, 201–206, 2022.
18. Dhiman, G., Juneja, S., Viriyasitavat, W., Mohafez, H., Hadizadeh, M., Islam, M.A., El Bayoumy, I., Gulati, K., A novel machine-learning-based hybrid CNN model for tumor identification in medical image processing. *Sustainability*, 14, 3, 1447, 2022.
19. Dhillon, A. and Verma, G.K., Convolutional neural network: A review of models, methodologies and applications to object detection. *Prog. Artif. Intell.*, 9, 85–112, 2020.

20. Vijayalakshmi, M.M., Melanoma skin cancer detection using image processing and machine learning. *IJTSRD*, 3, 4, 780–784, 2019.
21. Abdullah, D.M. and Abdulazeez, A.M., Machine learning applications based on SVM classification: A review. *QAJ*, 1, 2, 81–90, 2021.
22. Nallamala, S.H., Mishra, P., Koneru, S.V., Breast cancer detection using machine learning way. *IJRTE*, 8, 2S3, 1402–1405, 2019.
23. Sharma, T., Diwakar, M., Singh, P., Lamba, S., Kumar, P., Joshi, K., Emotion Analysis for predicting the emotion labels using Machine Learning approaches, in: *2021 IEEE 8th Uttar Pradesh Section International Conference on Electrical, Electronics and Computer Engineering (UPCON)*, IEEE, pp. 1–6, 2021, November.
24. Ambore, B., Gupta, A.D., Rafi, S.M., Yadav, S., Joshi, K., Sivakumar, R.D., A conceptual investigation on the image processing using artificial intelligence and tensor flow models through correlation analysis, in: *2022 2nd International Conference on Advance Computing and Innovative Technologies in Engineering (ICACITE)*, IEEE, pp. 278–282, 2022, April.
25. Aboamer, M.A., Sikkandar, M.Y., Gupta, S., Vives, L., Joshi, K., Omarov, B., Singh, S.K., An investigation in analyzing the food quality well-being for lung cancer using blockchain through CNN. *J. Food Qual.*, 2022, Article ID 5845870, 11 pages, 2022. https://doi.org/10.1155/2022/5845870
26. Negi, S.S., Memoria, M., Kumar, R., Joshi, K., Pandey, S.D., Gupta, A., Machine learning based hybrid technique for heart disease prediction, in: *2022 International Conference on Advances in Computing, Communication and Materials (ICACCM)*, IEEE, pp. 1–6, 2022, November.

17

Chili Pepper as a Natural Therapeutic Drug: A Review of Its Anticancer and Antioxidant Properties and Mechanism of Action Using the Machine Learning Approach

Rachana Joshi[1], Narinder Kumar[2*], B. S. Rawat[2], Reena Dhyani[2], Hemlata Sharma[2] and Rajiv Kumar[3]

[1]Department of Chemistry, School of Applied & Life Sciences, Uttaranchal University, Dehradun, Uttarakhand, India

[2]Department of Physics, School of Applied & Life Sciences, Uttaranchal University, Dehradun, Uttarakhand, India

[3]Department of Computer Science and Engineering, Uttaranchal Institute of Technology, Uttaranchal University, Dehradun, Uttarakhand, India

Abstract

As a spice, flavor enhancer, vegetable, and ingredient in herbal medicine, *Capsicum* spp. are significant. Numerous compounds found in different chili pepper genotypes have been identified and described, along with their medicinally significant effects. The main phytochemicals found in chili pepper fruits are capsaicinoids, carotenoids, vitamins, and flavonoids like anthocyanins. The most significant class of phytochemicals are capsaicinoids, which are spiciness-inducing analogs of capsinoids. Capsaicin and dihydrocapsaicin play a significant role in establishing pungency and therapeutic characteristics. In-depth research on the phytochemicals in chili pepper fruits using mice models and human cell lines has revealed a variety of anticancer effects on leukemia, myeloma, and other digestive tract carcinomas. Chili peppers also have antioxidant, antibacterial, anticholesteremic, anticlotting, anti-inflammatory, and antidiabetic properties. In order to give a thorough evaluation of the phytochemical profile and therapeutic benefits of chili pepper, this review was put together. Collectively, many research studies

**Corresponding author*: knarinder7@gmail.com

Kapil Joshi and Somil Kumar Gupta (eds.) Human Cancer Diagnosis and Detection Using Exascale Computing, (253–278) © 2024 Scrivener Publishing LLC

completed to date have shown the potential medical relevance of chili pepper for the creation of herbal medicines and to plan more investigations to reveal other hitherto unrecognized medicinal benefits.

Keywords: Phytochemicals, *Capsicum*, capsaicinoids, capsaicin, anticancer activity, machine learning

17.1 Introduction

Capsicum species, which include the chili pepper, are crucial to our daily diet. With a mean annual consumption of 3.5 million metric tonnes of dried fruit, it is the spice that the world consumes the most [1]. The distinctive flavor and pungency of chili pepper fruits add a special heat to meal preparations, and a variety of cuisines use this pungency in conjunction with salt and other spices to improve flavor [2]. There are 40 species in the very varied genus *Capsicum* [3]. The five species that people most commonly consume are *C. annuum* var. *annuum*, *C. frutescens*, *C. chinense*, *C. baccatum* variants *pendulum* and *umbilicatum*, and *C. pubescens* [4, 5].

In addition to its culinary applications, chili peppers have been employed in pharmaceutical formulations that offer nutritional and physiological benefits such analgesic, antibacterial, anticancer, anti-inflammatory, anticholesteremic, and anticlotting properties. According to numerous reports from India, chili pepper was used by the Mayans to treat microbial illnesses [6], headaches, gastrointestinal tract issues [7], toothache, extreme pain, wounds, ulcers, arthritis [8], and sleep disturbances. Using chili pepper as a remedy for rheumatism and hypersensitivity was also prevalent.

We may assume that the phytochemicals found in chili pepper fruits enhance and preserve human health because of the indigenous usage of chili pepper in folk medicine applications and the safe and extensive use of chili pepper as a spice throughout human history [9]. Numerous studies have shown the nutritional and therapeutic benefits of these phytochemicals. A few reviews on the bioavailability and metabolism of capsaicin, as well as its anticancer effects and general nutraceutical advantages, have been published [10–13]. The range of chili pepper's therapeutic characteristics has not, however, been examined all at once in order to understand all of its functions. This essay examines the therapeutic benefits of chili peppers for a variety of diseases, such as cancer, diabetes, cholesterolemia, and microbiological infections.

17.2 Machine Learning Technique

Researchers in the medical field and physicians are beginning to show a significant interest in the techniques of machine learning. We provide a conceptual introduction to machine learning as well as a practical guide to designing and assessing prediction algorithms for the development of cancer treatments in order to meet the demand for capacity development in this field.

17.3 Composition Profile

Numerous medicinally significant qualities of the phenolic compounds of chili peppers, including antidiarrheal, antioxidant, antimicrobial, antilithogenic, antihyperglycemic, and antimutagenic activities, are linked to this spice [14]. Flavonoids; β-catenin; capsaicinoids; carotenoids (capsorubin, capsanthin, and cryptocapsin); vitamins A, B, C, and E; glycerolipids; glycolipids; and esters are phenolic chemicals found in chili pepper fruits [15].

GC/MS spectrophotometry was used to analyze the chemical composition of chili pepper fruit extracts [16]. Capsaicin, nordihydrocapsaicin, homocapsaicin, dihydrocapsaicin, and homodihydrocapsaicin are the five main capsaicinoids found in chili peppers, and they are responsible for giving chili peppers its pungency [17] (Figure 17.1). Significant amounts of other capsaicinoids, including nonvamide and n-vanillyldecanamide, are also detected. Fruit extracts in acetone and hexane vary in total capsaicinoid concentration from 58.8% to 84.5% [19]. Ninety percent of the pungency of chili peppers comes from the dihydrocapsaicin [N-(4-hydroxy-3-methoxybenzyl)-8-methylnonenamide] and capsaicin [8-methyl-N-vaniloid-6-nonenamide] [18], which make up 37% and 29% of the total capsaicinoids, respectively [19].

Capsicum chinense, a member of the genus *Capsicum*, has the most capsaicin [20–22]. The species *C. annuum* has a greater vitamin E concentration than *C. frutescence*, even though the mean vitamin E level in chili peppers ranges from 1.98% to 2.10% [22]. For every 100 g of fresh fruit weight, the well-known chili pepper cultivar bell pepper provides 20.73 g of dietary fiber and 133 mg of vitamin C [23]. It has been discovered that *C. annuum* provides a reliable source of Zn, a crucial micronutrient [22].

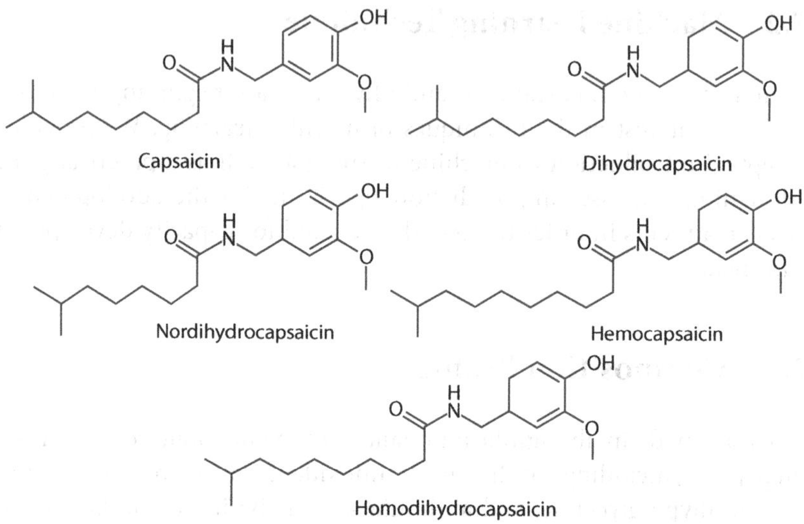

Figure 17.1 Structure of the five main capsaicinoids—capsaicin, dihydrocapsaicin, homocapsaicin, nordihydrocapsaicin, and homodihydrocapsaicin—found in chili peppers.

17.4 Reactions of Phytochemicals to Drying and Ripening

It has been established that traditional sun drying preserves capsaicin in the chili pepper fruits and that low-temperature drying ensures the excellent quality of chili pepper by protecting the phenolic components and vitamin C in the fruits [24]. The fact that chili peppers often contain more vitamin C than many other vegetables demonstrates the chili pepper's great nutritional worth [25]. It is also noteworthy to notice that drying maintains vitamin C. During ripening, the overall phenolic and carotenoid contents rise; the phenolic content doubles and the carotenoid content multiplies 10-fold. Even though the overall flavonoid concentration rises during initial ripening, it is subsequently decreased when fruits turn red [26]. When green chili peppers are dried, ascorbic acid level rises while total phenolic content falls, lowering the overall antioxidant potential [27]. However, Wangcharoen and Morasuk [28] observed that larger levels of phenolic components were maintained when chili pepper was dried at a temperature more than 100°C, leading to an improved antioxidant activity. It is also noteworthy that dried chili peppers retained their antioxidant activity for up to 18 months after harvest [29].

17.5 Antioxidant Activity

According to Chung *et al.* [30], the phytochemicals in chili peppers have anticancer activities. Among them, vitamin C and phenolic compounds can function as antioxidants to reduce the effects of reactive oxygen species (ROS) [31]. The cellular metabolic process that produces ROS has been linked to several illnesses, including cancer, diabetes, cardiovascular problems, and neurological issues [32]. Numerous enzymes found in the body and antioxidants received from dietary components, such as chili pepper, can detoxify ROS [33]. Among the frequently consumed fruits and vegetables, the antioxidant activity of chili pepper [34] is only second to spinach [35]. Numerous assaying systems have been used to measure and investigate the antioxidant activity of chili peppers, including the DPPH (2,2-diphenyl-1-picrylhydrazyl assay), DMPD (dimethyl-4-phenylenediamine assay), ABTS (2,2′-azino-bis [3-ethylbenzothiazoline-6-sulfonic acid] assay), and CuPRAC (cupric reducing antioxidant capacity assay) [36]. Chili peppers have antioxidant properties due to the presence of phenolic and anthocyanin chemicals [37–40]. Dietary phenolic compounds are helpful because they neutralize free radicals produced by the body by donating H atoms to them [37]. Additionally, aside from having potent antioxidants, chili peppers also contain vitamins C and E [32]. Consuming chili peppers in both dried and fresh forms may affect antioxidant levels, while research on the impact of drying has produced contradictory results [28].

The antioxidant content of various chili pepper species and cultivars varies as well. When the antioxidant activity of Turkish pepper cultivars was evaluated, the results showed a range of antioxidant activity of around seven times [41]. Bell and caribe, a type of yellow-fruited chili pepper, were discovered to have the greatest antioxidant activity out of the five chili pepper varieties studied. According to an estimate of 91.4% connection between phenolic content and antioxidant activity by Medina-Juarez *et al.* [42], the phenolic chemicals in chili peppers are primarily responsible for this antioxidant activity. Rahim and Mat [21] found that bell pepper had the greatest amount of phenolic content and the best antioxidant activity when compared with other species and cultivars, while Nadeem *et al.* [43] confirmed their findings. According to reports, *C. chinense* also has greater concentrations of antioxidants such ascorbate, carotenoids, and glutathione, and glutathione content rises with ripening [44]. The two main antioxidants that contribute to the Halliwell–Asada cycle, which allows H_2O_2 generated in chloroplasts to be detoxified without the need of the enzyme catalase, are glutathione and ascorbate [45].

17.6 Anticancer Activity

Hepatocellular carcinoma-derived HepG2 cell lines were treated with *C. chinense* fruit extracts, which showed to limit the growth of cancer cells. Utilizing tests for lactate dehydrogenase leakage, nitrous oxide (NO) generation, and methylthiazoltetrazolium (MTT), this inhibitory action was independently confirmed [46]. The phytochemicals in chili peppers cause cancerous cells to undergo apoptosis. By suppressing the mitochondrial plasma membrane NADH oxidoreductase enzyme, capsaicin triggers the apoptotic pathway [47, 48]. Additionally, capsaicin inhibits the action of the ATP-producing coenzyme Q by binding with it. This destabilizes the electron flow in the mitochondria, which leads to the production of ROS and the induction of death [49–52]. In human KB cancer cells (derived from the HeLa cell line), capsaicin agitated the mitochondria's membrane potential, which then activated the caspase signaling pathway. In pancreatic cancer cells, the ROS has been demonstrated to damage the mitochondrial membrane and activate apoptotic pathways [53]. Lin *et al.* [54] reported that capsaicin causes apoptosis in KB cancer cells and causes the cell cycle to be stopped in the G2/M phase. Caspases are activated and the mitochondrial membrane is permeabilized during the capsaicin-induced apoptosis in KB cells. These findings suggest that capsaicin may be helpful in preventing the spread of cancer cells [54]. Capsaicin may also suppress the NF-κB (nuclear factor kappa-light-chain-enhancer of activated B cells) pathway, which might reduce cancer-causing effects and trigger apoptosis [55, 56]. Studies using exogenous capsaicin in human cell cultures demonstrated apoptosis, autophagy, and suppression of cell metabolism [57–60]. Capsanthin, capsorubin, and cryptocapsin are three carotenoid pigments found in bell peppers that have strong free radical scavenging activity [61].

According to research employing derived human cutaneous squamous cell carcinoma, capsaicin has both preventative and curative effects against skin malignancies via inducing apoptosis and altering the epidermal growth factor receptor (EGFR) [62]. Capsaicin also inhibits Bcl-2 expression [63], which causes B16-F10 melanoma cells to undergo apoptosis. The ability of capsaicin to suppress chemically caused skin malignancies in animal models has also been demonstrated [64, 65]. In order to cure and prevent myeloma and other malignancies, capsaicin might be employed [66]. Capsaicin inhibits the growth of leukemia cells by degrading the TAX protein and increasing the NF-κB inhibitor alpha (I-B), which arrests the cell cycle and initiates apoptosis, according to *in vitro* studies using T-cell leukemia cell cultures. This illustrates the potential for employing capsaicin as a leukemia chemopreventive medication [67]. Additionally, oxidative stress caused by capsaicin is known to trigger the apoptotic pathway in leukemia cells [68]. Capsaicin causes apoptosis in glioma cells via binding to the transient receptor potential vanilloid type I (TRPV I) receptor [69]. Additionally, according to Gil and Kang [70], capsaicin causes apoptosis in human glioma cells via suppressing Bcl-2 expression. Additionally, it is known that capsaicin has inhibitory effects on the various digestive tract malignancies. According to Tanaka *et al.* [71], capsaicin has anticarcinogenic properties against tongue tumors via causing apoptosis by promoting the production of caspase-3 and caspase-9 activities [72]. According to Wu *et al.* [73], capsaicin causes CE 81T/VGH cells to go into apoptosis by activating caspase-3 and releasing ROS. Additionally, it has been observed that in the SNU-1 cell line, capsaicin increased the expression of protooncogenes, which initiate the apoptotic pathway, and the tumor-suppressor gene *p53* [74]. In hepatocarcinoma cells of the SK-Hep-1 human liver cell line, capsaicin promotes apoptosis by activating caspase-3 and downregulating Bcl-2, according to Jung *et al.* [75]. Capsaicin also promotes ROS-induced mitochondrial damage and triggers apoptosis in pancreatic cancer cells. Capsaicin is known to inhibit the β-catenin-dependent signaling pathway in colorectal cancer cells. Capsaicin inhibits the interaction between β-catenin and TCF-4 and limits the production of transcription factor 4 (TCF-4), suggesting the possibility of using chili peppers as a therapy for colorectal tumors [76]. Capsaicin inhibits cell growth in colorectal cancer cell lines, according to Lee *et al.* [77]. Capsaicin's anticancer effects are also shown in lung-related carcinomas. In mouse models, the usage of benzopyrene increases the risk of cancer, while capsaicin stabilizes the mitochondrial-related enzymes in the lungs and reduces that risk [81]. According to Jang *et al.* [79], capsaicin lowers the risk of lung tumor formation brought on by polycyclic aromatic hydrocarbons [80]. Brown *et al.* claim that capsaicin can be used to treat human small cell lung cancer because it has antiproliferative activity in both cell culture experiments and mouse models. This antiproliferative activity is triggered by inhibiting the E2F responses and proliferative gene expression. Ip *et al.* [81] describe the methods by which capsaicin produces endoplasmic reticulum stress, caspase-3 activation, and mitochondrial depolarization in NPC cell lines. Additionally, capsaicin inhibits the growth of prostate cancer by reducing the expression of the prostate-specific antigen (PSA) [82].

17.7 Activities that are Anti-Inflammatory and Relieve Pain

Chili pepper extracts have anti-inflammatory and anti-allergic effects [83, 84]. Capsaicin, one of the several phytochemicals found in chili peppers, has been shown to have the most anti-inflammatory effects [83], although anthocyanin, a color pigment, has also been linked to considerable anti-inflammatory effects [85]. According to Kang *et al.* [86], capsaicin suppressed the inflammatory reactions brought on by obesity in adipose tissue's macrophages, suggesting that it may be used as an analgesic. Capsaicin inhibits the production of pro-inflammatory cytokines including tumor necrosis factor (TNF) and interleukin 1 (IL-1), which lessens inflammatory reactions brought on by antigens [87]. Additionally, it was shown that lipopolysaccharide-stimulated peritoneal macrophages' ability to break down inflammatory mediators, IkB-a, was what really caused anti-inflammatory activity to occur rather than vanilloid receptor-1 [83]. An example of an early T-cell activation event that is inhibited by capsaicin and another form of capsinoid, nordihydrocapsiate, is NF-κB activation [88]. As it lessens the inflammatory heat, capsaicin can be used to treat osteoarthritis, rheumatoid arthritis, and peripheral arthritis [89]. Fraenkel *et al.* [90] reported that capsaicin was the most popular choice with 44% of the respondents surveyed preferring this option. Relatively few patients preferred nonselective NSAIDs (2%) and COX-2 inhibitors (7%), assuming patients are responsible for the full cost of their medications. The most preferred option was capsaicin, which was selected by 44% of survey participants. relatively few patients (2%) and COX-2 inhibitors (7%), preferring nonselective NSAIDs. Due to its capacity to regulate the secretion of pain-related neurotransmitters, it can also be employed to treat painful chemical hyperalgesia [91]. Capsaicin's analgesic effects can be utilized to lessen neuropathic pain problems. Capsaicin can be used as a short-term painkiller for oral mucositis that develops after chemo and radiation therapy for cancer patients [92]. According to Cruz [93], capsaicin helps lessen the bladder discomfort experienced by people with hypersensitive diseases.

17.8 Activities Controlling Diabetes and Hyperglycemia

The number of diabetes patients worldwide is predicted to reach 300 million by 2025 [92], necessitating the development of more effective and affordable therapies. Zhang *et al.* [94] reported that capsaicin exhibited hypoglycemic effects on rats with type 1 diabetes (T1D). Capsaicin activated the TRPV1 ion channel in the liver and increased the expression of TRPV1, LXR, and PDX-1. LXR and PDX-1 controlled glycometabolism balance by regulating the expression levels of GK, GLUT2, PEPCK, and G6pase, thereby inhibiting gluconeogenesis and promoting glycogen synthesis. Due to the presence of enzyme inhibitors for α-amylase and α-glucosidase, which are necessary for the breakdown of polysaccharides and disaccharides, chili pepper has shown to possess promising antidiabetic activity [95]. This means that it has a significant potential as a candidate plant for new drugs. Chili pepper has also been shown to reduce the absorption of D-glucose in the gut, making it useful for regulating the digestion of carbohydrates and the rise in blood sugar levels after meals [96]. Human volunteers were used to test capsaicin's effects on glucose metabolism during exercise and at rest. It was discovered that capsaicin elevates plasma norepinephrine and epinephrine by increasing oxygen consumption. This suggests that capsaicin is causing an increase in glucose oxidation [97]. Using human participants, Domotor *et al.* [98] further established that capsaicin raises blood glucagon levels and glucose absorption. By utilizing capsaicin, the metabolic condition caused by obesity-induced insulin resistance, which lowers the chance of developing type 2 diabetes, can be avoided. In animal models, capsaicin modifies gene expression, diminishes glucose resistance (hyperglycemia), and lowers fasting glucose levels [99]. In addition, the use of rat models allowed researchers to get a thorough understanding of the antidiabetic properties of chili peppers. Capsaicin is known to speed up the pace at which carbohydrates are metabolized in human beings. By inducing thermogenesis responses like lipid and glucose metabolism and reducing fatty acid storage in the body, the administration of chili pepper to rats lowers blood glucose level [100]. By stimulating the sympathetic nervous system, which encourages thermogenesis reactions, one can induce thermogenesis responses [95]. In this context, *C. frutescence* is always in demand due to research showing that it raises blood insulin levels in animals with type 2 diabetes [101]. According to Anthony *et al.*'s study [102], Capsicum frutescens supplementation at doses of 1g and 2g effectively decreased the fasting blood glucose level and body weight of alloxan-induced diabetic Wistar rats. Additionally, it was shown that *C. frutescence* increased the affinity of insulin toward its receptor (glucose), suggesting the possibility of employing chili pepper as a diabetic therapy [103].

17.9 The Impacts of Anticholesteremic Activity on Lipid Metabolism

According to reports, chili pepper has hypocholesteremic and hypolipidemic properties, making it useful for treating and preventing cardiovascular illnesses [104, 105]. By preventing the body from storing fatty acids [106], capsaicin can stimulate the thermogenesis and lipid metabolism pathways. Ahuja *et al.* [107] demonstrated its potential to be used as a therapy to manage obesity. Capsaicin promotes catecholamine production, which releases three adrenergic stimulation and causes a response known as thermogenesis [109–111]. By oxidizing dietary fats in the digestive system, capsaicin particularly modifies the lipid metabolism. According to Kempaiah *et al.* [112], capsaicin prevents low-density lipoprotein oxidation brought on by ferrous (*in vivo*) and copper (*in vitro*) ions. According to Ahuja *et al.* [107], serum lipoprotein oxidation caused by copper is inhibited by capsaicin and dihydrocapsaicin. In rats, capsaicin has been shown to have protective properties against hepatic lipid peroxidation [112]. Another rat research found that giving rats chili peppers combined with high-fat diets affected their levels of HDL and LDL cholesterol, total glycerides, and total lipids and that this drastically decreased blood cholesterol levels when compared with control treatments [100]. Similarly, it was noted that daily chili pepper meals in human subjects resulted in lower blood lipoprotein concentration [108]. Due to its stronger antioxidant activity than most other plants, chili pepper can be utilized to reduce lipid oxidation [113]. Human subject studies have also demonstrated that eating capsaicin causes belly fat reduction by boosting fat oxidation [114]. Ingestion of capsaicinoids boosted the body's rate of fat oxidation and energy expenditure, according to additional research with human individuals with higher body mass index (BMI), suggesting that it may be helpful to aid BMI reduction [115].

17.10 Anticlotting Effect

The phytochemicals in chili peppers have been shown to provide therapeutic benefits for mice with cardiovascular problems [116]. Research on rats indicated that chili peppers may lower the incidence of arthritis and cardiovascular problems [117]. Capsaicin was shown to prevent platelet aggregation by stabilizing red blood cell membranes and inhibiting the activity of the enzyme phospholipase A2 (PLA2) [118–120]. According to research using mouse models, capsaicin, which prevents platelet formation by blocking clotting factors VIII:C and IX, is superior to aspirin at preventing acute pulmonary thromboembolism [121]. As a result, capsaicin may one day be developed as a cardiovascular disease treatment and preventative.

17.11 Antimicrobial Activity

Historically, people have valued herbal products because of their known antibacterial benefits [122]. In addition to being used as a spice, chili peppers are frequently utilized as a food preservation agent [123]. Numerous investigations have documented the antibacterial properties of the chemicals found in *Capsicum* species [123, 124]. The pigment anthocyanin in chili peppers has both pungency-related compounds and antibacterial action [125]. The noxious pathogens *Pseudomonas aeruginosa, Escherichia coli, Sarcina lutea, Bacillus subtilis, Candida albicans, Bacillus cereus, Clostridium sporogenes, Clostridium tetani, Streptococcus pyogenes,* and *Vibrio cholera* have all been shown to be susceptible to the antibacterial properties of chili pepper [126]. The minimum inhibitory concentration (MIC) of capsaicin against the stomach pathogen *Helicobacter pyroli* was determined to be 10 g/ml [127] and verified by Zeyrek and Oguz [128]. Similar MIC values of 25 g/ml for *B. subtilis,* 200–300 g/ml for *E. coli,* 15 g/ml for *Salmonella typhimurium,* and 5–15 g/ml for *P. aeruginosa* were reported [129]. Additionally, capsaicin has inhibitory effects on a variety of microbiological strains that are resistant to antibiotics [128]. Antimicrobial activity against *Enterococcus faecalis, B. subtilis, P. aeruginosa, E. coli, S. aureus, Klebsiella pneumoniae,* and *C. albicans* was discovered in the acetonitrile extracts of dihydrocapsaicin, phytochemical chrysoeriol, and capsaicin from *C. frutescence* [130, 131]. Using DNA microarray technology, the mechanism of capsaicin's antimicrobial action was examined.

17.12 Immune Checkpoint Signaling

By suppressing T cells and promoting immune tolerance, immunological checkpoints, which are receptor-based signaling cascades, enable malignancies to evade immune surveillance and detection. The three most well-known of these checkpoints are CTLA-4, PD-1, and PD-L1.

As a revolutionary cancer therapy, monoclonal antibodies that disrupt immunological checkpoints have developed. After successfully treating advanced, incurable melanoma, immune checkpoint therapy has lately been expanded to treat other malignancies [67].

17.13 Suppression of Antitumor Immune Response

Certain tumor cells overexpress or generate immunosuppressive tumor products, such as transforming growth factor (TGF), which prevents lymphocyte and macrophage effector function and cell division. Fas ligand (FasL), which detects the Fas molecule on leukocytes, is expressed by additional tumor cells. The leukocytes die by an apoptotic process when FasL attaches to Fas [44].

17.14 Antigen Masking

Glycocalyx molecules like sialic acid may act as immune system shields for the cell surface tumor antigen. Since tumor cells have more glycocalyx (surface carbohydrate) molecules than normal cells, a process known as antigen masking takes place. Similar to normal cells, tumor cells can protect themselves from the immune system by triggering the coagulation cascade and covering themselves with fibrin. The tumor is immune-resistant because the antitumor antibodies or the generated specific T cells do not react with the hidden tumor cells [56].

17.15 Immune-Based Cancer Therapies

Immune-based cancer treatments can be clinically effective despite the self-regulatory challenges mentioned above, and certain immune-based strategies represent the gold standard for the treatment of cancer. As a therapy for superficial bladder cancer, intravesical bacillus Calmette–Guérin is thought to exert disease control through immune-mediated pathways. The Toll-like receptor 7 agonist imiquimod is frequently used to treat superficial skin malignancies. In these malignancies, topical imiquimod therapy causes an elevation of genes linked to tissue rejection [33]. Infusions of donor lymphocytes are now a common therapy for relapses following allogeneic transplant for hematologic malignancies. The clinical effectiveness of monoclonal antibody treatment with drugs like trastuzumab and rituxan is probably influenced by immune-mediated pathways to some extent. The fact that these methods are typically applied when cancers have a minimal disease burden and/or are non-invasive is a recurring theme important to the effectiveness of these techniques. Moreover, monoclonal antibody treatment is frequently administered together with cytoreductive chemotherapy, preventing the spread of the malignancy. The most effective use of immunotherapy is for the treatment of infectious diseases [67]. Yet, when a person receives a vaccine to prevent an infection, immunity is created before the pathogen is exposed. After an infection has taken hold, it is sometimes challenging to eradicate a disease that is quickly multiplying using a technique like active vaccination. Immunotherapy could also be challenging to use in cases with advanced cancer. Adoptive T-cell treatment, which involves reinfusing tumor-competent T cells that have grown to large numbers outside the body, has been found in clinical studies conducted at the National Cancer Institute to have a 50% response rate in patients with resistant advanced-stage melanoma [78]. Patients with melanoma that was resistant to both chemotherapy and immunotherapy received an injection of T cells that were isolated, cultured in culture, and taken from their tumors (IL-2). Although a high percentage of patients responded, some experienced prolonged disease stability, there have been a few reports of full responders, and the immune response given in the majority of patients did not completely eradicate the tumor [105].

17.16 Other Miscellaneous Medicinal Values

The digestive tract's correct operation and good health have long been associated with chili peppers. Saliva and gastric juice are necessary for effective food digestion and the treatment of gastrointestinal disorders, and capsaicin promotes their production [9]. By causing the stomach submucosal arteriolar dilatation, which is necessary for effective meal absorption, capsaicin also increases gastric blood flow. Since capsaicin suppresses the development of *H. pylori*, Zeyrek and Oguz [128] suggested that chili peppers may be useful for treating stomach and duodenal ulcers. According to Das *et al.* [132], capsaicin demonstrated hepatoprotective effect by promoting recovery from CCl_4-induced liver damage in rats. Chili pepper also displayed stomach ulcer protective activity [133]. Finally, research on mature red chili peppers has revealed its inhibitory effect against the angiotensin-1-converting enzyme, which lowers blood pressure [134].

The immune system defends the body against pathogenic microorganisms such as bacteria, fungi, viruses, and parasites. It consists of the body's responses to the damaged or diseased cells. Thus, the term "immunological response" is occasionally used to describe it. The immune system is crucial for people with cancer because cancer has been shown to damage the immune system. Immune system impairment may come from cancer therapy. The fight against cancer may benefit from the immune system. In general, the immune system in the body works to combat disease and injury, but it also targets body parts that do not function properly, such as cancer cells, which have developed their own strategies to evade the immune system, survive, and produce proteins that prevent any part of the immune system from fully eradicating the tumor that has formed. It scans the "non-self receptors" that are found on the cell membranes that are external to the body and shines on them. T lymphocytes, one of the body's immunological defense mechanisms, adhere to the tumor cell and produce weaponry and enzymes, which break down the tumor cell into tiny fragments that the body eventually gets rid of. As a tumor expands rapidly, the immune system nearly keeps up with it by obliterating the tumor cells.

When the immune system cannot keep up with the tumor's growth, the tumor grows larger and becomes cancerous. As the tumor grows, it develops various strategies to trick the immune system, including hiding or displaying receptors on its cell membranes that are similar to those found on normal cells to fool the immune system. The whole cell membrane of the receptors is present. Since certain tumors emit instructions directing immune cells to cease functioning, spreading, and defending the body, the immune system is not even aware of the presence of cancer, which permits it to progress. In order for a tumor to survive and spread, it must go through a number of evil processes to acclimatize to the body so that it does not identify it as a foreign body, and then it turns on it to take advantage of it by paralyzing it entirely and preparing a space for it to graze in as it pleases. As a result, tumor cells cooperate, comprehend, and fully integrate not only in maintaining their malignant tumor entity but also in developing numerous strategies to aid in their penetration into the body. These strategies include the secretion of enzymes that break down the barriers between cells to pass through and the secretion of proteins that stimulate the formation of blood vessels from which they can move into the bloodstream to the other members. Lastly, in order for tumor cells to survive at the expense of healthy cells while remaining immune system-safe, they produce molecules that both accelerate their growth and activity and other compounds that paralyze immune cell mobility and activity. One or more of the following pathways may arise, leading to the immune response's evasion process known as tumor escape.

Cancer-associated inflammation has a role in genomic instability, amplification of cancer anti-apoptotic pathways, epigenetic alteration, activation of cancer cell proliferation, stimulation of angiogenesis, and cancer spread. It is present at various stages of carcinogenesis. Research conducted over the past two decades has shown that inflammatory immune cells are crucial contributors to the inflammation associated with cancer. Understanding how immune cells affect tumor destiny at many phases of the illness, including early neoplastic transformation, clinically diagnosed tumors, metastatic spread, and therapeutic intervention, has been the focus of research. In this review, with a special emphasis on metastatic carcinomas, we concentrate on current discoveries, unified ideas, limitations, and future difficulties in investigating cancer-associated inflammatory cells.

17.17 Conclusion

The compounds found in chili peppers, such capsaicin, have the potential to have a wide range of therapeutic effects. It is evident that the most recent research on the therapeutic effects of chili pepper supports the ethnomedical uses described in historical sources. The anticancer efficacy is delivered through inducing apoptosis, stopping the cell cycle, and preventing cancer from proliferating. Human cancer cell lines and animal models were used to corroborate these behaviors. Additionally, reports of chili pepper's analgesic, antihyperglycemic, antifungal and antibacterial properties have been made. It has been extensively researched how chili peppers can treat different illnesses and problems such as ulcers of the digestive system, hypercholesterolemia, aging, obesity, and stroke. To demonstrate the mechanisms of action, the underlying phytochemicals and the related molecular pathways have been described. Although mostly restricted to the fruits of the two major species, *C. annuum* and *C. frutescence*, as well as the well-known cultivar bell pepper, which is also a *C. annuum*, the intergenera variability of the medicinal qualities has been examined. In order to investigate and define more effective bioactive chemicals from the underused *Capsicum* spp. in various geographical regions, more research is imperative. The amount of knowledge that is now accessible on the therapeutic benefits of chili pepper can be used to create brand-new medications to treat cancer and the other serious illnesses listed.

References

1. Nadeem, M., Anjun, F.M., Khan, M.R., Saeed, M., Riaz, A., Antioxidant potential of bell pepper (*Capsicum annum* L.)-A Review. *Pak. J. Food Sci.*, 21, 45–51, 2011.
2. Pino, J., Gonzalez, M., Ceballos, L., Centurión-Yah, A.R., Trujillo-Aguirre, M.J., Latournerie-Moreno, L., Sauri-Duch, E., Characterization of total capsaicinoids, colour and volatile compounds of Habanero chilli pepper (Capsicum chinense Jack.) cultivars grown in Yucatan. *Food Chem.*, 104, 1682–1686, 2007.
3. Krishna, A.G.G., Lokesh, B.R., Sugasini, D., Kancheva, V.D., Evaluation of the antiradical and antioxidant properties of extracts from Indian red chili and black pepper by *in vitro* models. *Bulg. Chem. Commun.*, 42, 62–69, 2010.
4. Moscone, E.A., Scaldaferro, M.A., Grabiele, M., Cecchini, N.M., Sánchez García, Y., Jarret, R., Daviña, J.R., Ducasse, D.A., Barboza, G.E., Ehrendorfer, F., The evolution of chili peppers (Capsicum - Solanaceae): A cytogenetic perspective. *ActaHorticulturae*, 745, 137–170, 2007.
5. Perry, L., Starch fossils and the domestication and dispersal of chili pepper (Capsicum spp. L.) in the Americas. *Science*, 315, 986–988, 2007.
6. Cichewicz, R.H. and Thorpe, P.A., The antimicrobial properties of chili peppers (Capsicum species) and their uses in Mayan medicine. *J. Ethnopharmacol.*, 52, 61–70, 1996.
7. Baruah, S., Zaman, M.K., Rajbongshi, P., Das, S., A review on recent research on Bhut jolokia and pharmacological activity of Capsaicin. *IJPSR.*, 15, 89–94, 2014.
8. Bhagowati, R.R. and Chankija, S., Genetic variability and traditional practices in Naga King Chilli landraces of Nagaland. *Asian Agri-History.*, 3, 171–180, 2009.
9. Bosland, P.W., Capsicum: Innovative uses of an ancient crop, in: *Progress in New crops*, J. Janick (Ed.), pp. 479–487, ASHS press, Arlington, Virginia, USA, 1996.
10. Rollyson, W.D., Stover, C.A., Brown, K.C., Perry, H.E., Stevenson, C.D., McNees, C.A., Ball, J.G., Valentovic, M.A., Dasgupta, P., Bioavailability of capsaicin and its implications for drug delivery. *JCR*, 196, 96–105, 2014.
11. Cao, S., Chen, H., Xiang, S., Hong, J., Weng, L., Zhu, H., Liu, Q., Anti-Cancer effects and mechanisms of capsaicin in chili peppers. *Am. J. Plant Sci.*, 6, 3075–3081, 2015.
12. Pawar, S.S., Bharude, N.V., Sonone, S.S., Deshmukh, R.S., Raut, A.K., Umarkar, A.R., Chillies as food, spice and medicine: A perspective. *IJPBS.*, 1, 311–318, 2011.
13. Milind, P. and Sushila, K., A hot way leading to healthy stay. *Int. Res. J. Pharm.*, 3, 21–25, 2012.

14. Adefegha, S.A. and Oboh, G., Phytochemistry and mode of action of some tropical spices in the management of type-2 diabetes and hypertension. *AJPP*, 7, 332–346, 2013.
15. Chu, Y.F., Sun, J., Wu, X., Liu, R.H., Antioxidant and antiproliferative activities of common vegetables. *J. Agric. Food Chem.*, 50, 6910–6916, 2002.
16. Wesolowska, A., Jadczak, D., Grzeszczuk, M., Chemical composition of the pepper fruit extracts of hot cultivars *Capsicum annuum* L. *Acta Scientiarum Polonorum Horticulture*, 10, 171–184, 2011.
17. Reyes-Escogido, M.L., Gonzalez-Mondragon, E.G., Vazquez-Tzompantzi, E., Chemical and pharmacological aspects of capsaicin. *Molecules*, 16, 1253–1270, 2011.
18. Surh, Y.J., Cancer chemoprevention with dietary phytochemicals. *Reviews*, 3, 768–780, 2003.
19. Giuffrida, D., Dugo, P., Torre, P., Bignardi, C., Cavazza, A., Corradini, C., Dugo, G., Characterization of 12 *Capsicum* varieties by evaluation of their carotenoid profile and pungency determination. *Food Chem.*, 140, 794–802, 2013.
20. Bosland, P.W. and Baral, J.B., 'BhutJolokia'-The world's hottest known chili pepper is a putative naturally occurring interspecific hybrid. *Hort Sci.*, 42, 222–224, 2007.
21. Rahim, R.A. and Mat, I., Phytochemical contents of Capsicum frutescens (Chili Padi), Capsicum annum (Chili Pepper) and Capsicum annum (Bell Peper) aqueous extracts. *Int. Conf. Biol. Life Sci.*, 40, 164–167, 2012.
22. Emmanuel-Ikpeme, C., Henry, P., Okiri, O.A., Comparative evaluation of the nutritional, phytochemical and microbiological quality of three pepper varieties. *JFNS*, 2, 74–80, 2014.
23. Durucasu, I. and Tokusoglu, O., Effect of grilling on luteolin (3', 4', 5, 7-tetrahydroxyflavone) content in sweet green bell pepper (*Capsicum annum*). *Pak. J. Biol. Sci.*, 10, 3410–3414, 2007.
24. Moraes, I.C.F., Sobral, P.J.D.A., Branco, I.G., Re, T.B., Gomide, C.A., Dehydration of "dedo de moça" pepper: Kinetics and phytochemical concentration. *Food Sci. Technol. (Campinas)*, 33, 134–141, 2013.
25. Kumar, O.A. and Tata, S.S., Ascorbic acid contents in chili peppers (*Capsicum* L.). *Notulae Scientia Biologicae*, 1, 50–52, 2009.
26. Shaha, R.K., Rahman, S., Asrul, A., Bioactive compounds in chilli peppers (Capsicum annuum L.) at various ripening (green, yellow and red) stages. *Ann. Biol. Res.*, 4, 27–34, 2013.
27. Ozgur, M., Ozcan, T., Akpinar-Bayizit, A., Yilmaz-Ersan, L., Functional compounds and antioxidant properties of dried green and red peppers. *Afr. J. Agric. Res.*, 6, 5638–5644, 2011.
28. Wangcharoen, W. and Morasuk, W., Antioxidant capacity changes in Chili Spur Pepper (*Capsicum annuum* Linn. var. acuminatumFingerh.) during drying process. *Asian J. Food Agro-Ind.*, 1, 68–77, 2008.

29. Ogiso, Y., Yabe, R.H., Kawamoto, Y., Kawamoto, T., Kato, K., Yabe, T., An antioxidant of dried chili pepper maintained its activity through postharvest ripening for 18 months. *Biosci. Biotechnol. Biochem.*, 72, 3297–3300, 2008.
30. Chung, S.Y., Sung, M.K., Kim, N.H., Jang, J.O., Go, E.J., P-glycoprotein by natural products in human breast cancer cells. *Arch. Pharmacal Res.*, 28, 823–828, 2005.
31. Podsedek, A., Natural antioxidants and antioxidant capacity of Brassica vegetables: A review. *LWT - Food Sci. Technol.*, 40, 1–11, 2007.
32. Sun-Hwa, H., Jung-Bong, K., Jong-Sug, P., Shin-Woo, L., Kang-Jim, C., A comparison of the carotenoid accumulation in *Capsicum* varieties that show different ripening colours: Deletion of the capsanthin-capsorubin synthase gene is not a prerequisite for the formation of a yellow pepper. *J. Exp. Bot.*, 58, 3135–3144, 2007.
33. Halliwell, B., Reactive species and antioxidants. Redox biology is a fundamental theme of aerobic life. *Plant Physiol.*, 141, 312–322, 2006.
34. Rosa, A., Deiana, M., Casu, V., Paccagnini, S., Appendino, G., Ballero, M., AssuntaDessiä, M., Antioxidant activity of capsinoids. *J. Agric. Food. Chem.*, 50, 7396–7401, 2002.
35. Pellegrini, N., Serafini, M., Colombi, B., Del Rio, D., Salvatore, S., Bianchi, M., Brighenti, F., Total antioxidant capacity of plant foods, beverages and oils consumed in Italy assessed by three different *in vitro* assays. *J. Nutr.*, 133, 2812–2819, 2003.
36. Krishna, A.G.G., Lokesh, B.R., Sugasini, D., Kancheva, V.D., Evaluation of the antiradical and antioxidant properties of extracts from Indian red chili and black pepper by *in vitro* models. *Bulg. Chem. Commun.*, 42, 62–69, 2010.
37. Borovsky, Y., Oren-Shamir, M., Ovadia, R., De Jong, W., Paran, I., The A locus that controls anthocyanin accumulation in pepper encodes a MYB transcription factor homologous to Anthocyanin2 of Petunia. *Theor. Appl. Genet.*, 109, 23–29, 2004.
38. Howard, L.R., Talcott, S.T., Brenes, C.H., Villalon, B., Changes in phytochemical and antioxidant activity of selected pepper cultivars (*Capsicum* species) as influenced by maturity. *J. Agric. Food. Chem.*, 48, 1713–1720, 2000.
39. Marín, A., Ferreres, F., Tomás-Barberán, F.A., Gil, M.I., Characterization and quantitation of antioxidant constituents of sweet pepper (*Capsicum annuum* L.). *J. Agric. Food. Chem.*, 52, 3861–3869, 2004.
40. Mennen, L.I., Walker, R., Bennetau-Pelissero, C., Scalbert, A., Risks and safety of polyphenol consumption. *AJCN*, 81, 326–329, 2005.
41. Frary, A., Keceli, M.A., Okmen, B., Sigva, H.O., Yemenicioglu, A., Doganlar, S., Water-soluble antioxidant potential of turkish pepper cultivars. *Hort Sci.*, 43, 631–636, 2008.
42. Medina-Juárez, L.A., Molina-Quijada, D.M.A., Toro-Sánchez, C.L.D., González-Aguilar, G.A., Gámez-Meza, N., Antioxidant activity of peppers (*Capsicum annuum* l.) extracts and characterization of their phenolic constituents. *Interciencia*, 37, 588–593, 2012.

43. Nadeem, M., Anjun, F.M., Khan, M.R., Saeed, M., Riaz, A., Antioxidant Potential of Bell Pepper (*Capsicum annum* L.)-A Review. *Pak. J. Food Sci.*, 21, 45–51, 2011.
44. Castro-Concha, L.A., Canche-Chuc, I., Miranda-Ham, M.D.L., Determination of antioxidants in fruit tissues from three accessions of habanero pepper (*Capsicum chinense*Jacq.). *J. Mex. Chem. Soc*, 56, 15–18, 2012.
45. Foyer, C.H. and Noctor, G., Redox regulation in photosynthetic organisms: Signaling, acclimation, and practical implications. *Antioxid. Redox Signaling*, 11, 861–905, 2009.
46. Amruthraj, N.J., Raj, J.P.P., Saravanan, S., Lebel, A., *In vitro* studies on anticancer activity of capsaicinoids from *capsicum chinense*against human hepatocellular carcinoma cells. *Int. J. Pharm. Pharm. Sci.*, 6, 254–558, 2014.
47. Morre, D.J., Chueh, P.J., Morre, D.M., Capsaicin inhibits preferentially the NADH oxidase and growth of transformed cells in culture. *Proc. Natl. Acad. Sci.*, 92, 1831–1835, 1995.
48. Morre, D.J., Sun, E., Geilen, C., Wu, L.Y., de-Cabo, R., Krasagakis, K., Orfanos, C.E., Morre, D.M., Capsaicin inhibits plasma membrane NADH oxidase and growth of human and mouse melanoma lines. *Eur. J. Cancer*, 32A, 1995–2003, 1996.
49. Macho, A., Blázquez, M.V., Navas, P., Muñoz, E., Induction of apoptosis by vanilloid compounds does not require de novo gene transcription and activator protein 1 activity. *Cell Growth Differ.*, 9, 277–286, 1998.
50. Macho, A., Calzado, M.A., Munoz-Blanco, J., Gomez-Diaz, C., Gajate, C., Mollinedo, F., Navas, P., Munoz, E., Selective induction of apoptosis by capsaicin in transformed cells: The role of reactive oxygen species and calcium. *Cell Growth Differ.*, 6, 155–165, 1999.
51. Macho, A., Lucena, C., Calzado, M.A., Blanco, M., Donnay, I., Appendino, G., Munoz, E., Phorboid 20-homovanillates induce apoptosis through a VR1-independent mechanism. *Chem. Biol.*, 7, 483–492, 2000.
52. Wolvetang, E.J., Larm, J.A., Moutsoulas, P., Lawen, A., Apoptosis induced by inhibitors of the plasma membrane NADH-oxidase involves Bcl-2 and calcineurin. *Cell Growth Differ.*, 7, 1315–1325, 1996.
53. Zhang, R., Humphreys, I., Sahu, R.P., Shi, Y., Sirivastava, S.K., *In vitro* and *in vivo* induction of apoptosis by capsaicin in pancreatic cancer cells is mediated through ROS generation and mitochondrial death pathway. *Apoptosis.*, 13, 1465–1478, 2008.
54. Lin, C., Lu, W., Wang, C., Chan, Y., Chen, M., Capsaicin induces cell cycle arrest and apoptosis in human KB cancer cells. *BMC Complement Altern. Med.*, 13, 46, 2013.
55. Han, S.S., Keum, Y.S., Seo, H.J., Chun, K.S., Lee, S.S., Surh, Y.J., Capsaicin suppresses phorbolesterinduced activation of NF-κB/Rel and AP-1 transcription factors in mouse epidermis. *Cancer Lett.*, 164, 119–126, 2001.
56. Patel, P.S., Varney, M.L., Dave, B.J., Singh, R.K., Regulation of constitutive and induced NF-κB activation in malignant melanoma cells by capsaicin

modulates interleukin-8 production and cell proliferation. *J. Interferon Cytokine Res.*, 22, 427–435, 2002.

57. Ghosh, A.K. and Basu, S., Fas-associated factor 1 is a negative regulator in capsaicin induced cancer cell apoptosis. *Cancer Lett.*, 287, 142–149, 2010.
58. Choi, C.H., Jung, Y.K., Oh, S., Selective induction of catalase mediated autophagy by dihydrocapsaicin in lung cell lines. *Free Radical Biol. Med.*, 49, 245–257, 2009.
59. Oh, S., Choi, C.H., Jung, Y.K., Autophagy induction by capsaicin in malignant human breast cells is modulated by p38 and ERK mitogen-activated protein kinase and retards cell death by suppressing endoplasmic reticulum stress mediated apoptosis. *Mol. Pharmacol.*, 78, 114–125, 2010.
60. Arora, R., Gill, N.S., Chauhan, G., Rana, A.C., An overview about versatile molecule Capsaicin. *IJPSDR*, 3, 280–286, 2011.
61. Matsufuji, H., Nakamuro, H., Chino, M., Mitsuharo, T., Antioxidant activity of capsanthin and the fatty acid esters in paprika (*Capsicum annuum*). *J. Agric. Food. Chem.*, 46, 3462–3472, 1998.
62. Hwang, M.K., Bode, A.M., Byun, S., Song, N.R., Lee, H.J., Dong, Z., Cocarcinogenic effect of Capsaicin involves activation of EGFR signaling but not TRPV1. *Therapeutics, Targets, Chem. Biol.*, 70, 6859–6869, 2010.
63. Jun, H.S., Park, T., Lee, C.K., Kang, M.K., Park, M.S., Kang, H.I., Surh, Y.J., Kim, O.H., Capsaicin induced apoptosis of B16-F10 melanoma cells through down-regulation of Bcl-2. *Food Chem. Toxicol.*, 45, 708–715, 2007.
64. Park, K.K. and Surh, Y.J., Effects of capsaicin on chemically induced two-stage mouse skin carcinogenesis. *Cancer Lett.*, 114, 183–184, 1997.
65. Yu, H., Pardoll, D., Jove, R., STATs in cancer inflammation and immunity: A leading role for STAT3. *Nat. Rev. Cancer*, 9, 798–809, 2009.
66. Bhutani, M., Pathak, A.K., Nair, A.S., Kunnumakkara, A.B., Guha, S., Sethi, G., Aggarwal, B.B., Capsaicin is a novel blocker of constitutive and Interleukin-6- inducible STAT3 activation. *Cancer Ther. : Preclinical*, 13, 3024–3032, 2007.
67. Zhang, J., Nagasaki, M., Tanaka, Y., Morikawa, S., Capsaicin inhibits growth of adult T-cell leukemia cells. *Leuk. Res.*, 27, 275–283, 2003.
68. Ito, K., Nakazato, T., Yamato, K., Miyakawa, Y., Yamada, T., Hozumi, N., Segawa, K., Ikeda, Y., Kizaki, M., Induction of apoptosis in leukemic cells by homovanillic acid derivative, capsaicin, through oxidative stress: Implication of phosphorylation of p53 at Ser-15 residue by reactive oxygen species. *Cancer Res.*, 64, 1071–1078, 2004.
69. Amantini, C., Mosca, M., Nabissi, M., Lucciarini, R., Caprodossi, S., Arcella, A., Giangaspero, F., Santoni, G., Capsaicin-induced apoptosis of glioma cells is mediated by TRPV1 vanilloid receptor and requires p38 MAPK activation. *J. Neurochem.*, 102, 977–990, 2007.
70. Gil, Y. and Kang, M., Capsaicin induces apoptosis and terminal differentiation in human glioma A172 cells. *Life Sci.*, 82, 997–1003, 2008.

71. Tanaka, T., Kohno, H., Sakata, K., Yamada, Y., Hirose, Y., Sugie, S., Mori, H., Modifying effects of dietary capsaicin and rotenone on 4-nitroquinoline 1-oxide-induced rat tongue carcinogenesis. *Carcinogenesis*, 23, 1361–1367, 2002.
72. Ip, S.W., Lan, S.H., Huang, A.C., Yang, J.S., Chen, Y.Y., Huang, H.Y., Lin, Z.P., Hsu, Y.M., Yang, M.D., Chiu, C.F., Chung, J.G., Capsaicin induces apoptosis in SCC-4 human tongue cancer cells through mitochondria-dependent and -independent pathways. *Environ. Toxicol.*, 27, 332–341, 2012a.
73. Wu, C.C., Lin, J.P., Yang, J.S., Chou, S.T., Chen, S.C., Lin, Y.T., Chung, J.G., Capsaicin induced cell cycle arrest and apoptosis in human esophagusepidermoid carcinoma CE 81T/VGH cells through the elevation of intracellular reactive oxygen species and Ca2+ productions and caspase-3 activation. *Mutat. Res.*, 601, 71–82, 2006.
74. Kim, J.D., Kim, J.M., Pyo, J.O., Kim, S.Y., Kim, B.S., Yu, R., Han, I.S., Capsaicin can alter the expression of tumor forming-related genes which might be followed by induction of apoptosis of a Korean stomach cancer cell line, SNU-1. *Cancer Lett.*, 120, 235–241, 1997.
75. Jung, M.Y., Kang, H.J., Moon, A., Capsaicin-induced apoptosis in SK-Hep-1 hepatocarcinoma cells involves Bcl-2 down-regulation and caspase-3 activation. *Cancer Lett.*, 165, 139–145, 2001.
76. Lee, S., Richardson, R.L., Dashwod, R.H., Baek, S.J., Capsaicin represses transcriptional activity of β-catenin in human colorectal cancer cells. *J. Nutr. Biochem.*, 23, 646–655, 2012.
77. Lee, S.H., Krisanapun, C., Baek, S.J., NSAID-activated gene-1 as a molecular target for capsaicininduced apoptosis through a novel molecular mechanism involving GSK3β, C/EBPβ, and ATF3. *Carcinogenesis.*, 31, 719–728, 2010.
78. Anandakumar, P., Kamaraj, S., Jagan, S., Ramakrishnan, G., Vinodhkumar, R., Devaki, T., Stabilization of pulmonary mitochondrial enzyme system by capsaicin during benzo (a) pyrene induced experimental lung cancer. *Biomed. Pharmacother.*, 62, 390–394, 2007.
79. Jang, J.J., Kim, S.H., Yun, T.K., Inhibitory effect of capsaicin on mouse lung tumor development. *In Vivo*, 3, 49–53, 1989.
80. Brown, K.C., Witte, T.R., Hardman, W.E., Luo, H., Chen, Y.C., Carpenter, A.B., Lau, J.K., Dasgupta, P., Capsaicin displays anti-proliferative activity against human small cell lung cancer in cell culture and nude mice models via the E2F pathway. *PLoS One*, 5, e10243, 2010.
81. Ip, S.W., Lan, S.H., Lu, H.F., Huang, A.C., Yang, J.S., Lin, J.P., Huang, H.Y., Lien, J.C., Ho, C.C., Chiu, C.F., Wood, W.G., Chung, J.G., Capsaicin mediates apoptosis in human nasopharyngeal carcinoma NPC-TW 039 cells through mitochondrial depolarization and endoplasmic reticulum stress. *Hum. Exp. Toxicol.*, 31, 539–549, 2012b.
82. Mori, A., Lehmann, S., O"Kelly, J., Kumagai, T., Desmond, J.C., Pervan, M., McBride, W.H., Kizaki, M., Koeffler, H.P., Capsaicin, a component of red

peppers, inhibits the growth of androgen independent, p53 mutant prostate cancer cells. *Cancer Res.*, 66, 3222–3229, 2006.

83. Kim, C.S., Kawada, T., Kim, B.S., Han, I.S., Choe, S.Y., Kurata, T., Yu, R., Capsaicin exhibits anti-inflammatory property by inhibiting IkB-a degradation in LPS-stimulated peritoneal macrophages. *Cell Signal.*, 15, 299–306, 2003.
84. Lee, J.J., Crosby, K.M., Pike, L.M., Yoo, K.S., Lescobar, D.I., Impact of genetic and environmental variation of development of flavonoids and carotenoids in pepper (*Capsicum* spp.). *Sci. Hortic.*, 106, 341–352, 2005.
85. Wang, H.B., Nair, M.G., Strasburg, G.M., Chang, Y.C., Booren, A.M., Gray, J.I., DeWitt, D.L., Antioxidant and antiinflammatory activities of anthocyanins and their aglycon, cyanidin, from tart cherries. *J. Nat. Prod.*, 62, 294–296, 1999.
86. Kang, J.H., Kim, C.S., Han, I.S., Kawada, T., Yu, R., Capsaicin, a spicy component of hot peppers, modulates adipokine gene expression and protein release from obese-mouse adipose tissues and isolated adipocytes, and suppresses the inflammatory responses of adipose tissue macrophages. *FEBS Lett.*, 581, 4389–4396, 2007.
87. Spiller, F., Alves, M.K., Vieira, S.M., Carvalho, T.A., Leite, C.E., Lunardelli, A., Polomi, J.A., Cunha, F.Q., Oliveira, J.R., Anti-inflammatory effects of red pepper (*Capsicum baccatum*) on carrageenan- and antigen-induced inflammation. *J. Pharm. Pharmacol.*, 60, 473–478, 2008.
88. Sancho, R., Lucena, C., Macho, A., Calzado, M.A., Blanco-Molina, M., Minassi, A., Appendino, G., Munoz, E., Immunosuppressive activity of capsaicinoids: Capsiate derived from sweet peppers inhibits NF- κB activation and is a potent anti-inflammatory compound *in vivo*. *EJI*, 32, 1753–1763, 2002.
89. Cordell, G.A. and Araujo, O.E., Capsaicin: Identification, nomenclature, and pharmacotherapy. *Ann. Pharmacother.*, 27, 330–336, 1993.
90. Fraenkel, L., Bogardus, S.T., Concato, J., Wittink, D.R., Treatment options in knee osteoarthritis: The patient's perspective. *Arch. Intern. Med.*, 164, 1299–1304, 2004.
91. Lynn, B., Capsaicin: Action on nocicepetive C-fibres and therapeutic potential. *Pain.*, 41, 61–69, 1990.
92. Berger, A., Henderson, M., Nadoolman, W., Duffy, V., Cooper, D., Sabersli, L., Bartoshuk, L., Oral capsaicin provides temporary relief for oral mucositis pain secondary to chemotherapy/radiation therapy. *J. Pain Symptom Manag.*, 10, 243–248, 1995.
93. Cruz, F., Mechanisms involved in new therapies for overactive bladder. *Urology*, 63, 65–73, 2004.
94. Sy, G.Y., Cissé, A., Nongonierma, R.B., Sarr, M., Mbodj, N.A., Faye, B., Hypoglycaemic and antidiabetic activity of acetonic extract of *Vernoniacolorata*leaves in normoglycaemic and alloxaninduced diabetic rats. *J. Ethnopharmacol.*, 98, 171–175, 2005.

95. Okumura, T., Tsukui, T., Hosokowa, M., Miyashita, K., Effect of caffeine and capsaicin on the blood glucose levels of obese/ diabetic KK-A(y) mice. *J. Oleo Sci.*, 61, 515–523, 2012.
96. Kwon, Y.I., Apostolidis, E., Kim, Y.C., Shetty, K., Health benefits of traditional corn, beans and pumpkin: *In vitro* studies for hyperglycemia and hypertension management. *J. Med. Food*, 10, 266–275, 2007.
97. Lim, K., Yoshioka, M., Kikuzato, S., Kiyonaga, A., Tanaka, H., Shindo, M., Suzuki, M., Dietary red pepper ingestion increases carbohydrate oxidation at rest and during exercise in runners. *Med. Sci. Sports Exercise*, 29, 355–361, 1997.
98. Domotor, A., Szolcsányi, J., Mózsik, G., Capsaicin and glucose absorption and utilization in healthy human subjects. *Eur. J. Pharmacol.*, 534, 280–283, 2006.
99. Kang, J.H., Tsuyoshi, G., Han, I.S., Kawada, T., Kim, Y.M., Yu, R., Dietary capsaicin reduces obesity-induced insulin resistance and hepatic steatosis in obese mice fed a high-fat diet. *Obesity*, 18, 780–787, 2010.
100. Magied, M.M.A., Salama, N.A.R., Ali, M.R., Hypoglycemic and hypocholesterolemia effects of intragastric administration of dried red chili pepper (*Capsicum annum*) in alloxan-induced diabetic male albino rats fed with high-fat-diet. *J. Food Nutr. Res.*, 11, 850–856, 2014.
101. Islam, M.S. and Choi, H., Dietary red chilli (*CapsicumfrutescensL.*) is insulinotropic rather than hypoglycemic in type 2 diabetes model of rats. *Phytother. Res.*, 22, 1025–1029, 2008.
102. Anthony, O.E., Ese, A.C., Lawrence, E.O., Regulated effects of *Capsicum frutescens* supplemented diet (C.F.S.D) on fasting blood glucose level, biochemical parameters and body weight in alloxan induced diabetic wistar rats. *Br. J. Pharm. Res.*, 3, 496–507, 2013.
103. Patel, D.K., Prasad, S.K., Kumar, R., Hemalatha, S., An overview on antidiabetic medicinal plants having insulin mimetic property. *Asian Pac. J. Trop. Biomed.*, 2, 320–330, 2012.
104. Kempaiah, R.K. and Srinivasan, K., Integrity of erythrocytes of hypercholesterolemic rats during spices treatment. *Mol. Cell. Biochem.*, 236, 155–161, 2002.
105. Srinivasan, K., Sambaiah, K., Chandrasekhara, N., Spices as beneficial hypolipidemic food adjuncts: A review. *Food Rev. Int.*, 20, 187–220, 2004.
106. Yoshioka, M., St-Pierre, S., Suzuki, M., Tremblay, A., Effects of red pepper added to high-fat and high-carbohydrate meals on energy metabolism and substrate utilization in Japanese women. *Br. J. Nutr.*, 80, 503–510, 1998.
107. Ahuja, K.D., Kunde, D.A., Ball, M.J., Geraghty, D.P., Effects of capsaicin, dihydrocapsaicin, and curcumin on copper-induced oxidation of human serum lipids. *J. Agric. Food. Chem.*, 54, 6436–6439, 2006.
108. Ahuja, K.D. and Ball, M.J., Effects of daily ingestion of chilli on serum lipoprotein oxidation in adult men and women. *Br. J. Nutr.*, 96, 239–242, 2006.

109. Kawada, T., Watanabe, T., Takaishi, T., Tanaka, T., Iwai, K., Capsaicin induced beta-adregenic action on energy metabolism in rats: Influence of capsaicin on oxygen consumption, the respiratory quotient, and substrate utilization. *Proc. Soc Exp. Biol. Med.*, 183, 250–256, 1986.
110. Jimenez, M., Leger, B., Canola, K., Lehr, L., Arboit, P., Seydoux, J., Russell, A.P., Giacobino, J.P., Muzzin, P., Preitner, F., β1 /β2 /β3 adrenoreceptor knockout mice are obese and cold sensitive but have normal lipolytic responses to fasting. *FEBS Lett.*, 530, 37–40, 2002.
111. Watanabe, T., Kawada, T., Yamamoto, M., Iwai, K., Capsaicin, a pungent principle of hot red pepper, evokes catecholamine secretion from the adrenal medulla of anesthetized rats. *Biochem. Biophys. Res. Commun.*, 142, 259–264, 1987.
112. Kempaiah, R.K., Manjunatha, H., Srinivasan, K., Protective effect of dietary capsaicin on induced oxidation of low-density lipoprotein in rats. *Mol. Cell. Biochem.*, 275, 7–13, 2005.
113. Embuscado, M.E., Spices and herbs: Natural sources of antioxidants – A mini review. *J. Funct. Foods*, 18, 811–819, 2015.
114. Snitker, S., Fujishima, Y., Shen, H., Ott, S., Pi-Sunyer, X., Furuhata, Y., Sato, H., Takahashi, M., Effects of novel capsinoid treatment on fatness and energy metabolism in humans: Possible pharmacogenetic implications. *AJCN*, 89, 45–50, 2009.
115. Inoue, N., Matsunaga, Y., Satoh, H., Takahashi, M., Enhanced energy expenditure and fat oxidation in humans with high BMI scores by the ingestion of novel and non-pungent capsaicin analogues (Capsaicinoids). *Biosci. Biotechnol. Biochem.*, 71, 380–389, 2007.
116. Ogunlade, I., Alebiosu, A.A., Osasona, A.I., Proximate, mineral composition, antioxidant activity, and total phenolic content of some pepper varieties (*Capsicum* species). *IJBCS*, 6, 2221–2227, 2012.
117. Kritchevsky, D., Antioxidant vitamins in the prevention of cardiovascular disease. *Nutr. Today*, 27, 30–33, 1992.
118. Adams, M.J., Effect of capsaicin and dihydrocapsaicin on *in vitro* blood coagulation and platelet aggregation. *Thromb. Res.*, 124, 721–723, 2009.
119. Hogaboam, C.M. and Wallace, J.L., Inhibition of platelet aggregation by capsaicin. An effect unrelated to actions on sensory afferent neurons. *Eur. J. Pharmacol.*, 202, 129–131, 1991.
120. Wang, J.P., Hsu, M.F., Teng, C.M., Antiplatelet effect of capsaicin. *Thromb. Res.*, 36, 497–507, 1984.
121. Wang, J.P., Hsu, M.F., Hsu, T.P., Teng, C.M., Antihemostatic and antithrombotic effects of capsaicin in comparison with aspirin and indomethacin. *Thromb. Res.*, 37, 669–679, 1985.
122. Alavijeh, P.K., Alavijeh, P.K., Sharma, D., A study of antimicrobial activity of few medicinal herbs. *AJPSKY*, 2, 496–502, 2012.

123. Omolo, M.A., Wong, Z.Z., Mergen, A.K., Hastings, J.C., Le, N.C., Reiland, H.A., Case, K.A., Baumier, D.J., Antimicrobial Properties of Chili Peppers. *Infect. Dis. Ther.*, 2, 145, 2014.
124. Careaga, M., Fernández, E., Dorantes, L., Mota, L., Jaramillo, M.E., Hernandez-Sanchez, H., Antibacterial activity of *Capsicum* extract against *Salmonella typhimurium* and *Pseudomonas aeruginosa* inoculated in raw beef meat. *Int. J. Food Microbiol.*, 83, 331–335, 2003.
125. Zhao, X.Y., Zhang, C., Guigas, C., Ma, Y., Corrales, M., Tauscher, B., Hu, X.S., Composition, antimicrobial activity, and anti-proliferative active capacity of anthocyanin extracts of purple corn (*Zea mays* L.) from china. *Eur. Food Res. Technol.*, 228, 759–765, 2009.
126. Chatterjee, S., Asakura, M., Chowdhury, N., Neogi, S.B., Sugimoto, N., Haldar, S., Awasthi, S.P., Hinenoya, A., Aoki, S., Yamasaki, S., Capsaicin, a potential inhibitor of cholera toxin production in *Vibrio cholera. FEMS Microbiol. Lett.*, 306, 54–60, 2010.
127. Jones, N.L., Shabib, S., Sherman, P.M., Capsaicin as an inhibitor of growth of the gastric pathogen *Helicobacter pyroli. FEMS Microbiol. Letters.*, 146, 223–227, 1997.
128. Zeyrek, Y.F. and Oguz, E., *In vitro* activity of capsaicin against *Heylicobacter pylori. Ann. Microbiol.*, 55, 125–127, 2005.
129. Molina-Torres, J., García-Chávez, A., Ramírez-Chávez, E., Antimicrobial properties of alkamides present in flavouring plants traditionally used in Mesoamerica: Affinin and capsaicin. *J. Ethnopharmacol.*, 64, 241–248, 1999.
130. Nascimento, P.L.A., Nascimento, T.C.E.S., Ramos, N.S.M., Silva, G.R., Gomes, J.E.G., Falcao, R.A.E., Moreira, K.A., Porto, A.L.F., Silva, T.M.S., Quantification, antioxidant and antimicrobial activity of phenolics isolated from different extracts of *Capsicum frutescens*(PimentaMalagueta). *Molecules.*, 19, 5434–5447, 2014.
131. Kurita, S.K., Kitagawa, E., Kim, C.H., Momose, Y., Iwahashi, H., Studies of the antimicrobial mechanism of Capsaicin using yeast DNA microarray. *Biosci. Biotechnol. Biochem.*, 66, 532–536, 2002.
132. Das, S., Deka, S., Gohain, K., A preclinical study on gastric ulcer protective activity of world"s hottest chilli *Capsicum frutenscenes. JCDR.*, 2, 1024–1027, 2008.
133. Hassan, M.H., Edfawy, M., Mansour, A., Hamed, A.A., Antioxidant and anti-apoptotic effects of capsaicin against carbon tetrachloride-induced hepatotoxicity in rats. *Toxicol. Health*, 28, 428–438, 2012.
134. Ranilla, L.G., Kwon, Y.I., Apostolidis, E., Shetty, K., Phenolic compounds, antioxidant activity and *in vitro* inhibitory potential against key enzymes relevant for hyperglycemia and hypertension of commonly used medicinal plants, herbs and spices in Latin America. *Bioresour. Technol.*, 101, 4676–4689, 2010.

18

Exascale Computing: The Next Frontier of High-Performance Computing

Rashmi M.[1], Girija D.K.[2] and Yogeesh N.[3]*

[1]*Faculty in Computer Science, GFGC, T. Dasarahalli, Bengaluru, Karnataka, India*
[2]*Department of Computer Science, Government First Grade College, Madhugiri, Karnataka, India*
[3]*Department of Mathematics, Government First Grade College, Tumkur, Karnataka, India*

Abstract

Exascale computing is the use of high-performance computing (HPC) devices capable of doing 10^{18} operations per second or one billion billion calculations per second. Applications of exascale computing are expanding quickly in many areas of science and engineering, including but not limited to weather prediction, drug discovery, climate modeling, and fusion energy research. Challenges in areas such as power consumption, data mobility, memory hierarchy, fault tolerance, and software scalability must be overcome in order to realize the full potential of exascale computing. Novel hardware architectures, innovative software algorithms, and machine learning techniques are all being investigated by researchers in the field as potential solutions to these difficulties. In this article, we discuss the state of exascale computing, covering recent developments in hardware and software and the most promising uses of exascale computing in science and engineering. We also explore the significant obstacles in the way of exascale computing and provide a roadmap for future research that will hopefully lead to the full promise of exascale computing being realized for scientific discovery and technological progress.

Keywords: Challenges, exascale, exaFLOPS, FLOPS, Frontier, high-performance computing, supercomputer, teraFLOPS

**Corresponding author*: yogeesh.r@gmail.com

Kapil Joshi and Somil Kumar Gupta (eds.) Human Cancer Diagnosis and Detection Using Exascale Computing, (279–304) © 2024 Scrivener Publishing LLC

18.1 Introduction

High-performance computing (HPC) is the use of extremely powerful computers to quickly and accurately solve complicated computational problems in a wide variety of industries, scientific disciplines, and technical domains. The United States ushered in the exascale era on 30 May 2022, when it unveiled the world's fastest supercomputer, Frontier, which could perform more than one quintillion (10^{18}) operations in a second. Aerospace, biotechnology, clean energy, and semiconductor design are just a few of the business and scientific disciplines that may see previously insurmountable problems resolved with the introduction of exascale computing. When it comes to industrial competitiveness, national security, and the ability to meet social concerns like earthquakes, hurricanes, and weather forecasting, national leadership in HPC constitutes a vital national strategic skill. Energy economy, scalability of hardware and software, data storage and administration, and robustness against hardware failures are just a few of the obstacles standing in the way of exascale computing. New technologies and methodologies, such as heterogeneous computing, enhanced memory and storage systems, and fault-tolerant computing, are being developed by researchers and engineers to meet these difficulties [1].

Overall, exascale computing is a giant leap forward in high-performance computing that could revolutionize many different disciplines of study and business. There has been a lot of focus from academics and business leaders on exascale computing lately, as it is a rapidly growing subject. In this survey of the literature, we will take a look at some of the most important articles and studies on exascale computing. The publication "The International Exascale Software Project: a Call to Coordinated Action by the Global High-Performance Community" by Jack Dongarra *et al.* is widely considered to be one of the most seminal works on exascale computing. The need for worldwide cooperation in the creation of exascale software was highlighted in a study released in 2011. The authors stressed the importance of a concerted effort to tackle the issues associated with exascale computing, such as low power, unreliability, and outdated programming approaches. The paper entitled "The Path to Exascale Computing" by Horst Simon and Thomas Sterling is another excellent read. This study from 2011 gives a high-level summary of the difficulties and potential benefits of exascale computing. New hardware and software architectures are discussed to support exascale computing, and the significance of interdisciplinary cooperation is emphasized in order to meet these difficulties. Many government investigations, corporate surveys, and academic analyses have also been published on exascale computing after the publication of these seminal works [2].

Exascale computing has the potential to revolutionize many fields, including energy, climate modeling, and materials science, as detailed in a 2016 report by the Office of Science at the United States Department of Energy. There is also the "Exascale Computing Study: Technological Issues in Delivering Exascale Systems" by the Advanced Scientific Computing Advisory Committee of the United States Department of Energy. This 2008 report analyzes the power requirements, memory bandwidth, and parallelism of exascale computing, as well as the difficulties and opportunities presented by this new technology. Recent works that investigate the applicability of exascale computing to climate modeling and analysis include "Exascale Deep Learning for Climate Analytics" by Prabhat *et al.* and "Exascale Computing and AI" by John Shalf *et al.* Generally, the literature on exascale computing underlines the substantial hurdles that must be overcome before this technology can realize its potential to enable advances in science and engineering. In order to overcome these obstacles and unlock the full potential of exascale computing, collaboration between researchers, the industry, and the government will be essential.

18.1.1 Literature Study

HPC has been increasingly important in recent years for driving forward scientific discovery, business innovation, and societal development (Council on Competitiveness, 2015). HPC has allowed researchers and organizations to simulate complicated systems, analyze large volumes of data, and solve computationally hard problems in fields as diverse as weather forecasting, drug discovery, and financial modeling [12]. However, the limitations of existing HPC systems are becoming more and more obvious as the demand for additional computing power continues to grow (Kogge, P., 2018). It is for this reason that exascale computing is being developed, a new class of supercomputers that promises to enhance processing power by a factor of 1,000 above petascale devices (Dongarra, J., *et al.*, 2011).

The term "exascale computing" refers to a level of performance that is orders of magnitude more than what is currently possible, with the ability to conduct a quintillion (10^{18}) calculations per second. This chapter introduces the reader to exascale computing and discusses its relevance, difficulties, and potential. Beginning with the first supercomputers and moving on to the most recent petascale systems, we trace the development of HPC and describe its current state of the art. We then provide an overview of exascale computing and discuss some of its potential uses. Power and energy usage, software development, and data management are just a few of the many obstacles standing in the way of creating exascale computing systems.

We elaborate on these difficulties and investigate the many strategies now under development to deal with them, including hardware and software advancements, co-design techniques, and heterogeneous architectural configurations (Alam, S., *et al.*, 2015). Exascale computing presents considerable prospects for scientific study, corporate innovation, and societal improvement, in addition to the technical hurdles. Here, we take a look at the ways in which exascale computing could be used in fields including materials research, genomics, climate modeling, and beyond. We also look toward the future of exascale computing and the trends and technologies that are shaping it (Norman, M., *et al.*, 2021).

The possible impact on society and industry underlines the significance of sustained investment and research in exascale computing (Office of Science and Technology Policy, 2016). In order to meet the challenges and embrace the opportunities given by this new frontier of high-performance computing, we urge interdisciplinary cooperation between academic institutions, businesses, and governments. This chapter lays the groundwork for future research and investigation in the realm of exascale computing by providing a detailed introduction to the topic that emphasizes its significance, problems, and prospects [10].

18.2 Exascale Computing

The ability of a computer system to conduct a billion billion computations per second, or one quintillion floating-point operations per second, is referred to as exascale computing (FLOPS). This offers a 1,000-fold improvement in processing power over today's state-of-the-art petascale systems. For several years, experts have been working on the notion of exascale computing, with the objective of enabling them to solve the most difficult scientific challenges, ranging from modeling the human brain to predicting climate change. Exascale computing system development is a big technical problem that requires the convergence of improvements in hardware, software, and system architecture. Power consumption is one of the most significant problems in reaching exascale computing [5].

A computer system would need a large amount of energy to do exascale-level calculations, which could be unsustainable with existing technologies. To address this, researchers are investigating a variety of creative energy-efficiency technologies, including better cooling systems, low-power processors, and alternative power sources such as renewable energy. The ability to handle vast amounts of data created by such systems is another hurdle in constructing exascale computing platforms. To attain exascale computing, systems must be built to efficiently handle massive volumes of data, from the input/output (I/O) subsystem to storage and memory management. To enable efficient data processing and storage, researchers are investigating new architectures and software solutions. Exascale computing involves serious ethical, privacy, and security issues in addition to technical challenges. Exascale systems' extraordinary computing capacity could be exploited for both useful and evil purposes. As a result, ethical aspects such as privacy, security, and data ownership must be considered during the creation of exascale computing systems. Exascale computing has a wide range of potential uses [13].

Exascale computing can help climate scientists estimate the effects of climate change on ecosystems, populations, and economies. Exascale computing can be used in medicine to simulate complicated biological systems, forecast drug efficacy, and devise individualized treatment strategies. Exascale computing can assist researchers in developing new materials with unique features and uses in materials science. Exascale computing systems require collaboration among academia, business, and government organizations. Numerous national programs, such as the US Department of Energy's Exascale Computing Project and the European Union's Horizon 2020 program, have been created in recent years to speed the development of exascale computing. These programs aim to encourage innovation and provide a venue for academics to create new applications and algorithms that can fully utilize the power of exascale computing. Exascale computing, in general, marks a significant milestone in the evolution of computing technology, allowing researchers to tackle the most challenging scientific concerns of our day. While reaching exascale computing is a big technical challenge, the possible benefits range from climate science and medicine to materials science and beyond. We can speed the development of exascale computing systems and realize the full promise of this disruptive technology by collaborating across academia, the industry, and the government [6].

18.2.1 Exascale Computers

To do at least 1 exaFLOPS, or one billion billion floating-point operations per second, exascale computers are the next generation of supercomputers. These machines will be significantly more powerful than current supercomputers, which are often measured in petaFLOPS (a thousand trillion floating-point operations per second). Climate modeling, nuclear fusion research, and drug discovery are just a few examples of the scientific and engineering challenges that exascale computing systems are expected to play a crucial role in solving. These tools will improve our understanding of the world by allowing scientists to reproduce complex occurrences on hitherto impossible scales. Construction of exascale computers, on the other hand, presents significant technical challenges. These systems will need not only new hardware architectures that can handle massive amounts of data but also new software tools and algorithms that can fully leverage these new hardware designs. The development of novel energy-efficient architectural designs and cooling techniques will be essential for exascale computer systems. Certain governments and organizations are working on exascale computing systems right now, and we can expect to see the first exascale systems implemented sometime in the early 2020s. Researchers and engineers in many disciplines hope that these systems will have a profound effect on their work, leading to new discoveries and innovations.

18.2.2 Case Study

Beginning with the creation of the first supercomputers in the 1960s and 1970s, exascale computing has come a long way. The information used is from the source Exascale-Reed-Dongarra.pdf, shown in Figure 18.1. These early systems required a lot of energy to run and were prohibitively expensive. On the other hand, they helped pave the way for modern high-performance computing by advancing scientific research and engineering.

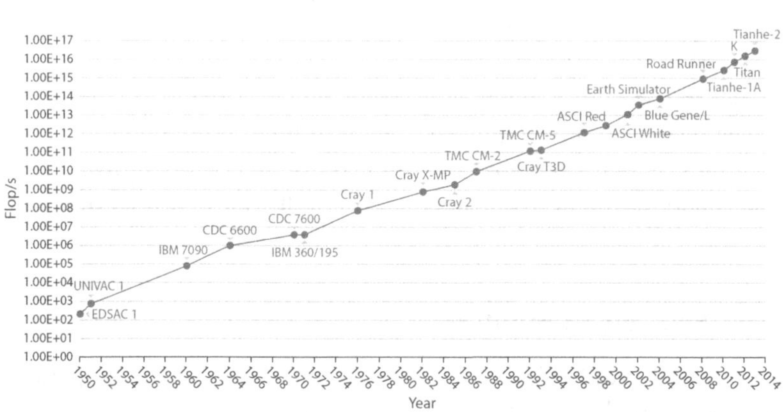

Figure 18.1 Evolution in computing performance measure.

Supercomputers have improved in speed, power, and efficiency during the decades after their inception. The ability to have numerous processors collaborate on a single task using parallel processing was a key step forward in this development. It was in the early 2000s that scientists started developing exascale computing devices, which could perform at least 1 exaFLOPS of computation. These machines were anticipated to be many times faster than existing supercomputers, necessitating novel hardware architectures, software systems, and algorithms.

Several nations and institutions committed resources to create exascale computers in the years that followed. These initiatives targeted the creation of software tools and programming languages that could take advantage of emerging hardware technology like central processing units (CPUs) and memory systems. By the year 2024, a number of exascale computer systems will either have been announced or will be in various stages of development. Breakthroughs in our understanding of the world may be possible as a result of the widespread application of these systems in sectors as diverse as science, engineering, and national security.

18.2.3 Measuring Computer Speed

One of the most used methods for measuring computer speed is floating-point operations per second (FLOPS). FLOPS is a unit of measurement for the number of mathematical operations that a computer can do in 1 s, specifically those involving floating-point numbers, which include integers with decimal points or those written in scientific notation. A computer, for example, may be capable of performing one billion (109) floating-point operations per second, which is referred to as a gigaflop (GFLOPS). A teraflop (TFLOPS) is equivalent to one trillion (10^{12}) floating-point operations per second, while a petaflop (PFLOPS) is equivalent to one quadrillion (10^{15}) floating-point operations per second. Other measures of computer speed, in addition to FLOPS, include instructions per second (IPS), which measures the number of instructions a computer can execute in a second, and bandwidth, which measures the amount of data that can be transferred between the computer's memory and its processor in a given time. It is crucial to remember that a computer's real performance is determined by numerous factors other than its raw processing speed, including memory, storage, and input/output (I/O) capabilities. As a result, benchmarks that assess overall system performance, such as the Standard Performance Evaluation Corporation (SPEC) benchmarks, consider parameters other than FLOPS or IPS, as seen in Figure 18.2.

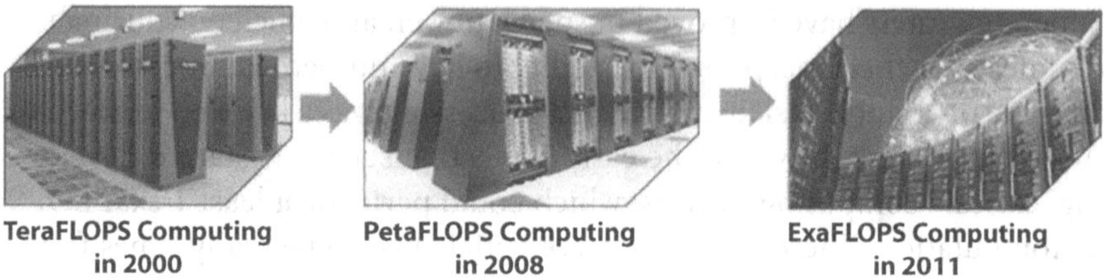
TeraFLOPS Computing
in 2000
PetaFLOPS Computing
in 2008
ExaFLOPS Computing
in 2011

Figure 18.2 Computer speeds: teraFLOPS, petaFLOPS, and exaFLOPS.

- **TeraFLOPS**: A teraFLOP is equal to one trillion (10^{12}) floating-point operations per second. This is a measure of computing performance that was achieved by the fastest supercomputers of the late 1990s and early 2000s. Today, many high-end workstations and servers can perform at least 1 teraFLOPS.
- **PetaFLOPS**: A petaFLOP is equal to one quadrillion (10^{15}) floating-point operations per second. This level of computing performance was first achieved by the Roadrunner supercomputer in 2008. Today, many of the world's fastest supercomputers are capable of performing at least 1 petaFLOPS.
- **ExaFLOPS**: An exaFLOP is equal to one quintillion (10^{18}) floating-point operations per second. This level of computing performance is currently at the forefront of HPC research and development, with several projects underway to build the first exascale supercomputers. The first exascale supercomputers are expected to become operational in the early to mid-2020s.

TeraFLOPS, petaFLOPS, and exaFLOPS represent different levels of computing performance, with each level being a thousand times more powerful than the previous one. While teraFLOPS and petaFLOPS are currently common in high-end computing, exaFLOPS is the next major milestone in HPC, and it is expected to enable new breakthroughs in science, engineering, and other fields [7].

18.2.4 Usage of FLOPS in Supercomputers

The Control Data Corporation (CDC) 6600, released in 1964, was widely regarded as the first successful supercomputer because of its ability to do three million floating-point calculations per second (FLOPS). In the year 2020, Sony released the PlayStation 5, which features hardware that can achieve up to 10.28 teraFLOPS. One teraFLOPS is equal to one trillion FLOPS. The definition of what constitutes a "supercomputer" and the workloads for which they are often deployed shift over time as both technology and the needs of businesses and governments change. The team at Frontier Enterprise has compiled a list of the top supercomputers in operation today and the problems they can solve.

1. Fugaku: The Fugaku supercomputer was created by the Fujitsu Group and the RIKEN Institute for Computational Science. In terms of hardware, it has a 512-bit ARM architecture with 7,630,848 cores and 5,087,232 GB of memory. The results on the benchmarks demonstrate why Fugaku is number 1: Their LINPACK score on the TOP 500s was 442.01 petaFLOPS. With a score of 16.00 petaFLOPS on the high-performance conjugate gradient test, it proves to be quite powerful. It achieved 2.004 exaFLOPS on the High-Performance LINPACK for Acceleration Introspection.

Fugaku is currently working mostly on coronavirus disease 2019 (COVID-19)-related fields, such as therapeutic candidate exploration, conformational dynamics prediction for proteins on the SARS-CoV-2 virus, and fragment molecular orbital (FMO) calculations for COVID-19 proteins. RIKEN's director Satoshi Matsuoka claims that "Fugaku has also contributed to the formulation of COVID-19 safety criteria for the government and commercial sector, and has helped lead a digital transition in the domain of infectious diseases." In addition, Matsuoka emphasized the supercomputer's speed in a practical scenario. FMO computations to analyze the COVID-19 spike protein, as referenced by Matsuoka, would have required "days, weeks, multiple weeks" on the K computer, Fugaku's predecessor. Three hours went by while Fugaku was at it. Fujitsu Chief Executive Officer Naoki Shinjo announced in March 2021 that the company's supercomputer Fugaku would be made available to researchers from other institutions. For example, "we expect Fugaku's utilisation to continue to play a significant role in the future in contributing to the realisation of the Japanese government's plan for Society 5.0 (a smart society programme), in fields like drug discovery, and guaranteeing a secure and safe society."

2. Cambridge-1: The British claim to have the world's fastest supercomputer with Cambridge-1. It can produce up to 400 petaFLOPS and was developed by the technology firm Nvidia. The vast majority of this energy is put toward improving human health. The following are examples of some of its work: Together, Nvidia and AstraZeneca have developed a generative AI model for chemical structures using transformers as part of their drug development study. There is also talk of using Cambridge-1 to teach AI algorithms for use in digital pathology. Using Cambridge-1, researchers at King's College London and Guy's and St. Thomas' NHS Foundation Trust are teaching artificial intelligence models to create synthetic brain images in order to better understand and treat neurological disorders like dementia, stroke, brain cancer, and multiple sclerosis.

3. Summit: Summit, a supercomputer developed by IBM and housed at ORNL in Tennessee, can perform 148.8 petaFLOPS, making it the fastest in the United States. In its present configuration, its 4,356 nodes are equipped with two 22-core Power9 Processors and six Nvidia Tesla V100 GPUs each (GPUs). Summit, which weighs more than 340 tons and takes up more than 5,600 square feet of area, is capable of 200 quadrillion FLOPS and 250 petabytes of storage. Wayne Joubert, a computational scientist at ORNL, claims that researchers may use Summit to tackle a problem that would take a desktop computer 30 years to complete in just one hour. IBM's senior vice president of cloud and cognitive software, Tom Rosamilia, has stated that Summit was designed with artificial intelligence workloads in mind and that it aims to solve problems like global warming, elucidating the genetic factors that contribute to opioid addiction, and foreseeing future weather disasters.

4. Sierra: The US Department of Energy's Stockpile Stewardship program relies heavily on Sierra, which was developed at California's Lawrence Livermore National Laboratory for use in predictive applications related to the safety of the nation's nuclear weapons stockpile. Each of the 4,474 nodes in the Summit and Sierra architectures has two Power9 central processing units and four Nvidia Tesla V100 graphics processing units. As a result, the Sierra supercomputer can achieve its maximum performance of 125 petaFLOPS.

5. Sunway TaihuLight: The Sunway TaihuLight is a massively parallel computing system with 40,960 nodes powered by SW26010 manycore 64-bit RISC processors, which were designed and built by the National Research Centre for Parallel Computing Engineering and Technology in China. With 256 processing cores and 4 additional cores dedicated to system management, the system has a total of 10,649,600 CPUs. The result is a processing speed of 93 petaFLOPS on the supercomputer. The National Supercomputing Centre in Wuxi is where TaihuLight is currently being operated. Applications include advanced manufacturing, climate, data analytics, earth systems modeling, and life science study.

6. Selene: Nvidia's Selene supercomputer uses rival company AMD's EPYC CPUs, A100 graphics processing units (GPUs), and Mellanox

HDR InfiniBand networking technologies. Selene can reach speeds of 63.60 petaFLOPS. Selene is utilized by Nvidia for a wide range of R&D, RD, and PD initiatives. Tools for quantum chemistry and genomics are included in this category, as are those for modeling languages on a large scale, driving autonomous vehicles, creating visuals, and analyzing genetic sequences.

7. JUWELS Accelerator Module: The Atos-built JUWELS Booster Module supercomputer at Germany's Forschungszentrum Jülich research center can perform at 85 petaFLOPS. To put it in perspective, this is the same as the processing power of nearly 300,000 state-of-the-art personal computers. With its AMD EPYC processors and Nvidia A100 GPUs, the JUWELS Booster Module is the most powerful supercomputer in Europe. Among the many ongoing projects in which JUWELS is engaged are:

- Examining drug binding over timescales of interest in biology.
- Using advanced machine learning techniques, we can make accurate predictions of the weather.
- Modeling plasma conditions for use in future particle accelerators.

8. HPC5: The HPC5, developed by the energy conglomerate Eni S.p.A., is capable of 51.7 petaFLOPS at its peak. In order to achieve this output, 1820 Dell EMC PowerEdge C4140 nodes are being used, each with two Intel Gold 6252 24-core CPUs and four Nvidia V100 GPUs. Almost 10 km of fiber optic cable are used to connect the nodes together utilizing a high-speed InfiniBand Mellanox HDR network technology capable of 200 Gbps. HPC5 includes a storage system with 15 petabytes and 200 GB/s of combined read/write speeds. Epi claims it uses the supercomputer for a wide range of technological, environmental, and academic tasks, such as analyzing subsoil data and creating subsoil models. The business really used this method to discover the Zohr gas resource in the Mediterranean. The HPC5 has also been made available by the business for the study of coronaviruses.

9. Frontera: With its 448,448 Intel Platinum Xeon processors, Frontera currently delivers 23.5 petaFLOPS and will be deployed in 2020 at The University of Texas at Austin's Texas Advanced Computing Center. Data can be transferred at rates of up to 200 Gbps using Mellanox HDR, just like the other supercomputers on this list. Frontera is tailored to academic use cases such as simulation, modeling, machine learning, and big data. It has been applied to studies including machine learning, modular modeling, and quantum mechanics, as well as research involving binary black hole mergers, brain cancer treatment, and chemical problem solving.

10. PARAM Siddhi-AI: With an Rpeak of 5.267 PFLOPS and an Rmax of 4.6 PFLOPS, PARAM Siddhi-AI is by far the fastest supercomputer ever created in India (Sustained). By facilitating more rapid simulations, medical imaging, and genome sequencing, AI aids investigation into cutting-edge materials, computational chemistry and astrophysics, healthcare systems, flood forecasting, and the COVID-19 application. As of November 2020, PARAM Siddhi-AI was ranked number 63 on the list of the world's most powerful supercomputers. The networking of this supercomputer is based on the Nvidia DGX SuperPOD reference architecture, while the HPC-AI engine, software frameworks, and cloud platform are all products of C-DAC's research and development.

18.2.5 Exascale Computing: A Crucial Technology

Some of the world's most complicated and critical problems cannot be solved with today's computing power, but exascale computing can. Scientific, technological, engineering, medical, and other advances can be fueled by the ability to handle massive volumes of data and conduct computations at lightning speed. Climate modeling is one area where exascale computing can improve our ability to foresee and comprehend weather events, natural disasters, and long-term climate trends. Furthermore, exascale computing can aid in the study of complicated genomes for medical research, paving the way for the development of tailored medicine and speeding up the creation of novel materials for energy storage, transmission, and production [9].

With real-time data analysis and decision-making made possible by exascale computing, sectors including finance, transportation, and logistics also stand to gain. It can help increase operational efficiency and lower costs by allowing for more precise simulations and predictions of market trends, traffic patterns, and supply chain logistics. More so, exascale computing can propel AI and ML forward by allowing for the development and training of increasingly complicated and sophisticated algorithms on larger datasets [16]. This has the potential to pave the way for advances in fields like natural language processing, computer vision, and robotics while also allowing for the development of smarter machines. Exascale computing has the potential to significantly impact many fields of study and business by facilitating the solution of previously intractable problems and the discovery of groundbreaking new information [15].

18.2.6 Requirements of High-Speed Computers

The teraFLOP, petaFLOP, and exaFLOP classifications of high-performance computers refer to their ability to do trillions, quadrillions, and quintillions of floating-point operations per second, respectively. In order to attain such high performance, these systems necessitate specialized hardware, software, and system design.

Hardware requirements: Hardware for teraFLOPS systems must have high-performance CPUs, memory, storage, and network interfaces. These parts must be available in considerably greater quantities and meet even more stringent performance requirements in order to power a petaFLOPS computer. More powerful and specialized hardware components, tuned and integrated to function together in a seamless fashion, are needed for exascale computers.

Software requirements: Prerequisites for software: Teraflop, petaflop, and exaflop machines require software designed specifically for high performance. Everything from the operating system to the programming language to the libraries and tools should be tailored to the specifics of the hardware. Also, the software needs to be highly parallel and scalable so that the system's abundant number of cores may be put to good use.

System architecture requirements: Designing the architecture of teraflops, petaflops, and exascale computers around the needs of immense parallelism, high-speed interconnects, and data-intensive applications is a need. This incorporates the use of various processing units, graphics processing units, and accelerators to get the desired results. Quantum processors, neuromorphic processors, and high-bandwidth memory are only some of the specialized hardware components needed for exascale computers.

Very high-performance computers, such as those with teraflops, petaflops, or exaflops, need massive amounts of electricity to run, in addition to elaborate cooling systems to keep them from melting down. These systems need to be built so that they can keep running even when under intense pressure, while also consuming as little power as possible. In general, the hardware, software, and system design of teraflops, petaflops, and exascale systems demand a great deal of expertise. These kinds of computers are frequently employed in high-performance computing tasks like scientific simulations and data analytics [2].

18.2.7 Milestones

Achieving exascale computing marks a significant step forward in the evolution of supercomputers (HPC). These computers can execute a billion computations per second or 1 exaFLOPS. The major steps toward exascale computing include:

- **First teraflop computer**: In 1996, the ASCI Red supercomputer was the first to consistently execute at 1 teraFLOPS (one trillion computations per second).
- **First petaflop computer**: In 2008, the Roadrunner supercomputer was the first to consistently perform at a rate of 1 petaFLOPS (one quadrillion calculations per second).
- **Exascale computing initiative**: The Exascale Computing Initiative (ECI) was established in 2011 by the US Department of Energy (DOE) to create exascale computing capabilities by the end of the decade.
- **DARPA exascale program**: The Defense Advanced Research Projects Agency (DARPA) started the High Productivity Computing Systems (HPCS) program in 2012 to create exascale computing power for military uses.
- **Aurora supercomputer**: The United States Department of Energy (DOE) has stated that Intel and Cray's Aurora supercomputer will be the country's first exascale supercomputer when it is completed in 2019. Timeline estimates put its launch around 2022.
- **Fugaku supercomputer**: The Fugaku supercomputer, jointly developed by Fujitsu and RIKEN, achieved exascale computing capabilities in June 2020 and is currently the world's fastest supercomputer, with a theoretical peak performance of 1.3 exaFLOPS and a LINPACK benchmark performance of 0.442 exaFLOPS.
- **Frontier supercomputer**: The Frontier supercomputer, a joint project of Cray and AMD located at Oak Ridge National Laboratory, achieved the distinction of being the world's first exascale computer in May 2022, with a peak performance of 1.5 exaFLOPS.

- **EuroHPC**: To better coordinate the creation of exascale computing capacities across Europe, the European Union formed the EuroHPC Joint Undertaking in 2018. At least two exascale supercomputers are planned to be completed by 2023 as part of this program.

These achievements are a reflection of the continued efforts of governments, academic institutions, and commercial firms to advance HPC and release the power of exascale computing for the advancement of science, national security, economic prosperity, and societal good [8].

18.2.8 Exascale Computing Processing

The term "exascale computing" is used to describe supercomputers with processing speeds of at least 1 exaFLOPS. Hardware, software, and system architecture are only a few of the essential parts of what makes exascale computing tick.

Hardware: Exascale computing calls for powerful computers capable of handling large datasets and intensive calculations with lightning speed. High-performance CPUs, memory, storage, and network connections are all part of this hardware.

Software: Exascale computing calls for tailored software that can take full advantage of the hardware's specific capabilities. System software, language software, library software, and development tools are all examples of this category of software.

System architecture: Exascale computing systems have an architecture that was developed to accommodate large amounts of parallel processing, fast data transfers, and resource-intensive programs. Processors, graphics processing units, and accelerators are all examples of heterogeneous computing systems that can be used in this context.

There are a few steps involved in getting to the end result of exascale computing:

Data processing: Phase 1 of exascale computing is data processing. For this, you will need high-powered computers and software designed for working with massive datasets.

Modeling and simulation: The second phase of exascale computing, modeling and simulation, entails simulating elaborate systems and phenomena using cutting-edge modeling and simulation tools. A high-performance computer system and specialized software designed for modeling complicated systems accurately are needed for this task.

AI and ML: The third phase of exascale computing is to use AI and ML to analyze massive datasets and draw conclusions or suggestions. To accomplish this, one needs high-powered computers and software designed for processing and analyzing massive data volumes quickly and effectively [14].

Visualization: Results from data processing, modeling and simulation, and machine learning and artificial intelligence approaches are visualized at the final step of exascale computing. For this purpose, you will need a computer and software that are up to the task of displaying massive amounts of data in an understandable format.

To enable huge data processing, modeling and simulation, machine learning and artificial intelligence, and visualization, exascale computing relies on a complex interplay between hardware, software, and system architecture [3].

18.2.9 Advantages of Exascale Computing

There are many benefits of using exascale computing over traditional systems. A few of the many benefits are as follows:

1. **Improved performance**: With exascale computing, calculations can be completed at unprecedented speeds, vastly outperforming traditional supercomputers. This is because of the development and widespread adoption of cutting-edge hardware, software, and algorithms that are specifically geared toward enhancing performance.
2. **Increased capacity**: Capacity increase: Exascale computers provide substantially more room for data storage and processing than traditional systems. This paves the way for the processing of far larger datasets and simulations, which can lead to advances in domains like climate modeling and drug discovery.
3. **Greater accuracy**: Accuracy improvements: The enhanced computing power and precision of exascale computing allows

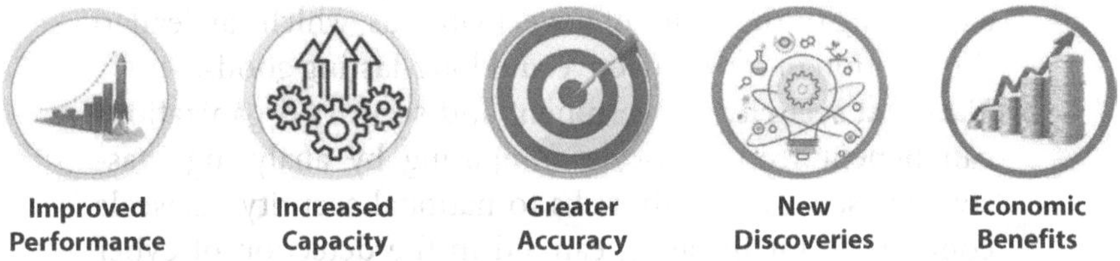
Improved Performance
Increased Capacity
Greater Accuracy
New Discoveries
Economic Benefits

Figure 18.3 Benefits of exascale computing.

for more precise simulations and forecasts. Applications in domains as diverse as meteorology and materials science stand to benefit from this.

4. **New discoveries**: By the analysis of massive datasets and simulations, exascale computing can pave the way for new discoveries in domains like astrophysics, cosmology, and particle physics.
5. **Economic benefits**: Advantages to the economy: There may be huge economic advantages to using exascale computing. One way it can benefit production is by facilitating more precise simulations of product designs, which in turn can lead to higher quality output at lower unit costs [4].

As a whole, exascale computing has several benefits that can help advance various fields of study, from science to economics as shown in Figure 18.3.

18.2.10 Exascale Computing in Various Domains

With exascale computing, you can do a billion billion computations per second, or an exaflop. Having access to such a large amount of computational power could have far-reaching implications for many areas of study and business. Exascale computing has many applications in many fields, including healthcare, energy, the economy, and national security [16].

1. **Scientific discovery**: Scientists and researchers can use exascale computing to run simulations and analyze data at breakneck rates, which can lead to groundbreaking discoveries. With exascale computation, astronomers may simulate the cosmos, learn about the workings of black holes, and delve deeper into the Big Bang theory. Furthermore, researchers in materials science can benefit from exascale computing by

simulating the behavior of novel materials, which can lead to the creation of more effective and long-lasting goods.

2. **National security**: Government and security organizations can benefit from exascale computing by analyzing massive datasets to identify risks to national security. Exascale computing, for instance, can aid in the detection of cyber threats and the prevention of harm to vital infrastructure. Furthermore, exascale computing can aid in the creation of cutting-edge encryption solutions to safeguard private information.
3. **Energy**: Exascale computing has the potential to facilitate the creation of cleaner, more reliable power sources. For instance, exascale computing can aid in the simulation of fusion reactions, which could lead to the creation of a new, clean, and abundant energy source. Wind and solar power generating optimization can benefit from exascale computing as well, leading to more efficient and cost-effective renewable energy.
4. **Economic growth**: It is believed that exascale computing would aid in the production of new products and services, which will in turn boost economic growth and create more employment opportunities. Exascale computing, for instance, can aid in the design of new pharmaceuticals and cures, leading to the discovery of effective new treatments for diseases. Exascale computing can also aid in the discovery of novel materials and manufacturing methods, which in turn can lead to the production of higher-quality, longer-lasting goods.
5. **Healthcare**: Exascale computing can help in the development of personalized medicine, leading to better outcomes for patients. For example, exascale computing can help in the analysis of large amounts of genomic data, leading to the development of new treatments for diseases. In addition, exascale computing can help in the simulation of complex biological systems, leading to a better understanding of the human body and the development of new treatments [11].

Hence, exascale computing is the next frontier of HPC that promises to deliver a 1,000-fold increase in computing power over existing systems. Exascale computing systems are capable of performing a quintillion (10^{18})

calculations per second and will enable scientific and engineering simulations at unprecedented levels of accuracy and detail.

The potential impact of exascale computing is vast, and it is expected to transform a range of fields, including climate science, energy research, drug discovery, materials science, and astrophysics, to name a few.

One of the most significant advantages of exascale computing is its ability to handle large-scale simulations and data-intensive applications that are beyond the capability of existing HPC systems. For example, in climate science, exascale computing can be used to create more accurate models of the Earth's climate and predict weather patterns with greater precision.

In energy research, exascale computing can be used to simulate the behavior of complex materials and chemical reactions, allowing researchers to develop more efficient energy storage systems, advanced batteries, and clean energy technologies.

In drug discovery, exascale computing can be used to simulate the behavior of molecules and predict how they will interact with biological systems, enabling the development of more effective and personalized drugs.

In materials science, exascale computing can be used to simulate the behavior of materials at the atomic and molecular levels, allowing researchers to design new materials with specific properties for use in advanced technologies.

In astrophysics, exascale computing can be used to simulate the behavior of galaxies, stars, and black holes, providing new insights into the structure and evolution of the universe.

Overall, exascale computing represents a significant advancement in HPC, and its impact will be felt across a range of fields, enabling researchers to tackle some of the most complex and challenging problems of our time.

18.2.11 Exascale Computer: A Supercomputer

An example of a high-performance computer, or supercomputer, is one that can perform massive computations at a rate significantly greater than that of a typical computer. The speed and accuracy with which these computers can do complicated computations make them perfect for use in fields like meteorology, CFD, and scientific modeling. The hardware and software that make up a supercomputer are often customized for speed and parallelism. Typically, they employ a network of interconnected processing nodes to handle enormous datasets in a single operation. The term "exascale computing" is used to describe the next generation of computing power, which will be a million times faster than the first terascale supercomputer.

There are more than a quintillion (10^{18}) possible floating-point operations per second on an exascale computer (FLOPS). Very large datasets may be quickly analyzed, and simulations of the intricate processes and relationships underlying the fundamental forces of the cosmos can be run. Precision medicine, climate research, and nuclear physics are just a few of the fields that have benefited from exascale computing [7].

FLOPS are used to quantify how quickly a computer can do basic arithmetic operations on numbers with decimals, such as adding or multiplying. The average human can do such an operation in 1 s, or 1 FLOPS, using only a pencil and paper. The standard laptop can perform a few trillion operations per second (teraFLOPS). In 1964, the first supercomputer was built, and it had a processing speed of 3 megaFLOPS. Ever since then, there has been an intense competition to develop ever-faster computers. The United States Department of Energy's Intel ASCI Red supercomputer attained the terascale benchmark of 1.06 teraFLOPS in 1996. In 2008, when 1.026 petaFLOPS was recorded on the Roadrunner supercomputer, the petascale milestone (15 zeros) was officially accomplished. A million times faster than ASCI Red is exascale computing. More than 1 exaFLOPS, or 1 quintillion FLOPS, is possible on an exascale computer. In May of 2022, the Frontier supercomputer at Oak Ridge National Laboratory in Tennessee achieved the distinction of being the world's first exascale computer, with a performance of 1.1 exaFLOPS. Eventually, it may theoretically reach a high of 2 exaFLOPS in the future years.

18.2.12 Exascale Computing Different from Quantum Computing

There are many different ways to increase a computer's processing power, with each having their own advantages and disadvantages. Classical computing, which processes data using digital bits, forms the foundation of exascale computing. There are just two possible values for these bits: 0 and 1. For difficult issues, traditional computers just cannot keep up, but exascale computers are built to do an unprecedented number of operations per second.

Yet, qubits, the building blocks of quantum computing, can only be created in accordance with the laws of quantum physics. In contrast to classical bits, qubits are capable of existing in more than one state at once. This allows quantum computers to do multiple calculations simultaneously, rather than just one calculation at a time like classical computers. In particular, this method shines when used for issues that necessitate intensive data analysis or elaborate simulations. One of the fundamental contrasts between exascale computing and quantum computing is the types of issues they are best suited to solve. If a problem can be decomposed into a large number of smaller jobs that can be run in parallel, then exascale computing is the way to go. This makes it ideally suited for use in applications like simulating the weather, fluid dynamics, and material research. Instead, quantum computers excel at optimization problems and quantum system simulations that require intricate statistical analysis. As a result, it is a useful resource for researchers in areas such as cryptography, pharmaceuticals, and AI [4].

Another distinction is the technology that goes into making an exascale computer versus a quantum computer. As opposed to exascale computing, which uses traditional digital hardware like transistors and circuits, quantum computing makes use of quantum bits, which are inherently more difficult to manipulate and control. Exascale and quantum computing are still in their infancy, but they hold great promise for tackling hard challenges. Several nations and businesses are already investing extensively in this field; thus, it is likely that exascale computing will become a reality within the next few years. Meanwhile, the field of quantum computing is just getting started, with just a small number of businesses and academic institutions devoting resources to its development thus far. In conclusion, there are two unique methods for creating more powerful computers: exascale computing and quantum computing. Classical digital technology forms the basis of exascale computing, which excels at problems amenable to being partitioned into a large number of smaller, independently solvable tasks. Yet, issues that require complicated statistical analysis lend themselves to the principles of quantum physics, which form the basis of quantum computing. While both approaches have the potential to be highly productive in the long run, they are still in their infancy and it is unclear which will show to be the more efficient in the long run as time goes on [11].

18.3 Exascale Computing Challenges

Before exascale computing can truly change many fields, it must first overcome considerable obstacles. Among the many difficulties associated with exascale computing are the following:

- **Power consumption**: Exascale computers will have a very high power need, perhaps as high as 100 MW. We need to find better ways to manage power and conserve energy if we are ever going to reach that level of electricity use.

- **Memory and storage**: Many petabytes or more of memory and storage space will be needed for exascale computing. This suggests that new memory and storage designs will be required if current storage technologies are to keep up.
- **Algorithms and software**: Exascale computing necessitates novel software and algorithms that take full advantage of the enormous datasets and processing power at their disposal. A lot of money needs to be put into R&D for this to happen.
- **Data movement and communication**: Transferring the massive amounts of data produced by exascale machines to other portions of the system will be a difficult task. It will be necessary to create brand new means of communication and data transfer protocols.
- **Fault tolerance and reliability**: The complexity of exascale computing systems means that errors and breakdowns will occur frequently. It will be difficult to create systems that can keep running even if some of their components fail.
- **Security**: Since exascale computing is likely to be a valuable target for cyberattacks, it is crucial that safe solutions be developed [3].
- **Interdisciplinary collaboration**: Exascale computing will necessitate interdisciplinary work involving academics from many different disciplines, such as computer science, physics, chemistry, biology, and many more. Success will need the formation of efficient interdisciplinary teams and the promotion of cooperation.

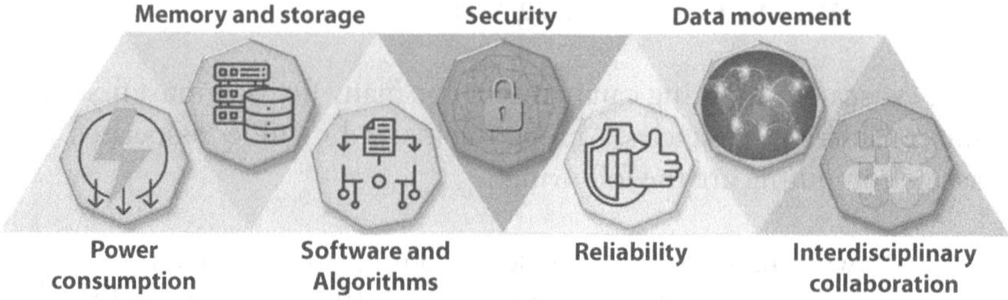

Figure 18.4 Challenges of exascale computing.

Dealing with these issues calls for heavy spending on R&D and cooperation between private enterprises, universities, and governments as seen in Figure 18.4. Nonetheless, many experts think the expense will be justified because of the enormous benefits that could be gained from exascale computing.

18.4 Future Lookup

Integrating quantum computing technologies is one future improvement that could be made to exascale computing. When applied to difficult problems in fields like materials science, cryptography, and optimization, quantum computing has the potential to vastly improve computational speed and efficiency. However, there are significant technical challenges associated with integrating quantum computing with classical HPC systems, such as the need to develop hybrid software architectures that can effectively combine classical and quantum computing resources and the need to address issues related to data movement and memory hierarchy.

The development of hybrid classical–quantum algorithms, the incorporation of quantum co-processors into classical HPC systems, and the creation of new software frameworks able to effectively orchestrate computation across classical and quantum resources are just some of the avenues being explored by researchers to meet these challenges. The combination of quantum and exascale computing has the potential to drive the development of new computational techniques and algorithms and to push the boundaries of what is possible in terms of computational complexity and scalability, in addition to its benefits for scientific discovery and engineering innovation. It is a step in the right direction for the field of exascale computing, and that is exciting.

18.4.1 Needed Improvements

Because of its infancy, exascale computing has a lot of space for improvement and expansion. A few possible upgrades to exascale computing are as follows:

1. **Software and algorithms**: Tapping into the full potential of exascale computers will require the development of software and algorithms suited for exascale computing. To make the most of the exascale systems' parallelism and memory,

researchers will need to create new algorithms and programming models.

2. **Hardware**: While exascale computing is currently tremendously powerful, it still has opportunity for development in hardware design. Further improvements in exascale system performance may be possible with advancements in CPU and memory design.
3. **Energy efficiency**: The massive amount of energy needed to run exascale devices is a potential barrier to its widespread use. To make exascale systems more widely available, improvements in energy-efficient hardware and cooling technologies are needed.
4. **Interconnect technology**: The success of exascale systems hinges on how well their many parts can exchange information and coordinate their efforts to achieve a common goal, and this is where interconnect technology comes in. There is room for significant performance gains in exascale systems with the help of enhanced interconnect technology.
5. **Integration with AI and machine learning**: It is possible that the development and implementation of AI and ML systems could be considerably accelerated with the help of exascale computing. Advances in both software and hardware have the potential to further enhance the utility and effectiveness of these systems, which might eventually pave the way for significant progress in areas like medicine, finance, and robotics.

Exascale computing has a very bright future full of opportunities for innovation and progress. New discoveries and improvements in sectors as diverse as science and engineering, healthcare, and finance might be anticipated as researchers continue to test the limits of exascale computing.

18.5 Conclusion

The advent of exascale computing will undoubtedly be a watershed moment in the history of high-performance computing, with far-reaching implications for the fields of science and engineering. The article has also shown the existence of significant technical obstacles in the creation of exascale computing systems, such as those related to power consumption, data transfer, memory hierarchy, fault tolerance, and software scalability.

Researchers in this area are making great strides toward resolving these issues by creating novel hardware architectures, sophisticated software algorithms, and cutting-edge machine learning methods. Future research in exascale computing could benefit from incorporating quantum computing with classical high-performance computing systems; doing so could spur the development of novel computational techniques and algorithms while also expanding the bounds of what is possible in terms of computational complexity and scalability. It is becoming increasingly evident that as exascale computing systems continue to develop and mature, they will play a crucial role in advancing scientific inquiry, technological advancement, and engineering creativity. Exascale computing has the potential to be a tremendous instrument for addressing some of the most important concerns confronting our society today, and ongoing investment in research and development will ensure that this is the case.

References

1. Council on Competitiveness, *High-performance computing: The engine of discovery*, Council on Competitiveness, Washington, DC, 2015.
2. Kogge, P., Exascale computing and big data. *J. Comput. Inf. Sci. Eng.*, 18, 2, 020801, 2018.
3. Dongarra, J. *et al.*, The international exascale software project roadmap. *Int. J. High Perform. Comput. Appl.*, 25, 1, 3–60, 2011.
4. Alam, S. *et al.*, The exascale computing challenge: Hardware, software, and co-design. *Proc. IEEE*, 103, 8, 1287–1308, 2015.
5. Norman, M. *et al.*, Exascale computing and the future of science. *Front. Res. Metrics Anal.*, 6, 671151, 2021.
6. Office of Science and Technology Policy, *National strategic computing initiativestrategic plan*, Executive Office of the President, Washington, DC, 2016.
7. Dongarra, J., Beckman, P., Moore, T., Aerts, P., Aloisio, G., Andre, J.-C., Yelick, K., The international exascale software project roadmap. *Int. J. High Perform. Comput. Appl.*, 25, 1, 3–60, 2011.
8. Geist, A. and Lucas, R., Major computer science challenges at exascale. *IJHPCA*, 23, 4, 427–436, 2009.
9. Esmaeilzadeh, H., Blem, E., Amant, R.S., Sankaralingam, K., Burger, D., Dark silicon and the end of multicore scaling. *Proceedings of the 38th Annual International Symposium on Computer Architecture*, pp. 365–376, 2011.
10. Schroeder, B. and Gibson, G.A., A large-scale study of failures in high-performance computing systems. *Proceedings of the International Conference on Dependable Systems and Networks*, 2006.

11. Pinheiro, E., Weber, W.-D., Barroso, L.A., Failure trends in a large disk drive population. *5th USENIX Conference on File and Storage Technologies (FAST'07)*, 2007.
12. William, P., Yogeesh, N., Vimala, S., Gite, P., Selva Kumar, S., Blockchain technology for data privacy using contract mechanism for 5G networks, in: *2022 3rd International Conference on Intelligent Engineering and Management (ICIEM)*, IEEE, pp. 461–465, 2022, https://doi.org/10.1109/ICIEM54221.2022.9853118.
13. Mishra, S., Choubey, S., Choubey, A., Yogeesh, N., Durga Prasad Rao, J., William, P., Data extraction approach using natural language processing for sentiment analysis, in: *2022 International Conference on Automation, Computing and Renewable Systems (ICACRS)*, IEEE, pp. 970–972, 2022, https://doi.org/10.1109/ICACRS55517.2022.10029216.
14. William, P., Yogeesh, N., Tidake, V.M., Gondkar, S.S., Vengatesan, K., Framework for implementation of personality inventory model on natural language processing with personality traits analysis, in: *2023 International Conference on Intelligent Data Communication Technologies and Internet of Things (IDCIoT)*, IEEE, pp. 625–628, 2023, https://doi.org/10.1109/IDCIoT56793.2023.10053501.
15. Gupta, K., Choubey, S., Yogeesh, N., William, P., Vasanthakumari., T.N., Kale, C.P., Implementation of motorist weariness detection system using a conventional object recognition technique, in: *2023 International Conference on Intelligent Data Communication Technologies and Internet of Things (IDCIoT)*, IEEE, pp. 640–646, 2023, https://doi.org/10.1109/IDCIoT56793.2023.10052783.
16. Yogeesh, N., Mathematical approach to representation of locations using K-Means clustering algorithm. *IJMAA*, 9, 1, 127–136, 2021.

Index

Printed in the USA/Agawam, MA
February 28, 2024

861872.001